Surgery Morning Report: Beyond the Pearls

Surgery Morning Report:
Beyond the Pearls

Series Editors
RAJ DASGUPTA, MD, FACP, FCCP, FAASM

Assistant Professor of Clinical Medicine
Division of Pulmonary/Critical Care/Sleep Medicine
Associate Program Director of the Sleep Medicine Fellowship
Assistant Program Director of the Internal Medicine Residency
Keck School of Medicine of the University of Southern California
Los Angeles, California

R. MICHELLE KOOLAEE, DO

Rheumatologist, Healthcare Partners Medical Group
Assistant Professor of Medicine
Division of Rheumatology
University of Southern California
Los Angeles, California

Volume Editors
AUSTIN D. WILLIAMS, MD, MSEd

General Surgery Resident
Department of Surgery
Lankenau Medical Center
Wynnewood, Pennsylvania

JONATHAN Y. GEFEN, MD

Associate Program Director, Lankenau Surgical Residency
Department of Surgery
Lankenau Medical Center
Wynnewood, Pennsylvania

BARRY D. MANN, MD

Chief Academic Officer, Main Line Health
Vice Chairman for Education, Department of Surgery
Program Director, Lankenau Surgical Residency
Lankenau Medical Center
Wynnewood, Pennsylvania
Professor of Surgery, Sidney Kimmel College of Medicine
Thomas Jefferson University
Philadelphia, Pennsylvania

ELSEVIER

Elsevier
3251 Riverport Lane
St. Louis, Missouri 63043

SURGERY MORNING REPORT: BEYOND THE PEARLS ISBN: 978-0-323-59759-3

Library of Congress Control Number: 2019937964

Content Strategist: James Meritt
Content Development Manager: Rebecca Gruliow
Content Development Specialist: Ann Ruzycka Anderson
Publishing Services Manager: Deepthi Unni
Project Manager: Janish Ashwin Paul
Design Direction: Bridget Hoette

Printed in China

Last digit is the print number: 9 8 7 6 5 4 3 2 1

Working together
to grow libraries in
developing countries

www.elsevier.com • www.bookaid.org

Volume Editors

For Brandon
Without whose unconditional patience and support
my surgical training would not be possible.

Austin D. Williams, MD MSEd

For Marisa, my love and inspiration.

Jonathan Y. Gefen, M.D., FACS

For Tilda
Without whose love, wisdom, and strength
work and life would have been unbalanced.

Barry D. Mann, MD, FACS

Series Editors

We would like to dedicate this book to my father, Arabinda
Dasgupta. He is a loving grandfather to our two children,
Mina and Aiden. We are very proud of his courage to overcome
recent challenges with his health. Even with these challenges,
he continues to smile and make others happy. Thank you for
your love and support and for being a great dad.

Raj Dasgupta, MD, FACP, FCCP, FAASM

PREFACE

Medical education is unique in that the balance one must strike between learner and teacher shifts regularly depending on the day, the hour, or even the minute. Residents, who themselves are learners and for the first time are viewed by medical students as teachers, must find a way during their busy clinical day to provide an effective educational experience. Whereas lectures, textbooks, and journal articles are all important to the educational process, most educators ultimately find that it is the informal conversations during patient care which are the moments that most effectively crystallize students' understanding of surgical disease and treatment.

The case-based approach of *Surgery Morning Report: Beyond the Pearls* is specifically meant to highlight the learning process that occurs at the bedside: development of broad differential diagnoses, reliance upon history and physical examination to tailor the differential, and consideration of the therapeutic options that are most appropriate for the individual. The question-and-answer format, in the context of a clinical scenario, mimics the bedside conversations that are so central to medical education. Similar to these conversations, the chapters herein are short and quick to the point. This makes for efficient reading, affords the opportunity to review a broad base of surgical topics within the brief duration of a clerkship, and enables easy retention for the learner. For the teacher, it provides a framework to guide the conversation.

SERIES EDITOR PREFACE

It is with great pleasure once again that we present our fourth book, *Surgery Morning Report: Beyond the Pearls*, first edition. Writing the "perfect" review text has been a dream of mine ever since I was a first-year medical student. Dr. Koolaee and I envisioned a text that incorporates the United States Medical Licensing Examination (USMLE) steps 1, 2, and 3 along with up-to-date evidence based clinical medicine. We wanted the platform of the text to be drawn from a traditional theme such as the "morning report" format that many of us are familiar with from residency. This book is geared toward a wide audience, from medical students to attending physicians practicing general surgery. Each case has been carefully chosen and covers scenarios and questions frequently encountered on the surgery boards, shelf exams, and wards, integrating both basic science and clinical pearls.

We would like to sincerely thank all of the many contributors who have helped to create this text. Your insightful work will be a valuable tool for medical students and physicians to gain an in-depth understanding of surgery. It should be noted that, although a variety of clinical cases in surgery were selected for this book, it is not meant to substitute a comprehensive surgical reference.

Dr. Koolaee and I would like to thank our volume editors, Dr. Williams, Dr. Gefen, and Dr. Mann, for all their hard work and dedication to this book. It was truly a pleasure to work with all of you, and we look forward to our next project together.

FOREWORD

Drs. Dasgupta and Koolaee are to be congratulated for developing the new and much needed series of case-based books for in-training and practicing medical professionals, *Surgery Morning Report: Beyond the Pearls*. With *Surgery*, volume editors Drs. Austin Williams, Jonathan Gefen, and Barry Mann, the team has succeeded in delivering what every surgeon can use: in-depth, user-friendly, clinical cases with practical take-home facts. Whether for the medical student, the resident, or the clinician in practice, *Surgery Morning Report* will keep us fresh, current, and sharp. "Dr. Raj" is not only our go-to sleep medicine and pulmonary specialist for *The Doctors* television show for the last six seasons, but he has also been a clinical educator for my son at the University of Southern California and my daughter during her preparation for the USMLE. "Dr. Raj" always brings positive energy to the show and truly personifies the core elements of a great teacher: engaging personality, great work ethic, and amazing knowledge of medicine. This book is as passionate, energetic, and informative as his segments on the show.

Andrew Ordon, MD
Emmy®-nominated cohost of award-winning talk show *The Doctors*
Board-certified plastic surgeon
Associate Professor of Plastic Surgery
USC Keck School of Medicine

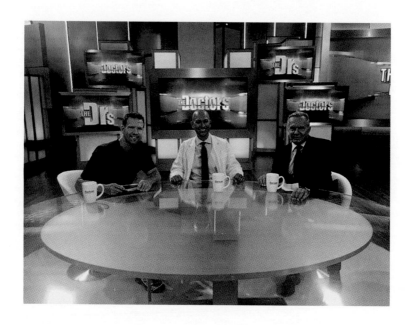

Healthcare has traditionally been perceived as silo-based hospital systems. However, over the last several years the importance of a team-based approach has become more apparent, especially in the intensive care unit (ICU). Contrary to a *Grey's Anatomy* television episode showcasing different arrogant doctors competing to "own" a surgical patient's case, our healthcare teams are thankfully looking to each other with respect and leaning on each other's expertise.

During my surgical ICU fellowship, I learned quickly how symbiotic relationships among surgeons could benefit patient safety and quality of care. Although I was trained in internal medicine, my fellowship was through the department of surgery, and I mostly worked in the surgical and neurosurgical ICUs. To some, it might seem odd that a nonsurgeon physician would take full care of postoperative patients, but this made complete sense to me. For a majority of the day, my surgical colleagues were working hard in the operating room and relied on me to provide excellent bedside medical care to the sickest postoperative patients. We relied on each other's expertise and respected various viewpoints.

Now as the codirector of a neurosurgical ICU, I work closely with neurologists, neurointensivists, and neurosurgeons. Last year a young man with unexplained status epilepticus was admitted to our ICU. All of the services worked diligently to save his life and find his diagnosis. He was placed in an induced coma and required mechanical ventilation for several weeks. Finally, after weeks of being on autoimmune disease treatments, his condition turned around. He spent 4 months in the ICU but was finally able to walk out of the hospital to spend Thanksgiving Day with his family. This is in large part due to the alignment of values and complementary skills that each team member brought to the table.

The days of "command and control" type of leadership from one doctor are long gone—thankfully. We are at the precipice of advancing the way we deliver healthcare with more emphasis on team-based, multidisciplinary approaches. Excellent outcomes in healthcare depend on teamwork and collaborative efforts. I'm happy to be a part of the leadership evolution of medicine and surgery as it integrates and prioritizes physician collegiality.

Roozehra Khan, DO, FCCP
Assistant Professor of Clinical Medicine
Keck School of Medicine at USC
Director of Keck Hospital Neurosurgical ICU
Director of Bedside Ultrasound

CONTRIBUTORS

Cary B. Aarons, MD
Associate Professor of Surgery
Department of Surgery
Hospital of the University of Pennsylvania,
    Philadelphia
Pennsylvania
United States

Shannon Acker, MD
Pediatric Surgery Fellow
Pediatric Surgery
Children's Hospital Colorado, Denver
Colorado
United States

Emily C. Alberto, MD
General Surgery Resident
Christiana Care Health System, Newark
Delaware
United States

Steven R. Allen, MD
Associate Professor of Surgery
Surgery
Penn State Milton S. Hershey Medical Center,
    Hershey
Pennsylvania
United States

Adnan Alseidi, MD, Ed.M, FACS
HPB fellowship Director, Assoc PD Surgery
HPB & Endocrine Surgery
Virginia Mason Medical Center, Seattle
Washington
United States,
Assistant Professor
Department of Surgery
University of Washington, Seattle
Washington
United States

Sourodeep Banerjee, BS
Student
Lewis Katz School of Medicine
Temple University, Philadelphia
Pennsylvania
United States

Loren Berman, MD, MHS
Associate Professor of Surgery and Pediatrics
Sidney Kimmel Medical College at Thomas
    Jefferson University
Philadelphia, Pennsylvania
Pediatric Surgeon
Nemours - Alfred I. duPont Hospital for
    Children
Wilmington, Delaware
United States

Matthew Boelig, MD
Pediatric Surgery Fellow
Pediatric General, Thoracic and Fetal Surgery
Children's Hospital of Philadelphia,
    Philadelphia
Pennsylvania
United States

Christopher Brandt, MD
Chairman
Department of Surgery
The MetroHealth System, Case Western
    Reserve University, Cleveland
Ohio
United States

L.D. Britt, MD, MPH, DSc (Hon), FACS, FCCM
Henry Ford Professor and Edward J.
    Brickhouse Chairman
Department of Surgery
Eastern Virginia Medical School, Norfolk, VA
Virginia
United States

Elizabeth Carlson, MD
General Surgery Resident
Virginia Mason Medical Center, Seattle
Washington
United States

Ned Carp, MD
Campus Chief of Surgery Lankenau Medical
    Center
Barbara Brodsky Chief of Surgery Chair
    Lankenau Medical Center
Lankenau Medical Center, Wynnewood
Pennsylvania
United States

Daniel Choi, BS, MSE
Medical Student
Thomas Jefferson Medical College,
   Philadelphia
Pennsylvania
United States

Robin M. Ciocca, DO
Department of Surgery
Lankenau Medical Center
Wynnewood, Pennsylvania
United States

George Cybulski, MD
Associate Professor
Department of Neurosurgery
Northwestern University, Chicago
Illinois
United States

Raj Dasgupta, MD, FACP, FCCP, FAASM
Assistant Professor of Clinical Medicine
Department of Medicine Division of
   Pulmonary, Critical Care and Sleep
   Medicine
Keck School of Medicine of the University
   of Southern California,
   Los Angeles
California
United States
Associate Program Director
Sleep Medicine Fellowship
Keck School of Medicine of the University of
   California, Los Angeles
California
United States
Assistant Program Director
Internal Medicine Residency
Keck School of Medicine of the University of
   California, Los Angeles
California
United States

Dan M. DePietro, MD
General Surgery Resident
Lankenau Medical Center, Wynnewood
Pennsylvania
United States

Courtney Lee Devin, MD
General Surgery Resident
Department of Surgery
Thomas Jefferson University, Philadelphia
Pennsylvania
United States

Vincent DiGiovanni, DO, FACOS
Division of Vascular Surgery
Lankenau Medical Center, Wynnewood
Pennsylvania
United States

Colin Doyle, MD
Surgical Critical Care Fellow
Department of Surgery
University of Hawaii, Honolulu
United States

Rebecca Evangelista, MD
Associate Professor of Surgery
MedStar Georgetown University Hospital,
   Washington
District of Columbia
United States

Kelly Fan, MD
Pulmonary and Critical Care Medicine Fellow,
   Pulmonary and Critical Care Medicine
University of Southern California, Los Angeles
California
United States

Abbey Fingeret, MD
Assistant Professor
Department of Surgery
University of Nebraska Medical Center,
   Omaha
Nebraska
United States

Derek Freitas, MD, MSPH
General Surgery Resident
NYU Langone Health, NYC
New York
United States

Matthew A. Fuglestad, MD
General Surgery Resident
University of Nebraska Medical Center,
   Omaha
Nebraska
United States

Royd Fukumoto, MD
Clinical Assistant Professor of Surgery
Surgery, University of Vermont
Danbury Hospital, Danbury
Connecticut
United States

Roberto Gedaly
Director, Transplant Center
Professor of Surgery
University of Kentucky, Lexington
Kentucky
United States

Jonathan Gefen, MD
Associate Program Director
Department of Surgery
Lanknau Medical Center, Wynnewood
Pennsylvania
United States

Julia Glaser, MD
Assistant Professor of Clinical Surgery
Department of Surgery
University of Pennsylvania Health System,
    Philadelphia
Pennsylvania
United States

Amy Goldberg, MD
Professor and Chair
Department of Surgery
Lewis Katz School of Medicine at Temple
    University, Philadelphia
Pennsylvania
United States

Scott M. Goldman, MD
Department of Surgery
Lankenau Medical Center
Wynnewood, Pennsylvania
United States

Christopher E. Greenleaf, MD, MBA
Fellow
Congenital Cardiac Surgery
Texas Children's Hospital, Houston
Texas
United States

Erin K. Greenleaf, MD, MS
General Surgery Resident
Penn State Health M.S. Hershey Medical
    Center, Hershey
Pennsylvania
United States

Kevin L. Grimes, MD
Assistant Professor
Department of Surgery
University of Cincinnati, Cincinnati
Ohio
United States

Sriharsha Gummadi, MD
General Surgery Resident
Lankenau Medical Center, Wynnewood
Pennsylvania
United States

Meera Gupta, MD, MSCE
Assistant Professor of Surgery
Surgery, Abdominal Transplant Program
University of Kentucky, Lexington
Kentucky
United States

Rebecca L. Hoffman, MD, MSCE
General Surgery Resident
University of Pennsylvania, Philadelphia
Pennsylvania
United States

Celeste Hollands, MD
Associate Professor
Department of Surgery
Texas Tech University Health Sciences Center,
    Lubbock
Texas
United States

Mary Ann Hopkins, MD, MPhil
Associate Professor of Surgery
Surgery
NYU School of Medicine, New York
New York
United States
Director of Global Health Initiatives
NYU School of Medicine, New York
New York
United States

Gary Nace, MD
Assistant Professor of Surgery
Pediatric General and Thoracic Surgery
Children's Hospital of Philadelphia,
    Philadelphia, Pennsylvania
United States

Kei Nagatomo, DO
General Surgery Resident
Lankenau Medical Center, Wynnewood
Pennsylvania
United States

Susanna Matsen Nazarian, MD, PhD
Assistant Professor
Department of Surgery
University of Pennsylvania, Philadelphia
Pennsylvania
United States
Staff Surgeon
Corporal Michael J. Crescenz Veterans Affairs
    Medical Center
Pennsylvania
United States

Madalyn Neurwirth, MD
General Surgery Resident
Hospital of the University of Pennsylvania,
    Philadelphia
Pennsylvania, United States

Robert B. Noone, MD
Department of Surgery
Lankenau Medical Center
Wynnewood, Pennsylvania
United States

Kristin Ojomo, MD
General Surgery Resident
Brigham and Women's Hospital, Boston
Massachusetts
United States

D. George Ormond, MD
General Surgery Resident
Danbury Hospital, Danbury
Connecticut
United States

Colette Pameijer, MD
Associate Professor of Surgery
Surgery
Penn State College of Medicine, Hershey
Pennsylvania
United States

James C. Pendleton, MD, PhD
General Surgery Resident
Lankenau Medical Center, Wynnewood
Pennsylvania
United States

Roy Phitayakorn, MD, MHPE (MEd), FACS
Director of Medical Student Education and
    Surgery Education Research
General and Endocrine Surgery
Massachusetts General Hospital, Boston
Massachusetts
United States

Konstadinos Plestis, MD
Chief, Cardiac Surgery
Lankenau Medical Center, Wynnewood
Pennsylvania
United States

Michael J. Pucci, MD
Associate Professor of Surgery
Surgery
Thomas Jefferson University, Philadelphia
Pennsylvania
United States

Michael J. Qaqish, MD
General Surgery Resident
Lankenau Medical Center, Wynnewood
Pennsylvania
United States

Stephanie Lynn Rakestraw, BS
Medical Student
Sidney Kimmel Medical College
Thomas Jefferson University, Philadelphia
Pennsylvania
United States

Kaitlin Ritter, MD
General Surgery Resident
Cleveland Clinic Foundation, Cleveland
Ohio
United States

Jonathan P. Roach, MD
Assistant Professor
Pediatric Surgery Children's Hospital
    Colorado Aurora
Colorado
United States

Reza Ronaghi, MD, MS
Pulmonary and Critical Care Fellow
University of Southern California,
    Los Angeles
California
United States

Patrick Ross, MD, PhD
Chairman, Department of Surgery
Lankenau Medical Center
Wynnewood, Pennsylvania
United States

Ahmad Safra, MD
General Surgery Resident
Lankenau Medical Center, Wynnewood
Pennsylvania
United States

Jean F. Salem, MD
General Surgery Resident
Lankenau Medical Center, Wynnewood
Pennsylvania
United States

Adam Jude Santoro, DO
Medical Research Assistant
General Surgery
Einstein Medical Center, Philadelphia
Pennsylvania
United States

Dane Scantling, DO, MPH
General Surgery Resident
Drexel University College of
    Medicine/Hahnemann University Hospital,
    Philadelphia
Pennsylvania
United States

Paul Schenarts, MD
Professor & Chief of Acute Care Surgery
University of Nebraska, Omaha
Nebraska
United States

Henry P. Schoonyoung, MD
Department of Surgery
Lankenau Medical Center
Wynnewood, Pennsylvania
United States

Ashesh Shah, MD
Assistant Professor
Department of Surgery

Thomas Jefferson University, Philadelphia
Pennsylvania
United States

Vishal Shah, DO
General Surgery Resident
Lankenau Medical Center, Wynnewood
Pennsylvania
United States

Hui Yi Shan, MD
Assistant Professor of Clinical Medicine,
    Nephrology Fellowship Program Director
Medicine
Keck School of Medicine of University of
    Southern California, Los Angeles
California
United States

Viri Siripurapu, MD
General Surgeon
Huntsville Hospital Valley Surgical Associates,
    Huntsville
Alabama
United States

Lars Sjoholm, MD
Director of Trauma and Surgical Critical Care
Department of Surgery
Lewis Katz School of Medicine at Temple
    University, Philadelphia
Pennsylvania
United States

Douglas Smink, MD, MPH
Program Director,
    General Surgery Residency
Department of Surgery
Brigham and Women's Hospital, Boston
Massachusetts
United States

Alycia So, BA, MD
General Surgery Resident
Icahn School of Medicine at Mount Sinai,
    New York
New York
United States

Drew Allan Spencer, MD
Health System Clinician
Neurosurgery
Northwestern Medicine, Chicago, Illinois
United States

Anna Spivak, DO
Resident
Surgery
Lankenau Medical Center, Wynnewood
Pennsylvania
United States

Susan Steinemann, MD
Associate Professor
Surgery
University of Hawaii, Honolulu
Hawaii
United States
The Queen's Medical Center, Honolulu
Hawaii
United States

Julia Tchou, MD, PhD
Co-Director, Rena Rowan Breast Center
Section Chief, Breast Surgery
Associate Professor of Clinical Surgery
Perelman School of Medicine
Hospital of the University of Pennsylvania,
    Philadelphia
Pennsylvania
United States

Erin Teeple, MD
Pediatric Surgeon
AI Dupont Hospital for Children, Wilmington
Delaware
United States

Amanda Teichman, MD
General Surgery Resident
Hahnemann University Hospital, Philadelphia
Pennsylvania
United States

Kyla Terhune, MD, MBA
Associate Professor
Department of Surgery
Vanderbilt University, Nashville, Tennessee
United States

Madeline B. Torres, MD
General Surgery Resident
Penn State Milton S. Hershey Medical Center,
    Heryshey
Pennsylvania
United States

Natalie Tully, BS
Medical Student
Texas Tech University Health Sciences Center,
    Lubbock
United States

Alexander Uribe, MD
Chief, Division of Vascular Surgery
Department of Surgery
Lankenau Medical Center, Wynnewood
Pennsylvania
United States

Michael Walker, MD
Chief, Thoracic Surgery
Main Line Health System, Bryn Mawr
Pennsylvania
United States

Michael Weingarten, MD, MBA
Professor and Assistant Dean
Department of Surgery
Drexel University College of Medicine,
    Philadelphia
Pennsylvania
United States

Austin D. Williams, MD, MSEd
General Surgery Resident
Lankenau Medical Center, Wynnewood
Pennsylvania
United States

Carl Winkler, MD
General Surgery Resident
Mount Sinai St. Luke's - Roosevelt, New York
New York
United States

Ujwal Yanala, MBBS
General Surgery Resident
University of Nebraska Medical Center,
    Omaha
Nebraska
United States

Yan Zhong, MD, PhD
Clinical Assistant Professor
Division of Nephrology
Keck School of Medicine
University of Southern California, Los Angeles
California
United States

CONTENTS

SECTION 10   *Pediatric Surgery*   *409*

Surgery Morning Report: Beyond the Pearls

General Principles

CHAPTER 1

Medical Student and Resident Survival at Morning Report

Paul J. Schenarts ■ Matthew A. Fuglestad

So why should you care if you perform well at morning report, and how does this relate to your survival? After all, there are many other clinical and academic venues in which you can demonstrate your clinical skills and fund of factual knowledge. Morning report, however, is a particularly unique educational experience. Unlike other conferences, morning report does not allow for an extended period of preparation, usually is directly related to care of a current patient, and requires you to articulate your critical thinking skills in real time. It is one of the best opportunities to practice the question-and-answer format of oral examinations and may be the most educational conference you can attend.

The format, focus, and conduct of morning report may differ among hospitals. However, there are three typical formats. The first is a morning report in which the primary focus is the exchange of clinical information during the transition from the night team to the day team. The second is primarily focused on education, utilizing a case or patient who was admitted the previous day as the starting point for the discussion. The third type is a hybrid of the first two in which a period of time is devoted to an educational discussion, using the Socratic method, followed by an exchange of clinical information also known as "running the patient list." Regardless of the style used at your hospital, the following survival keys will help you be successful.

The vast majority of the faculty will not remember your in-service or board scores. Rather, they will base their evaluation of you in large measure on how well you orally articulate your clinical decision making. Remember: reputations are established early and are difficult to reverse. Therefore it is important to do well right from the beginning.

Unfortunately, there are no evidence-based guidelines or randomized trials on how to be successful. The survival tips that follow are based on the experiences of the two authors, one a resident and the other a senior faculty member.

Survival Tip 1: "Do Not Be a Bleeder"

In other words, don't sabotage yourself before you even begin. When you are surrounded by "sharks" (a.k.a. attendings and senior residents), the most important thing to do is to avoid bleeding. Once blood is in the water, morning report turns into a feeding frenzy. One example of bleeding from a self-inflicted wound is to arrive late—or worse, late with breakfast or coffee in hand. There are only two good reasons for being late to a scheduled conference: giving or receiving cardiopulmonary resuscitation.

Another common self-sabotage technique is not dressing up when you have been asked to. We know that everyone is tired. If you want to be the first on the hot seat, a good way to get there is to be in scrubs when your chief, who was up all night operating, is in dress clothes and white coat. Remember, you are in a select company of individuals who are dedicated to the art and traditions of surgery. Dressing up is a sign of good time management and respect. In some programs you can expect the majority of challenging questioning to come your way if you can't be bothered to dress appropriately.

If you want to avoid the "shark's appetite," know what is expected of you at morning report. Be sure that before the rotation starts you clearly understand the expectations. Asking the attending or senior resident about expectations in advance may also have the added benefit of starting the rotation off right.

Survival Tip 2: Honesty First

Trustworthy communication is a cornerstone of surgical residency. When discussing patients and their medical care, there are only two acceptable answers: #1—the truth; and #2—"I don't know; I will go look it up." It is unacceptable to present partially correct information to any member of the healthcare team. There are few things more devastating to a resident's career than a reputation of partial truths or outright lies. If you cannot be trusted to report the correct white blood cell count, your ability to be given autonomy is compromised. Inevitably, we all forget to look up a laboratory value or a detail of a pathology report. It is okay to admit you don't know what is being asked of you and go find the information. It isn't enough to believe the creatinine is normal! Just go look it up.

Survival Tip 3: Be Prepared

Depending on the format and focus of the morning report, your ability to prepare may be difficult. Regardless, it is possible to *appear* well prepared. One of the falsities of the electronic medical record is ease of data acquisition. True, the electronic medical record is a comprehensive repository of current and old medical records. However, it is nearly impossible in real time to find the information you need immediately, as it is often buried in a pile of other notes and data points.

One solution for this dilemma is to write down the pertinent information on your patient list or have an index card for each patient for whom you are responsible. The index card is nice because it is less bulky than the full patient list and can serve as a handy way to recall data from previous days. Also, it can serve as another record of operations or procedures that you will need for board certification.

If your morning report is more education or a hybrid, preparation may be particularly challenging in that you may not know the case or topic of discussion in advance. There are several strategies that may help here. First, by arriving early you may overhear the faculty talking about the case or topic. Then you can quickly use a handheld device to review the topic. This isn't cheating—it is using good sense. Another method is to write down on an index card or your handheld device the pathophysiology, basic diagnostic steps, treatment options, common complications, and follow-up plan for the 20 most common diseases you will encounter on the service. Cards or notes can be added as needed as you progress through residency. This approach has several advantages. First, the process of writing out this information provides cognitive reinforcement. Second, these cards can be used as flash cards or study notes during periods of down time, such as waiting for conferences or rounds to start. Third, these can serve as an outline when presenting a case or when teaching students.

Survival Tip 4: Be Concise but Full of Information

Time is the most valued commodity, so do not waste it. When presenting information, be concise and make every word or data point count. Be the person who presents only the important facts and avoids the drama and silliness that often accompanies verbal presentations. No doubt some stories are funny, but being all business at morning report will pay dividends. It is also recommended that you read the room and the attending. There are times when the service and patient needs are pushing back against the educational. Recognize those times and be ready to expand or contract your presentations accordingly. More does not always equal better. Know how to distill the data and your presentations to the most essential elements. But importantly, when you are asked for more information after your presentation, be the resident who knows the patient from head to toe. A quick way to lose autonomy and trust of your superiors is to not know your patients. Again, be concise but have the fully history available when needed.

Survival Tip 5: Be Polished

As stated previously, very few of your faculty or senior residents know or even care about your scores on examinations. Your clinical reputation is primarily established by how you present yourself verbally. One of the best ways to establish yourself is to be organized, concise, and polished during morning report. Let's take the case of two residents, both presenting a case of acute cholecystitis. Resident A: "Patient is a 47-year-old woman with a 'hot gallbladder'. She is scheduled for a 'lap chole' this afternoon." Resident B: "47-year-old female, without previous medical history, presents with right upper quadrant pain, emesis, and fever. On examination she has no jaundice but has right upper quadrant tenderness and Murphy's sign suggestive of acute cholecystitis, which is supported by a leukocytosis and ultrasound findings of gallstones, pericholecystic fluid, and wall thickening." In as little as one more sentence Resident B is more polished. An unseen benefit of Resident B's description is that she has reinforced her own learning by including the ultrasonic findings of acute cholecystitis. Residents can do the same by including reports of specific organisms, the chosen antibiotic coverage, or the particular cardiac vessels occluded based on the ECG findings.

Survival Tip 6: How to Successfully Navigate Case Conference

During morning report you will be expected to walk through theoretical case scenarios aimed at testing your fundamentals of patient evaluation and management. There are key pitfalls that younger residents tend to make, and avoiding these makes conference more enjoyable and limits embarrassment. Here are a couple tips.

Don't Repeat the Details of the Case Out Loud. Take a deep breath and take a moment to silently synthesize the information you are given. There is nothing wrong with taking a moment to organize your thoughts. These cases are often challenging and require you to think on the fly. Don't get caught in the trap of trying to stall by repeating information (*Everybody knows what you're up to!*). Likewise, limit the amount of additional questions you ask in regard to the presentation. The point of case conference is to teach, not to trick. You will be given enough information to answer the questions you are asked.

Don't Default to Consulting Another Team. In case conference *you* are the emergency department, interventional radiologist, surgeon, infectious disease, and medicine attending. Take the patient's care as far as you reasonably can with the knowledge you have. If you do need to call a consult, make sure you know what you are asking the consulting team to do, and think about how you would manage the problem if your consultants happen to not be available.

Hedging Your Bets. It is never right to support two or more competing treatment plans that cannot be performed at the same time. An example would be suggesting, "You could admit the patient to the ICU for serial hemoglobins or take her to IR for embolization of her splenic injury or take her to the OR for splenectomy." If you present your case in this fashion, you can expect the response: "No, doctor, the question asked was what do *you* want to do." The best part about morning report is only your ego can be injured; the patients are 100% safe. Now is the time to make mistakes and learn from them without harm. Better now than presenting them at the M&M podium.

Don't Offer Up More Information Than Is Needed to Answer a Question Asked of You. If your attending asks you how you would treat an intracranial bleed in a patient with known von Willebrand disease, treat it and move on. Now is not the time to attempt to describe the intricacies of the disease process. If you go down this route, the next question will surely be to describe the pathophysiology of the subtypes of von Willebrand and more specific questioning that you may not know the answer to. The attending will give you the information you need to know. Just answer the question and get ready for the next one.

Admit When You Don't Know the Next Step and Read About It. Now isn't the time to invent a new operation or create a new treatment regimen. Admit what you don't know and learn from it. Morning report is the great revealer of the unknown in your surgical knowledge. Make sure to reflect on the case and read as much as you can. The time spent will pay high dividends over the years and on your in-service examination. And lastly, if your attending hands something out to be read, be sure to *read it.* No attending enjoys being greeted with blanks stares when asking, "What did you think of the article?"

Survival Tip 7: Do Not Be Offended by Critical Questioning

Don't get upset if you don't know an answer. Many residents become offended when asked difficult or critical questions. This is unfortunate, because the purpose of all education is to improve the breadth and depth of understanding. This is really only possible by first determining what residents know and then pushing them to the next level. Although growth is not always a comfortable feeling, it is a fair price to be paid to increase learning. The greatest form of engagement is for an attending or senior resident to ask these questions. Although it may make you happy if you are not asked any questions, you are probably in grave trouble or the attending really does not care a bit about your education.

Survival Tip 8: Cut Them Off at the Pass

One of the basic concepts in argumentation is to anticipate questions and to address them before the question can even be asked. This has two benefits. First, you will be able to demonstrate your comprehensive fund of factual knowledge and how you incorporate it into your daily clinical decision making. A second benefit is that the attending will not be able to waste your time by asking questions to which you already know the answer.

Survival Tip 9: Gamification

Have fun and view morning report as a game. Yes, it is a very important forum for you to demonstrate your critical thinking skills, but have fun with the process. View morning report as a game that you will sometimes win and sometimes lose. This attitude will keep this occasionally high-stress experience in proper perspective.

Survival Tip 10: Be a Leader

Our final pearl: lead by example. Never be late, know your patients better than anyone else, read any chance you get, and be dedicated to becoming a better doctor every day. Pass along these pearls to medical students and to new incoming residents. It is never too early or too late to make changes.

It's easy to slide through conference when you're tired or distracted. But remember, you only have a few years to obtain the vast knowledge required to be called a surgeon. Your future patients will depend on the skills you learn now. Give it all you've got every day and you won't regret it.

In conclusion, morning report is a unique opportunity for a student or resident to demonstrate a fund of factual knowledge, attention to detail, professionalism, and critical decision-making skills while, more importantly, benefiting the patients.

CHAPTER 2

Preoperative and Postoperative Patient Care

Kaitlin Ritter ■ Jeremy M. Lipman

Standard Preoperative Evaluation

Presurgical assessment is an essential component of preoperative care and helps assure the safe delivery of anesthesia and proposed operation. However, it is not appropriate to subject all patients to an extensive preoperative evaluation due to the increased patient risk and lack of cost effectiveness of such a strategy. Appropriate evaluation must be individualized, selecting only the preoperative testing that will affect patient management. Although many guidelines exist, a useful approach is provided in Table 2.1. Perhaps the most important component of the evaluation is the history and physical examination performed in the surgeon's office. This should be done with a focus on identifying findings that may alter a patient's risk for surgery or anesthesia.

A number of tools exist to evaluate a patient's risk for perioperative complications. One of the most straightforward is the American Society of Anesthesiology (ASA) Physical Status Classification (Table 2.2). The ASA classification is not only easy to use but has been shown to correlate with the incidence of postoperative morbidity and mortality across many surgical specialties and operations. Typically, patients with an ASA 3 or higher should be referred for a formal preanesthesia evaluation by the anesthesiology team or a physician specializing in internal medicine.

When planning preoperative testing, a useful strategy is only ordering tests that will alter how the patient is managed. For patients with low ASA classification undergoing routine surgical procedures that carry low risk, there is little workup that needs to be completed. A female patient of childbearing age would be recommended for a urine HCG test to assure she is not pregnant, usually performed on the day of surgery. Recommendations for other specific preoperative testing will vary between institutions.

PREOPERATIVE PATIENT COUNSELING

The preoperative teaching performed in the surgeon's clinic is extremely important for assuring a safe operation and perioperative course. This should include a detailed discussion of what will happen before, during, and after the operation. Preoperative counseling can help set appropriate expectations and prepare patients for potential complications. When the patient and surgeon have mismatched expectations, even a perfect recovery in the surgeon's view can be unsatisfactory to the patient.

The discussion should include information regarding preoperative preparation such as additional required testing and involvement of other providers such as ostomy nurses or consulting physicians. When to stop eating, how to complete a bowel prep (if required), how the location and time of arrival will be communicated, and how additional testing will be arranged should also be discussed. Perhaps the most important element of this conversation should be identifying a point person whom the patients can contact with questions as they move through the surgical process. Patients should be allowed the opportunity to ask questions and express any concerns they may have

TABLE 2.1 ■ **Clinical Indications for Preoperative Laboratory Testing**

Complete blood count (CBC)	Perform for patients with high preoperative risk for anemia including: • Chronic kidney disease • Chronic liver disease • Chronic inflammatory condition • Clinical signs and symptoms of anemia Perform if significant surgical blood loss anticipated Patients with known bleeding/hematologic disorders
Type and screen	Perform if significant surgical blood loss anticipated
Coagulation testing	Patients with known coagulation/bleeding disorders Patients with known liver/renal dysfunction Patients with concern for undiagnosed clotting disorder including: • Family history of heritable coagulopathy • Personal history of easy bruising • Personal history of excessive posttrauma/postsurgical bleeding Patients on anticoagulation therapy
Serum chemistries	Patients with known endocrine disorders Patients with known liver/renal dysfunction Patients using medications with known renal/hepatic effects including but not limited to: • Diuretics • ACE inhibitors/ARBS • Digoxin Consider for: • All patients over age 65 • Patients at increased risk for acute kidney injury
Pregnancy testing	Offer to all females of childbearing age Perform if clinical concern for pregnancy
Urinalysis	No routine testing Consider for: • Patients with symptoms of urinary tract infection • Patients undergoing prosthesis implantation (heart value, prosthetic joint) • Patients undergoing urologic procedures
Glucose	No routine testing Consider for: • Patients at high risk for undiagnosed diabetes mellitus • Patients with signs and symptoms or a history of diabetes mellitus

preoperatively. Common concerns often include pain control, dietary modifications, and activity restrictions postoperatively.

Explanations should be conducted without unnecessary medical jargon, and written directions should be provided as required. When counseling patients, it is important to remember patients have varied educational backgrounds, and medical literacy can be limited. Even if the patient has a medical background, preoperative discussions should abandon all assumptions to prevent unnecessary confusion and unrealistic expectations. At the conclusion of the visit, the patient should be able to describe the expected perioperative course, broad steps of the operation, and potential complications.

Careful consideration must be taken when formulating a perioperative plan regarding the cessation or continuation of a patient's home medications. A guide is provided in Table 2.3 outlining which medications are usually safe to continue and which should be altered before an operation.

TABLE 2.2 ■ American Society of Anesthesiology Physical Status Classification

	Characteristics	Example
ASA 1	Normal healthy patient	Fit, nonobese, nonsmoker with good exercise tolerance
ASA 2	Patient with mild systemic disease	No functional limitations with a well-controlled disease (such as treated hypertension)
ASA 3	Patient with severe systemic disease that is not life-threatening	Some functional limitations as a result of disease process (poorly controlled hypertension or diabetes)
ASA 4	Patient with a severe systemic disease that is a constant threat to life	Functional limitations from severe, life threatening disease (unstable angina, poorly controlled COPD)
ASA 5	Moribund patient who is not expected to survive without the operation	Not expected to survive beyond the next 24 hours without surgery (ruptured AAA, massive trauma)

Adapted from the American Society of Anesthesiologist Physical Status Classification System, published October 2014.

TABLE 2.3 ■ Preoperative Management of Common Medications

	Day before Surgery	Day of Surgery
Cardiovascular		
Beta blockers	Continue	Continue
Calcium channel blockers	Continue	Resume with oral intake
Statins	Continue	Continue
ACE Inhibitors/ARBs	Continue	Continue If held, restart as soon as possible
Anticoagulants		
Warfarin	Hold 5 days before Bridge as needed	Hold
Direct Thrombin Inhibitors (CrCl ≥ 30)	Hold 48–96 hours	Hold
Factor Xa Inhibitors (CrCl ≥ 30)	Hold 24–48 hours	Hold
Antiplatelets		
Aspirin	Hold 7–10 days before Continue if high CV risk	Hold
ADP Receptor Inhibitors	Hold 7–10 days before	Hold
Antihyperglycemic Agents		
Oral Antihyperglycemic		
Secretagogues	Continue	Hold
SGLT-2 Inhibitors	Hold	Hold
Thiazolidinediones	Continue	Hold
Metformin	Continue	Hold
DPP-4 Inhibitors	Continue	Continue
Injectable Insulin Therapy		
Glargine/Detemir	80% of pm dose	80% of am dose
NPH/ 70–30 Insulin	80% of am and pm dose	50% of am dose Hold for blood glucose less than 120 mg/dL
Lispro, Aspart, Glulisine, Regular	Regular dose	Hold

CV, Cardiovascular; CrCl, Creatinine Clearance.

A number of factors go into such decisions, particularly when it comes to patients on therapeutic anticoagulation or antiplatelet therapy. One must consider the indication for the medication, the duration of treatment, and the associated health factors for each patient. Creating a perioperative plan for all home medications, including herbal supplements and over-the-counter medications, is an important part of the preoperative visit with an anesthesia or internal medicine provider. The plan must be clearly explained to the patient preoperatively, and compliance must be ensured the morning of surgery by the operative team. Failure to continue or hold key medications may result in cancelation of the surgical case.

> **CLINICAL PEARL**
>
> At the end of each preoperative visit, ask patients to explain back what they understand about how they should prepare for surgery, what the operation will entail, and what to expect if things go well or if complications develop. Identifying errors or misconceptions early prevents problems later.

INFORMED CONSENT

In order to be "informed" the patient must understand the proposed procedure, as well as its purpose, benefits, risks, and alternative options. Achieving this requires a basic discussion of how the operation is performed, including the approach (open versus laparoscopic) and summary of the general concepts of what will be done. The patient should be given realistic expectations for the outcome of the procedure, including which benefits should and should not be anticipated.

A review of the surgical risks should include a discussion of the most common complications and an estimated percentage of their frequency if known. It is impossible to cover every adverse outcome, but the focus should be on the most common events (wound infections, urinary retention) or those that are or may be of greatest concern to the patient (common bile duct injury, inadvertent bowel injury).

Additionally, alternative therapies should be discussed. For example, a discussion of elective cholecystectomy for gallstones should include diet modification as an alternative means to minimize symptoms. The patient should also understand what would be expected if he or she elects not to have the operation. Ultimately, the patient should come to the decision to proceed with surgery after considering all of this information together.

Once the patient understands all of these factors, the informed consent form will need to be physically filled out. This must include the full name of the operation, the provider who will be performing the procedure, the laterality when applicable, and the signature with date and time of both the patient and the person obtaining the consent. No abbreviations should be used, and the form must be legible. The form and content will vary between institutions, but these elements are included in recommendations from the Centers for Medicare and Medicaid Services and thus are widely adopted.

The Day of Surgery

When the patient arrives in the preoperative holding area, the care plan should be reviewed with the patient and the operative team, including any relevant imaging and office notes. The patient should be interviewed to determine whether there have been any relevant changes in their medical condition or history since they were seen in the clinic. The anesthesia team will obtain IV access and meet with the patient to review the anesthetic plan and obtain informed consent for their portion of the procedure.

The operative site should be marked by the surgeon. Although policies vary, in general this is accomplished by initialing the site of the planned incision in an area that will be visible after the patient is prepped and draped in the OR. This should be done with the patient awake and alert ensuring they agree with the location and laterality of the mark. It is important to verify the marked side matches the side indicated in the informed consent, as applicable.

Based on his/her perioperative risk, the patient may receive venous thromboembolic (VTE) chemoprophylaxis such as unfractionated or low-molecular-weight heparin. Sequential compression devices may also be applied.

The nursing team will meet with the patient and confirm that all of the necessary documentation and laboratory evaluations have been completed, such as an up-to-date history and physical examination, appropriately completed informed consent, operative site marking, and pregnancy test as needed. They will also introduce themselves as members of the team and assure that the patient understands the role of everyone participating in the OR.

Routine Postoperative Care

Although most hospitals now employ an electronic health record with prebuilt order sets, it is imperative that postoperative orders be entered correctly to assure the patients receive the intended care. The mechanism by which these are entered will vary by system and the specific health record, but the overall content is consistent.

Admit: To which floor, service, and attending will the patient be admitted? This is also an opportunity to provide contact information including the name/team(s) and number(s) to be called to reach the covering physician during the day, night, or on the weekends.

Diagnosis: The primary reason for admission.

Condition and code status: Is the patient stable? Is a "Do Not Resuscitate" order in place?

Vitals: How often should they be obtained? Anything special such as measuring a drain output or nasogastric tube should be listed as well.

Activity: Is the patient free to ambulate? Should he/she have assistance with movement? Is he/she at risk for falling?

Nursing: Should the nurses change the patient's dressings? Are there special drain care instructions? Is the patient hard of hearing or requiring special assistance otherwise? What vital signs and findings should the physician be notified about?

Diet: Should the patient be kept NPO (nothing by mouth) for a period of time, or is a diet appropriate? Does the patient have specific dietary restrictions or requirements (i.e., low sugar diet for diabetics)?

Allergies: Be sure these are appropriately updated.

Labs: Think carefully about what needs to be checked and when. How will these results affect the management of the patient?

IV fluids: What solution? What rate?

Special: Think about anything else the patient may need. This is the place to order sequential compression devices for VTE prophylaxis or incentive spirometry to decrease atelectasis. Does the patient need to see physical therapy, nutrition, occupational therapy, or another specialized service?

Medications: Carefully review the patient's home medications and decide which should be started right away and which should be held. Many patients will benefit from VTE chemoprophylaxis. If antibiotics are being ordered, think about how long the course will be and order as such. What medications will be used for analgesia?

In the outpatient surgery setting, these orders are replaced by discharge instructions given to the patient and their caregivers. It is important to be as specific as possible about any deviations from normal daily activities, how and when the patient should contact the physician's office, their medication regimen, and when they should be seen in follow-up.

POSTOPERATIVE ANALGESIA

Ideally, patients should be on an oral regimen that minimizes opiates, though the nature of the patient's operation may preclude this type of regimen initially (patients who are NPO or who remain intubated). Acetaminophen and/or an NSAID should be initiated as the first line for pain control, with extra precaution for patients with liver disease, renal impairment, or elevated bleeding risk. Opiates should be reserved for breakthrough pain. It is important to be mindful of opiates combined in a single pill with acetaminophen or ibuprofen. Overlooked duplications can rapidly lead to drug toxicity.

For patients who are unable to tolerate oral medications, an IV analgesic regimen is appropriate. Nonopiate medications are also available in intravenous formulations and may be preferable via this route. When significant postoperative pain is encountered, a patient-controlled analgesic (PCA) machine can be a useful adjunct. This allows the patient to self-administer IV opiate at a prescribed dose through the push of a demand button. Although the patient may press the button for medication delivery often, a prescribed "lock-out" period prevents them from receiving the medication too frequently. A maximum hourly dose can also be set. PCAs have significant advantages for postoperative pain control. They provide the patient with control over when they receive their medication, they decrease the need for nursing visits to the room to administer medications, and they decrease the risk for overdose as the patient is unable to press the button if they become too sedated.

If significant postoperative pain is anticipated or pain is difficult to control, it can be beneficial to involve an acute pain service if one is available at your institution. This is typically a group of anesthesia providers with special training in pain management. They may employ epidural analgesics or regional blocks such as a transversus abdominus plane (TAP) block.

POSTOPERATIVE ASSESSMENT

Typically, 4 to 6 hours after an operation is completed, it is good practice to perform a "postoperative check" on the patient. This should include seeing the patient at the bedside to inquire about pain or nausea, and assessing for any immediate complications that can develop in the perioperative period such as bleeding or acute cardiovascular or pulmonary events. The operative site should be examined, though usually dressings are left in place until at least the next day. Note should be made of the dressing's appearance and any skin changes around the surgical wound.

Any laboratory evaluations or images that were ordered postoperatively should be reviewed. The patient may also have questions about the conduct or findings of the operation which should be discussed. The postoperative check is an opportunity to identify issues before they become problems. Anything outside the expected postoperative course should be communicated to a more senior

TABLE 2.4 ■ **Signs and Symptoms That May Indicate the Development of Some Common Postoperative Complications**

Sign/Symptom	Possible Causes
Incisional pain	Inadequate pain control, wound infection (acute/necrotizing, delayed), wound disruption/dehiscence
Nausea/vomiting	Reaction to medications (including anesthesia), paralytic ileus
Acute confusion	Medications, sleep disturbances, dehydration, hemorrhage, sepsis
Tachycardia	Pain, volume depletion, hemorrhage, atrial fibrillation (or other conduction abnormality)
Hypotension	Volume depletion, hemorrhage, atrial fibrillation (or other conduction abnormality)
Hypertension	Pain, baseline hypertension (home medications not resumed)
Chest pain	Myocardial ischemia, reactive airway
Dyspnea	Atelectasis, reactive airway, pneumonia, failure to clear secretions, fluid overload, pulmonary embolism, myocardial ischemia
Leg swelling	Fluid overload, venous thromboembolism
Low urine output	Volume depletion, urinary retention, hemorrhage, urinary tract infection
Fever	Atelectasis, surgical site infection, urinary tract infection, drug reaction

member of the team right away. It is important to note that if the person who was present for the operation will not be the one performing the postoperative check, all relevant information about the patient and his or her operation must be related to that person.

Throughout the postoperative period, it is important to evaluate the patient for the development of common postoperative complications by regularly completing thorough physical examinations and assessments of the patient. A list of signs and symptoms that may indicate the development of some common postoperative complications is found in Table 2.4. Additionally, each operation will have its own set of specific possible complications related to the anatomic and physiologic alterations caused by the operation, and patient medical comorbidities may modify the risk of developing these complications.

Discharge From the Hospital

For patients to be safely discharged, they must be able to function in an environment where they will not have access to hospital resources. This means they must be able to maintain their nutrition and hydration enterally, their pain must be controlled with an oral regimen, they must be ambulatory without significant risk for falling, and they must be able to care for their wound and perform other basic activities of daily living. If there are questions about the patient's safety for going home, consultation with physical and occupational therapists can help determine whether a patient would benefit from additional rehabilitation in an inpatient or outpatient setting.

If a patient will have a complicated wound, a drain, a stoma, or another medical issue requiring care, it may be helpful to arrange for a visiting nurse to come to the patient's home. It is important to identify the patient's support structure and any assistance that will be available to the patient in regard to homecare needs. Alternatively, patients can be transferred to a skilled nursing facility (SNF) where they can continue to receive care, though at a lower acuity than is available in the hospital.

WHAT INSTRUCTIONS SHOULD A PATIENT RECEIVE WHEN LEAVING THE HOSPITAL?

Discharge instructions after hospitalization for surgery should be clear and specific. The discharge day is often a stressful time for patients, as they are still recovering from their operation and often have concerns about their safety and care at home. Carefully written instructions, however, can alleviate much of this anxiety, help assure patient safety, and prevent potential problems.

The instructions should include dietary recommendations, including what foods to avoid. Prehospitalization medications should be carefully reviewed and any changes to these regimens noted. If medications are to be held, it should be clear when they will be restarted and at what dose and frequency. Some medications may no longer be required, and it should be clearly noted that they should be stopped indefinitely. If the patient is going to be prescribed analgesics, these should be reviewed to assure proper usage. Patients should be counseled regarding the side effects of these and any other new medications initiated during hospitalization or at discharge. Interactions of prescribed medications with common over-the-counter medications and supplements should also be discussed.

Any limitations in activity should be clearly stated. Patients often want to know when they can shower, when they can drink alcohol, when they can drive a vehicle, and when they can return to work. Patients should be reminded to check with their employers for any documentation that might be required, such as disability claim forms, Family Medical Leave Act (FMLA) forms, or medical certifications for return to work.

The patient must also have clear instructions for outpatient follow-up. The location, time, and place of the postoperative appointments should be clearly explained and documented. Discussing the discharge instructions provides a good opportunity to identify any barriers to attending these appointments and to help arrange for transportation or rescheduling at a more convenient time.

Lastly, the patient should be given the specific phone numbers or mechanisms for getting help if there are any questions or concerns. It is useful to provide specific parameters, such as fever or vomiting, that should prompt a phone call. Spelling out what defines a fever, what kind of wound drainage is concerning, and what is an expected level of pain will align expectations and enhance identification of problems in a timely manner.

Suggested Readings

Bilimoria, K. Y., et al. (2013). Development and evaluation of the universal ACS NSQIP Surgical Risk Calculator: A decision aid and informed consent tool for patients and surgeons. *JACS, 217*(5), 833–842.

Castanheira, L., et al. (2011). Guidelines for the management of chronic medication in the perioperative period: Systematic review and formal consensus. *Journal of Clinical Pharmacy and Therapeutics, 36*(4), 446–467.

Committee on Standards and Practice Parameters. (2012). Practice advisory for preanesthesia evaluation: an updated report by the American Society of Anesthesiologists Task Force on Preanesthesia Evaluation. *Anesthesiology, 116*(3), 522–538.

Douketis, J. D., et al. (2015). Perioperative bridging anticoagulation in patients with atrial fibrillation. *NEJM, 373*(9), 823–833.

Kearon, C., et al. (2017). Antithrombotic therapy for VTE disease. *Chest, 149*(2), 315–352.

CHAPTER 3

Surgical Techniques

Sriharsha Gummadi   ■   Veeraiah Siripurapu

Surgical Fundamentals of Anesthesia

Although an in-depth discussion of anesthesia principles is outside the scope of this book, there are several important concepts that are important for surgeons-in-training to understand to safely perform any operation. Having a thorough understanding of every phase of the operation will allow the surgeon to predict potential pitfalls and complications before they occur.

PATIENT POSITIONING

In preparation for any operation, the first consideration is patient positioning. Considerations with choice of positioning include adequate airway management,access to the operative field, and ability to manage catastrophic complications. At best, unexpectedly having to reposition a patient in the middle of an operation can be laborious and possibly dangerous. However, sometimes one is forced to change patient position as part of a combined procedure and the process and logisits should be well thought out ahead of time. Considerations for choice of positioning include adequate airway management, access to the operative field, and ability to manage catastrophic complications. Common surgical positions are illustrated in Fig. 3.1.

SEDATION PHARMACOLOGY

Sedation agents can be divided into three general groups based on their functional goal: hypnosis, analgesia, and neuromuscular blockade. Hypnosis refers to lack of awareness or memory around the time of and during the operation. Analgesia refers to pain control. Finally, neuromuscular blockade refers to pharmacologic acetylcholine blockade preventing striated muscle contraction. In certain operations, this is required to allow for adequate muscle relaxation (such as in laparoscopic surgery or hernia surgery). However, in other operations, minimizing neuromuscular blockade is important because it allows for normal muscle stimulation and contraction, allowing the surgeon to identify nerves, such as in dissection of the axilla. Commonly used sedative agents are listed in Table 3.1.

TYPES OF ANESTHESIA

There are three types of anesthesia administration. In order from the "deepest" to "lightest," these include **general anesthesia** (GA), **monitored anesthesia care** (MAC), and **local/regional anesthesia**.

General anesthesia (GA) is the deepest form of anesthesia and involves complete sedation. Consequently, GA requires definitive airway control and mechanical ventilation. Compared with other forms of anesthesia, GA has the greatest effect on physiologic homeostasis and must be used with caution in patients with significant cardiopulmonary comorbidities. All procedures that require endotracheal intubation, neuromuscular blockade, or abdominal insufflation of gas (such as laparoscopic or robotic surgery) should be performed under GA.

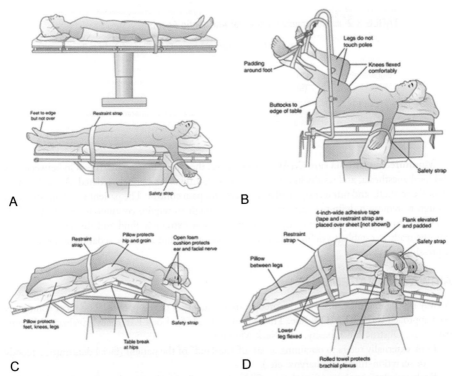

Fig. 3.1 Common positions for abdominal surgeries are depicted. (A) Supine position is used for most abdominal procedures and can be used with the patient's arms out or tucked to the side. (B) Lithotomy position is used for many urogynecologic and anorectal procedures. (C) Prone (jackknife variation) position may be used for anorectal procedures. (D) Lateral position can be used for retroperitoneal operations and thoracoabdominal procedures. (Images adapted from Fuller, JK: *Surgical Technology: Principles and Practices*, ed 6, St. Louis, MO, 2013, Elsevier Health Sciences.)

TABLE 3.1 ■ **Commonly Used Agents for Sedation**

Hypnosis	Analgesia	Neuromuscular Blockade
Propofol	Ketamine	Succinylcholine
Etomidate	Ketorolac	Rocuronium
Ketamine	Acetaminophen	Cisatracurium
Nitrous Oxide	Opioid narcotics	Vecuronium
Sevoflurane		
Benzodiazepines		

Contrastingly, **local and regional anesthesia** involves the infusion or injection of local anesthetic agents (such as lidocaine) directly into the operative area. Common local anesthetic agents are detailed in Table 3.2. Surgeons may infiltrate the actual tissue to be incised or may perform a "field block" in which all the cutaneous nerves around the incision are anesthetized. Both techniques are frequently utilized for bedside procedures. For more complex procedures, a regional block may be performed by instilling local anesthetic agents directly into the innervating nerve (peripheral nerve block), into the spinal fluid (spinal anesthesia) or around the spinal cord (epidural anesthesia).

TABLE 3.2 ■ Commonly Used Local Anesthetic Agents

	Maximum Dose (mg/kg)[a]	Duration of Action (hr)
Lidocaine	4 (7)	2
Bupivacaine	2 (3)	6
Procaine	7 (9)	1.5

[a]Epinephrine may be added for vasoconstriction, allowing for the administration of a higher dose with less systemic absorption and longer duration of effect.

Monitored anesthesia care (MAC) encompasses the wide range of anesthesia in between GA and local anesthesia, and results in the patient being lightly or moderately sedated. A combination of local anesthetic and intravenous analgesic is used for pain control. The patient is not anesthetized enough to require a definitive airway but deeply enough to require continuous monitoring. It is important to note that a patient's depth of anesthesia is extremely fluid and the anesthesiologist must be ready to establish a definitive airway (intubation) should excessive sedation and respiratory depression occur.

AIRWAY MANAGEMENT

Airway management begins with the preoperative evaluation of the patient. The most commonly used approach is the **LEMON** rule. This acronym stands for Look Externally, Evaluate, Mallampati score, Obstruction/Obesity, and Neck Mobility.

Look externally refers to obtaining a "lay-of-the-land" of the patient (facial deformities, bloody or secretion-filled oropharynx, etc.).

Evaluate relates to the predicted ease of laryngoscopy for intubation. A variety of rules exist, but all are predicated on assessing whether the patient's mouth is geometrically favorable for direct laryngoscopy. The modified **M**allampati score (Table 3.3 and Fig. 3.2) allows for an estimation of oral crowding (which prevents visualization).

Obstruction/**O**besity refers to upper away obstructive processes that can make laryngoscopy difficult.

Neck mobility refers to the ability of the practitioner to place the patient in the "sniffing position" (neck flexion and head elevation) for easier intubation.

A variety of airway devices are available (Fig. 3.3). The most fundamental is bag-mask ventilation (BMV). If a patient is adequately ventilated via BMV, there is time to obtain a more definitive airway. The endotracheal tube (ETT) provides a definitive airway as it lies directly within the trachea. However, in limited (less than 3 hour) GA procedures among low-risk patients, anesthesiologists may elect for a laryngeal mask airway (LMA) instead, which is a supraglottic alternative to the endotracheal tube. Although this does not provide a classical definitive airway, it is easier to place and may cause less oral and airway irritation. Adjuncts include oropharyngeal and nasopharyngeal airways—devices placed in the patient's pharynx to keep the airway open (particularly under

TABLE 3.3 ■ Modified Mallampati Score

	Hard Palate	Soft Palate	Uvula	Tonsillar Pillars
Class I	Visible	Visible	Visible	Visible
Class II	Visible	Visible	Only Base Visible	Not Visible
Class III	Visible	Visible	Not Visible	Not Visible
Class IV	Visible	Not Visible	Not Visible	Not Visible

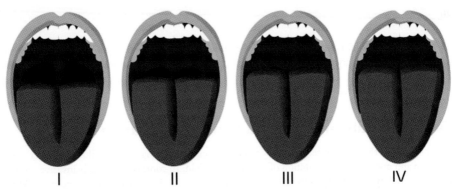

Fig. 3.2 Modified Mallampati Score to assess oral crowding based on external examination of the tongue, tonsils and uvula.

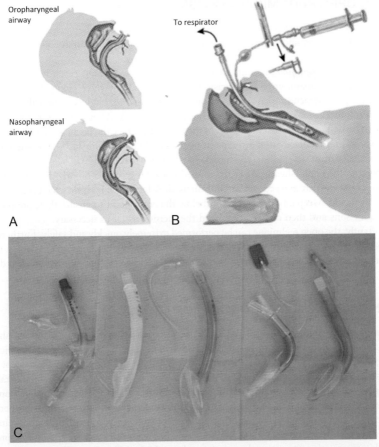

Fig. 3.3 (A) Common airway adjuncts include oropharyngeal and nasopharyngeal airways. (B) Endotracheal tubes extend below the vocal cords (subglottic) and provide a definitive airway when the cuff is inflated. (C) A variety of supraglottic devices such as the laryngeal mask airway (LMA) exist and can be a less invasive option for the appropriate patient. (Image (A) and (B) adapted from Delaney, CP: *Netter's Surgical Anatomy and Approaches*, Philadelphia, PA, 2014, Elsevier Health Sciences. Image (C) adapted from Metterlein, T, Dintenfelder, A, Plank, C, Graf, B, Roth, G: A comparison of various supraglottic airway devices for fiberoptical guided tracheal intubation, *Brazilian Journal of Anesthesiology* (English Edition) 67(2): 166–171, 2017.)

MAC anesthesia). Neither of these options is considered a definitive airway as they do not protect against aspiration or laryngospasm. Importantly, if a patient cannot be adequately ventilated via BMV and a definitive airway cannot be established, the patient requires a surgical airway—a tracheostomy, or in a true emergency, a cricothyroidotomy.

Fundamentals of Open and Minimally Invasive Surgery

Open surgery is the classical technique by which a fascial incision is made to allow for direct visualization and manual instrumentation of the operative field. In contrast, minimally invasive surgery includes a variety of techniques for minimizing or eliminating the skin and fascial incisions. Minimally invasive techniques include laparoscopic surgery, robotic surgery, endoscopic surgery, and natural orifice surgery.

GAINING OPEN ABDOMINAL ACCESS

One of the keys to any successful operation is adequate exposure of the operative field. Making the appropriate incision and adequately retracting are both necessary for successful exposure in an open case.

Common open abdominal incisions are detailed in Fig. 3.4. The most well-known open incisions is the midline laparotomy. This incision can be carried anywhere along the line from the xiphoid to the pubis depending on the extent of exposure required. Understanding abdominal wall anatomy is important for safe open abdominal access (Fig. 3.5). After the skin incision is made, dissection is carried to the decussating fascia of the linea alba. Once the fascia is incised, only a loose areolar layer of preperitoneal fat and the peritoneum should be encountered. If the surgeon inadvertently deviates from the midline, the muscle of the rectus abdominis will be seen with concomitant entry into the rectus sheath. After the preperitoneal fat has been bluntly dissected away, the peritoneum can be gently grasped and carefully incised. After abdominal entry has been confirmed, the surgeon should sweep a finger above and below the entry point to ensure there are no intrabdominal adhesions and then proceed to extend the incision as far as necessary.

Importantly, the open technique can be performed extremely quickly and safely. Furthermore, a generous midline incision allows access to almost the entire abdomen. For these reasons, a midline laparotomy incision (as opposed to minimally invasive approaches) should be considered for all patients who are unstable or suffering from major intraabdominal catastrophe.

TECHNICAL CONSIDERATIONS OF LAPAROSCOPY

Laparoscopy is the use of a camera (laparoscope) and long instruments inserted into the abdomen through a series of small (frequently less than 10 mm) working ports (Fig. 3.6). Laparoscopic procedures are performed within the peritoneal cavity. However, the fundamentals of laparoscopy can be applied to any potential space, including the preperitoneal space, retroperitoneum, and pleural space.

Whereas open surgery relies on retraction to create a working space, laparoscopy relies on pneumoperitoneum and "pneumodissection." That is, the surgeon insufflates air into the peritoneal space, grossly separating the parietal and visceral peritoneum. Consequently, the abdominal wall is lifted away from the intraabdominal organs, providing a working space. CO_2 is the preferred gas for this purpose because it is relatively inert, has a high diffusion coefficient, and is rapidly cleared from the body. Any insufflated CO_2 not evacuated at the end of the procedure is absorbed by the blood and cleared by ventilation.

Modern laparoscopic equipment continually monitors the peritoneal insufflation pressure and maintains it at a set point, typically 15 mm Hg. A pressure consistently lower than the set point suggests an air leak that can make the operation difficult by limiting visualization. In contrast, a pressure higher than the set point can signal the presence of abdominal muscle contraction in the patient.

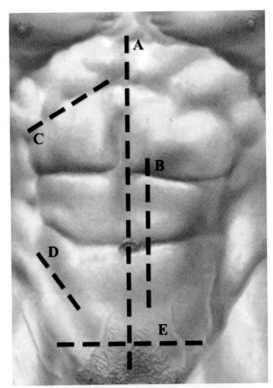

Fig. 3.4 Common abdominal incisions. (A) The midline incision allows for excellent exposure for most abdominal operations and is the incision of choice in trauma. (B) The paramedian incision to either side can be used as an alternative to the midline incision for select patients. (C) The Kocher (subcostal) incision allows for exposure of the gallbladder and liver. The incision may be performed on the left side for access to the spleen or bilaterally (Chevron incision) for exposure of the entire upper abdomen. (D) The McBurney incision is the incision of choice for appendectomies. (E) The Pfannenstiel incision allows access to pelvic organs and is frequently utilized by urologists and gynecologists. (Image adapted from Delaney, CP: *Netter's Surgical Anatomy and Approaches*, Philadelphia, PA, 2014, Elsevier Health Sciences.)

This can be the first sign that an additional dose of anesthetic is required to achieve full neuromuscular blockade. A variety of pressure (and gas flow) settings can be used depending on the patient's age, pathology, medical comorbidities, and technical considerations of the procedure.

The standard laparoscope is a rigid fiberoptic camera with a diameter ranging between 2 to 10 mm. The camera (and working instrumentation) is inserted into the abdomen through one of several ports inserted through the abdominal wall. Newer cameras can provide high-resolution images and are small enough to fit through smaller (5 mm or less) ports. The laparoscope is fitted with a lens at the end of its shaft to allow for an angled view of the working field (0–135 degrees). This allows for flexibility to look up, down, or sideways around obstructing structures.

Port placement can be highly variable depending on surgeon preference and the operation. However, several key principles must be followed. First, the surgeon should aim for triangulation. That is, the angle between two lines each drawn from each working port to the target area should be at least 30 degrees. This allows for freedom of movement of the instruments without collision. Additionally, the ports should be far enough from the target pathology to be ergonomic for the surgeon but close enough to be reachable by the instruments. This can be difficult to achieve in obese patients or when working deep in the pelvis.

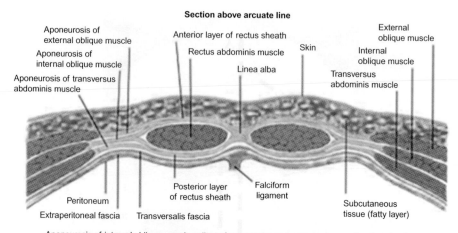

Aponeurosis of internal oblique muscle splits to form anterior and posterior layers of rectus sheath, Aponeurosis of external oblique muscle joins anterior layer of sheath: aponeurosis of transversus abdominis muscle joins posterior layer. Anterior and posterior layers of rectus sheath unite medially to form linea alba.

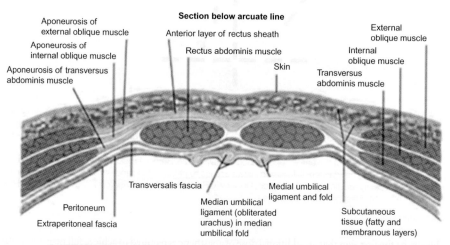

Aponeurosis of internal oblique muscle does not split at this level but passes completely anterior to rectus abdominis muscle and is fused there with both aponeurosis of external oblique muscle and that of transversus abdominis muscle. Thus, posterior wall of rectus sheath is absent below arcuate line and is composed of only transversalis fascia.

Fig. 3.5 Standard abdominal wall anatomy. Importantly, there is no posterior layer to the rectus sheath below the arcuate line. (Image from Netter, FH: *Atlas of Human Anatomy*, Philadelphia, PA, 2011, Elsevier Health Sciences.)

CARDIOPULMONARY CONSIDERATIONS OF LAPAROSCOPY

Modern laparoscopy can have several secondary cardiopulmonary effects. These effects are predominantly mediated by the increased intraabdominal pressure exerted by the pneumoperitoneum and the use of CO_2 as the insufflating gas. These effects tend to be more pronounced in patients with existing cardiopulmonary disease and limited reserve. Importantly, intraoperative hemodynamic perturbations related to laparoscopy can be easily reversed with immediate desufflation.

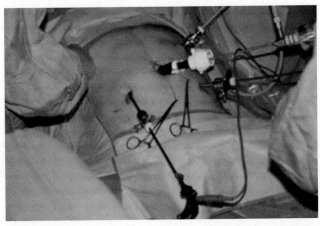

Fig. 3.6 Laparoscopic surgery is performed using long instruments passed into the abdominal cavity via trocars. (Image from Townsend, CM, et al: *Sabiston Textbook of Surgery*, ed 20, Philadelphia, PA, 2016, Elsevier Health Sciences.)

The cardiac effects of laparoscopy are generally transient, but patients with extensive cardiac disease must be monitored very closely. Insufflation pressure can compress the abdominal vasculature, leading to decreased venous return and increased afterload, both of which can lead to decreased cardiac output. Additionally, CO_2 absorption can result in transient hypercarbia, leading to increased systemic vascular resistance (SVR) and cardiac arrhythmia.

The pulmonary effects of laparoscopy tend to last the duration of the operation. Hypercarbia from CO_2 insufflation triggers an increase in minute ventilation in the patient to maintain acid–base balance. However, in patients unable to adequately hyperventilate (such as in chronic obstructive pulmonary disease or asthma), the anesthesiologist must account for this rise in P_{CO_2}. Additionally, the patient's own functional residual capacity (FRC) may decrease with the elevation of diaphragm and increased intraabdominal pressure.

GAINING LAPAROSCOPIC ABDOMINAL ACCESS

When gaining safe abdominal access for laparoscopy one must take care not to inadvertently injure bowel or solid organs during trocar insertion. Since initial access to the abdomen can be largely blind, the first trocar has the greatest potential to cause intra-abdominal injury, and great care must be taken to avoid this. Three common techniques for primary port placement have been described: **open or Hasson, Veress needle**, and **optical trocar**.

The **open technique** (also known as the Hasson technique) begins with a small incision frequently near the umbilicus. The subcutaneous tissues are dissected away and the linea alba is visualized. After incising the linea alba, sutures may be placed to mark the fascial edges to make final fascial closure easier ("stay sutures"). The preperitoneal fat is bluntly dissected, and the peritoneum is sharply and carefully incised enabling the trocar to be inserted under direct visualization. Many surgeons choose this technique for patient's who are expected to have a large volume of intraabdominal adhesions due to previous abdominal surgeries since it allows for more direct visualization compared with the other techniques.

Contrastingly, the **Veress needle technique** utilizes a 14- to 18-gauge spring-loaded needle, which is inserted somewhat blindly. This needle is small enough that any inadvertent bowel or solid organ injury can be mitigated. After a small (5 mm) incision is made in the desired location (often umbilical or "Palmer's point," 2 cm below the costal margin at the left midclavicular line), the needle is inserted into the abdomen. Every "click" of the spring in the device represents passing from a high- to low-resistance tissue. Specifically, this occurs when passing through the abdominal fascia and parietal peritoneum. Frequently, there will be two "clicks" through an umbilical incision—one for the linea alba and one for the peritoneum. There may be three clicks or more with other incisions wherein the falciform ligament or additional fascial layers are encountered. Once the needle tip is presumed to be in the peritoneal space, it is aspirated to confirm there is no blood return (which would indicate intravascular placement) or enteric contents (which would indicate placement in the bowel lumen). A small volume of saline is then instilled by gravity through the Veress needle. If fluid passes easily, the needle is confirmed to be in a low-resistance space, presumably the peritoneal cavity, rather than the abdominal wall. Of note, if the needle inadvertently punctures the bowel wall, there may be no resistance to the flow of saline because the tip is within the bowel lumen. After confirmation of intraperitoneal placement, air is insufflated, the needle is removed and a trocar can be safely (albeit blindly) inserted.

A newer technique that is available is referred to as the **optical trocar technique**. First, a small (5 mm) incision is made in the desired trocar location. Using a compatible laparoscope–trocar system, the trocar is inserted into the abdomen with the camera inside it. The surgeon is able to visualize each layer of the abdominal wall as it passes with advancement of the optical trocar until peritoneal entry is achieved. Some have suggested utilizing a combination of this technique with the Veress needle technique for the safest entry. Compared with the open technique, the Veress needle and optical trocar technique allow the surgeon to make the smallest incision possible for the primary port placement. This is particularly beneficial for obese patients.

SUTURE

Suture is used in both open and laparoscopic surgery to approximate tissues, mark locations of interest, and close incisions. A variety of suture types are available to surgeons (Table 3.4). They are frequently classified by their absorbability and the number of filaments within a strand. Although nonabsorbable suture may have increased durability, there can be a long-term concern for chronic foreign body reaction or infection. Additionally, multifilament (braided) suture may increase knot security, but the multifilament nature in and of itself may serve as a nidus for infection. Additional characteristics to consider in suture selection include memory (tendency to unravel to its original state), tensile strength, and tissue reactivity. Furthermore, surgeons may specify the diameter and length of the suture, the size and type of the needle, and even whether there are needles on both ends of the suture. Frequently, the choice of suture is dependent on surgeon familiarity.

TABLE 3.4 ■ **Commonly Used Suture Material in the Operating Room**

Suture Material	Absorbability	Number of filaments
Catgut	Absorbable	Multifilament
Chromic catgut	Absorbable	Multifilament
Poliglecaprone 25	Absorbable	Monofilament
Polyglactin 910	Absorbable	Multifilament
Polydioxanone	Absorbable	Monofilament
Silk	Nonabsorbable (very slow)	Multifilament
Polypropylene	Nonabsorbable	Monofilament
Polyamide	Nonabsorbable	Mono- or Multifilament

ELECTROSURGERY

The advent of electrosurgery has allowed for simultaneous precise dissection and hemostatic control. The two most frequently encountered systems are monopolar and bipolar electrosurgery instrumentation. In monopolar electrocautery, current passes from a pencil-like tip into the operative site, travels through the patient to a grounding pad adhered to the skin, and exits back to the generator. The thermal effect of the electric current is limited to the small area at the tip of the instrument, rather than the large area of the grounding pad. In bipolar electrocautery, a dual-pronged instrument applies a current between its heads, applying the current only to interposed tissue. The bipolar method allows for even more precise application of energy.

Surgeons can also specify the level of modulation of the current passing through their instrument. A minimally/unmodulated, continuous current ("cut" mode) rapidly heats tissues at its tip and tends to cause immediate and precise tissue vaporization. Conversely, a highly modulated, noncontinuous "coagulate" mode tends to result in more charring at the cut tissue margin due to simultaneous protein desiccation and coagulation. Despite these categorizations, the bioeffect of electrosurgery can be quite variable and is dependent on the actual level of modulation, application distance, power output of the unit, and tissue characteristics. Surgeon experience and familiarity play a significant role in electrosurgery parameter optimization during an operation.

Advanced energy devices are becoming increasingly more prevalent, particularly for minimally invasive applications. These bipolar devices are tissue responsive and sense the rise in impedance created by coagulation to control the exact amount of energy and duration of the current cycle, allowing for more precise vessel sealing. There are multiple advanced energy devices, each of which has its own functional parameters. Additional sources of energy now include ultrasonic and laser devices.

BEYOND THE PEARLS

- When planning an operation, considerations include patient positioning, type of anesthesia, and whether to pursue an open or minimally invasive approach.
- The only definitive airway is an endotracheal tube. However, it is worth considering a less invasive alternative in the appropriate patient.
- Laparoscopic surgery should be considered when appropriate—it allows for smaller incisions and may expedite postoperative recovery compared with open surgery.
- If a patient is unstable or if obtaining laparoscopic abdominal access is hazardous, there should be no hesitation to convert to an open technique.
- The choice of suture is highly dependent on surgeon familiarity and circumstance.
- Electrosurgery has become integral to modern surgery. Familiarity with its application and safety profile is paramount to safely performing most operations.

Suggested Readings

Fleisher, L. A., Fleischmann, K. E., Auerbach, A. D., Barnason, S. A., Beckman, J. A., Bozkurt, B., et al. (2014). 2014 ACC/AHA guideline on perioperative cardiovascular evaluation and management of patients undergoing noncardiac surgery. *Circulation*.

Neudecker, J., Sauerland, S., Neugebauer, E., Bergamaschi, R., Bonjer, H., Cuschieri, A., et al. (2002). The European Association for Endoscopic Surgery clinical practice guideline on the pneumoperitoneum for laparoscopic surgery. *Surgical Endoscopy, 16*(7), 121–1143.

Philips, P. A., & Amaral, J. F. (2001). Abdominal access complications in laparoscopic surgery. *Journal of the American College of Surgeons, 192*(4), 525–536.

CHAPTER 4

Radiology: Basic Methods and Modalities

Daniel M. DePietro   ■   Anton Mahne

Introduction

Medical imaging plays an integral role in the care of surgical patients, and has revolutionized the way in which surgery is practiced. Diagnostic imaging studies have become one of the most powerful tools a surgeon can utilize to help make a diagnosis, plan an operation, follow up on expected postprocedure findings, or reveal unexpected complications. It is imperative for the surgical trainee to become familiar with various imaging modalities commonly used in the diagnosis and treatment of surgical disease, develop a sense of when and why to order an imaging study when pursuing a diagnosis, and begin to develop the skills necessary to interpret such imaging studies. Together with a sound history and physical examination, a properly selected imaging study helps navigate the differential and hopefully confirm the underlying diagnosis.

In order to achieve this, it is important to actively work toward understanding the indications for different imaging studies and develop an ability to interpret imaging findings, which is not an easy task in the busy life of a surgical trainee! To aid in this endeavor, here are some words of advice:

- **Interpret the patient's imaging studies:** Throughout this section, we will introduce various imaging modalities commonly used when managing the surgical patient, and discuss some common pathologic imaging findings. Remember that the greatest benefit comes from actively interpreting a patient's imaging studies throughout training. Always read a patient's studies, and seek expert consultation for confusing or advanced studies.
- **Normal versus abnormal**: In order to properly interpret images, begin developing an idea of what "normal" versus "abnormal" imaging findings look like. This seemingly simple first step is not as easy as it sounds and takes time to develop. Once normal versus abnormal imaging findings are easily distinguished, begin to focus on the different types of abnormal findings, which will help lead to making a diagnosis.
- **Appropriate versus inappropriate:** Appropriateness in imaging can have many interpretations. Is this the appropriate study that will provide the data needed to make a medical decision? Is this the appropriate time for an imaging study? Is ordering this study an appropriate use of hospital resources? The list goes on. Trainees must learn to think critically about ordering imaging studies at the appropriate time and for the appropriate reason. Whether a study is appropriate can often be answered by asking one simple question: *How will the results of this test change the care of this patient?* If the study will aid in making a diagnosis, guide decision making in the care of a patient, or help safely plan the approach to an operation, the study is rendered appropriate. Developing a sense of when an imaging study is appropriate requires the trainee to continually question why an imaging study is being performed and how the results will be used to guide patient care.

Although this section is not a comprehensive review of all the relevant imaging modalities and studies that a surgeon-in-training will have to be familiar with, let it serve as a brief introduction to the most common modalities, and illustrate a number of imaging findings that one should learn to recognize.

Contrast Agents

Before considering the types of imaging studies, it is important to understand that their interpretation relies on understanding that the images generated are due to different densities of tissues and other materials in the body. Contrast agents are utilized to accentuate the visibility of internal organ systems by creating differences in density in structures that otherwise do not have an inherent difference in density compared with their surroundings.

Iodinated contrast agents: Iodinated contrast agents are ionic or nonionic, water-soluble solutions utilized in many radiologic, interventional, and endovascular procedures. They are commonly used in contrast-enhanced computed tomography (CT) studies. These contrast agents must be used with care, as many patients have allergies to iodine, and they may also cause renal impairment. Patients may need to be premedicated to prevent a potentially life-threatening allergic reaction or kidney damage.

Barium: Barium, a white powder suspended in a liquid to allow for its ingestion, is used as a water-insoluble, high-density contrast agent for fluoroscopic studies of the gastrointestinal tract. Barium is contraindicated when intestinal perforation is suspected, as there is no way for the body to remove the barium suspension if there is extraluminal spillage into the peritoneal cavity. Barium should also be avoided if a GI tract operation is anticipated in the near future.

Gastrografin: Gastrografin is a high-osmolality, water-soluble iodinated contrast agent used in GI studies when barium is contraindicated. Being water-soluble, it may be absorbed by the body if extraluminal spillage occurs. The disadvantages of gastrografin include its lower density compared with barium, limiting its ability to delineate anatomic structures, and its high osmolality, which may cause a fluid shift into the bowel lumen when used, resulting in hypovolemia. There is also a potential risk of pulmonary edema if gastrografin is aspirated.

Carbon Dioxide: Carbon dioxide may be utilized as an intravascular contrast agent in patients with impaired renal function or contraindications to iodinated contrast administration.

Plain Radiographs

Radiographic imaging is based on the concept that objects of different densities absorb light of a certain wavelength differently. X-rays, whose wavelength is less than that of visible light and ultraviolet light, are able to penetrate through objects that are opaque to visible light. This allows one to see through otherwise opaque objects and provides a window into the human body. X-rays represent a two-dimensional image of a complex object that represents the sum of the densities of the object being imaged and is therefore dependent on the varying densities of the object being imaged. This allows for plain radiographs to delineate among gas, fat, soft tissue, bone, and metal. Air and gas is black; fat is dark gray; soft tissue is light gray; bone is white; metal is bright white. In addition to the density of the organs and objects being imaged, the thickness of the various components and how they are layered together within the human body must also be taken into account during image interpretation.

COMMON SURGICAL USES OF PLAIN RADIOGRAPHS

Chest radiograph—the common chest radiograph—is a fast, easy, and inexpensive way to evaluate for a number of different disease states. The ease at which it can be obtained makes it useful in simple decision making: *Does the patient need to emergently go to the OR? Is the patient short of breath*

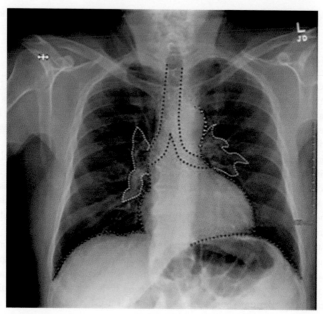

Fig. 4.1 Normal chest radiograph. Note the trachea and main stem bronchi *(blue)*, the hila *(white)*, the aortic knob *(yellow)*, the heart border *(red)*, and the diaphragm *(green)*.

due to a collapsed lung or pulmonary edema? Is a central line in the correct position? All of these questions can be quickly answered by obtaining a chest radiograph, more commonly known as a "chest x-ray" (Fig. 4.1). The surgeon-in-training should develop a system for evaluating and reading a chest radiograph and be able to identify common pathologies.

EVALUATION OF THE CHEST RADIOGRAPH

- **A**irway: trachea, carina, bronchi, hilar structures
- **B**reathing: lungs (opacities, absence/presence of lung markings, air bronchograms), pleural spaces
- **C**ardiac: heart, mediastinum, aorta, pulmonary vasculature
- **D**iaphragm: free air (pneumoperitoneum), costophrenic angles (pleural effusions)
- **E**verything else: bones and soft tissue (spine, ribs, clavicle, scapula, subcutaneous air), tubes (nasogastric, endotracheal, and chest tubes), catheter positions (central lines, Mediports, PICCs, etc.), pacemakers, the upper abdomen, foreign bodies, prostheses

Abnormal Chest Radiograph Findings of Interest for the Surgeon-in-Training

Abnormal chest radiograph findings are referred to as "The Ps."

Pneumoperitoneum: Defined as free air under the diaphragm, it is best evaluated on an upright chest x-ray (Fig. 4.2). Free air is a perforated viscus until proven otherwise and constitutes a surgical emergency. There are, however, a number of benign causes of free air that one should be familiar with as well (Table 4.1).

Pneumothorax: Defined as an abnormal collection of air between the lung and the chest wall (Fig. 4.3). The presence of air in the pleural space prevents proper expansion of the lung, leading to respiratory distress. Absent lung markings and a visible line marking the border of the compressed lung can be noted on a chest x-ray. A pneumothorax is treated by inserting a chest tube into the pleural space to evacuate the air and allow the lung to reinflate.

CLINICAL PEARL

Tension pneumothorax is the progressive buildup of air within the pleural space and is an immediately life-threatening situation. Venous return to the heart is obstructed due to the increased pressure within the chest and resulting mediastinal shift. Tension pneumothorax results in hypotension, hypoxia, and absent breath sounds on the affected side. Imaging will show pneumothorax and tracheal/mediastinal shift toward the contralateral hemithorax. Treatment is emergent needle decompression (needle thoracostomy) to release the air and pressure followed by chest tube placement.

TABLE 4.1 ■ Causes of Pneumoperitoneum

Causes of Pneumoperitoneum Requiring Surgical Intervention	Causes of Pneumoperitoneum Without Perforated Viscus
Patients will have peritonitis	Patients will not have peritonitis
Perforated gastric/duodenal ulcer	Postoperative (air may be present for days after laparotomy/laparoscopy)
Perforated cancer	Mechanical ventilation
Ischemia (embolus primary ischemia, strangulated bowel) leading to perforation	Pneumothorax
Perforated diverticulitis	Pelvic manipulation
Perforated appendicitis	Benign pneumatosis intestinalis
Anastomotic breakdown	Cardiopulmonary resuscitation

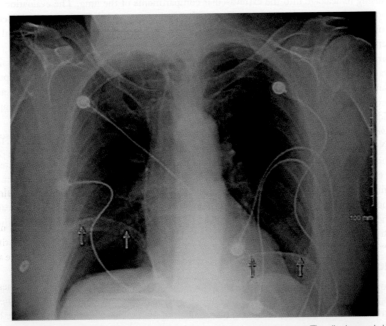

Fig. 4.2 Pneumoperitoneum is seen under both the right and left hemidiaphragms. The diaphragm is indicated by the yellow arrows. This patient had a colonic perforation.

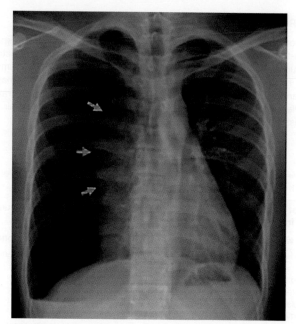

Fig. 4.3 Right-sided pneumothorax. Notice the lack of pulmonary vasculature on the right side and the increased density of the compressed right lung *(yellow arrows)*.

Pulmonary edema: There are many causes of fluid accumulation in the pulmonary vasculature, causing its leakage into the extravascular compartments of the lung. The evaluation of pulmonary edema on a chest x-ray is often used to evaluate a patient's fluid status in the setting of fluid overload, resuscitation, and diuresis (Fig. 4.4). Serial chest x-rays can be useful in this setting.

Pleural effusions: The buildup of fluid within the pleural space. The fluid may be classified as transudative or exudative, and may commonly consist of serous fluid, blood, chyle, or pus. The fluid is usually gravity dependent and will blunt the costophrenic angles when small and will present as a "white-out" on a chest x-ray when large (Fig. 4.5). A lateral chest radiograph may aid in the diagnosis of a small pleural effusion.

Proper tube placement: Proper central venous catheter, endotracheal tube (ETT), nasogastric (NGT), and Dobhoff tube positioning is commonly evaluated by chest x-ray (Fig. 4.6). In the adult, proper ETT placement is in the middle third of the trachea, approximately 5 to 7 cm above the carina, around the T2–T4 level, with the neck in neutral position. NGT and Dobhoff tubes are evaluated for proper positioning within the GI tract, ensuring that they are not improperly placed within the trachea or bronchial tree. Central venous catheters should have their tip residing at the distal superior vena cava where it joins with the right atrium, known as the cavoatrial junction.

CLINICAL PEARL

The position of any tube into which something is to be infused (central venous catheter, Dobhoff feeding tube, nasogastric tube for oral contrast, etc.) should be evaluated with imaging post placement to ensure proper positioning before use.

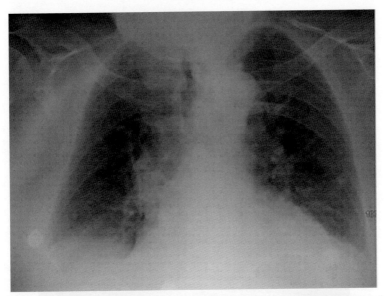

Fig. 4.4 Pulmonary edema is suggested by increased congestion (cephalization) of the pulmonary veins, making them more prominent on x-ray, and patchy opacities with air bronchograms. Air bronchograms are noticeable due to the increased difference in density between the fluid-filled lung tissues compared with the air-filled bronchi. Compare this image to the normal lung in Fig. 4-1.

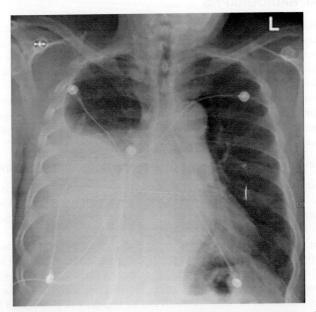

Fig. 4.5 A large, right-sided pleural effusion, the lung is "whited out" by the buildup of fluid within the pleural space.

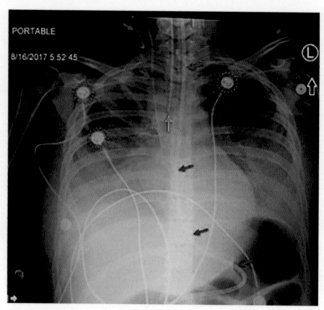

Fig. 4.6 Multiple lines and tubes are present in this x-ray. A central venous catheter inserted in the right internal jugular vein is properly positioned with its tip at the cavoatrial junction *(blue arrows)*. An endotracheal tube terminates superior to the carina *(yellow arrow)*. A Dobhoff feeding tube is seen passing through the stomach and beyond the pylorus *(green arrows)*. ECG leads, commonly seen on x-ray, are highlighted in red.

ABDOMINAL RADIOGRAPHS

The abdominal radiograph is a useful and easy study to obtain in the initial workup of abdominal pain or distention, but inherently suffers from low sensitivity and accuracy for many disease processes. It is often used to help delineate a bowel obstruction versus an ileus in the surgical patient and can be utilized to evaluate for free air, foreign bodies, calculi and volvulus. The most common abdominal radiograph is the kidney, ureter, bladder radiograph, or KUB.

Interpretation of a KUB or other abdominal film includes analysis of the gas pattern, soft tissues, bones, calcifications (stones, calcific deposits in organs), and "everything else." A normal bowel gas pattern is defined as small bowel loops filled with gas or fluid less than 3 cm in size; the colon can be larger in size, and air may be seen in the stomach and rectum.

Abnormal Findings of Interest on a KUB to the Surgeon-in-Training

Pneumoperitoneum: Defined earlier, when pneumoperitoneum is present, it is observed on a KUB similarly to how it is observed on a chest x-ray, with free air present underneath one or both hemidiaphragms (Fig. 4.7). Note that air under the diaphragms will only be observed in the KUB is performed in the upright position.

Pneumatosis intestinalis: Defined as the presence of gas tracking within the bowel wall. This imaging finding indicates intestinal ischemia and, if the condition is severe, infarcted bowel (Fig. 4.8). The presence of portal venous gas may be present in severe cases as well.

Bowel obstruction: Dilated loops of bowel will be observed proximal to an obstruction. Air–fluid levels may be observed in an upright KUB and are especially suspicious for a bowel obstruction; they help distinguish an obstruction from an ileus on KUB (Fig. 4.9). A small bowel obstruction will have a nondistended colon on KUB, as the bowel is decompressed distal to the obstruction, whereas one should see dilated colon in a large bowel obstruction.

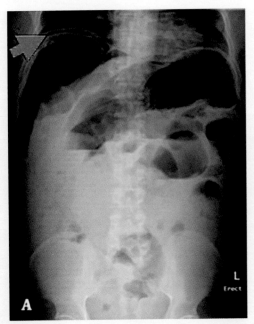

Fig. 4.7   Pneumoperitoneum *(yellow arrow)* observed on a KUB along with dilated loops of bowel and air-fluid levels.

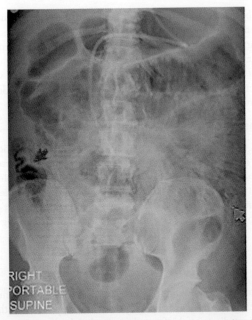

Fig. 4.8   Pneumatosis intestinalis observed on a KUB. Intramural gas *(red arrow)* and linear air streaks *(yellow arrow)* can be seen tracking within the bowel wall.

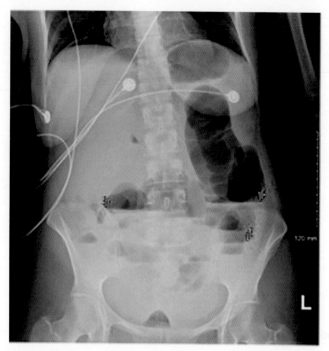

Fig. 4.9   Evidence of large bowel obstruction on a KUB. The yellow arrows highlight multiple air fluid levels within the dilated small and large bowel proximal to the obstruction.

Ileus: Defined as bowel without peristalsis in the absence of a mechanical obstruction, commonly encountered after any intraabdominal surgery. Loops of gas-filled bowel will be present on imaging (Fig. 4.10). Air–fluid levels are generally absent or minimal, distinguishing an ileus from a true bowel obstruction.

Volvulus: Volvulus is the result of the bowel twisting on itself. Sigmoid volvulus is more commonly encountered than cecal volvulus and is typically seen in the elderly. Radiographs will show a large, extremely dilated, air-filled loop of colon (Fig. 4.11).

Obstruction Series

An obstruction series, once the go-to imaging study for the evaluation of abdominal pain and distension, is comprised of three radiographs including: 1) an upright chest radiograph; 2) a supine abdominal radiograph; and 3) an erect or left lateral decubitus radiograph (Fig. 4.12). CT has largely replaced the obstruction series as the first test a patient would undergo in such a clinical setting. It is still commonly used as a follow-up study to evaluate a patient's progression after an initial diagnosis of bowel obstruction is made and is useful in delineating an obstruction from an ileus.

Fluoroscopy

Fluoroscopy can be simply described simply as real-time, continuous x-ray imaging that is sent to a monitor rather than being developed as a radiograph. Fluoroscopy allows for the study of the motion of internal structures, providing useful information regarding both anatomy and function. Contrast agents are commonly used to highlight the structures of interest on fluoroscopic studies. Common

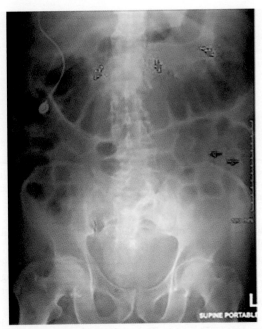

Fig. 4.10 KUB of a patient with a postoperative ileus. The red arrows highlight gas-filled loops of small bowel; the yellow arrows highlight an air-filled large bowel, specifically the transverse colon. Note the absence of air-fluid levels compared with Fig. 4.9.

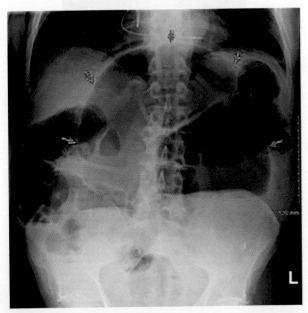

Fig. 4.11 KUB of a patient with sigmoid volvulus. The sigmoid colon has twisted on itself and has become grossly dilated, now residing in the upper abdomen *(yellow arrows)*.

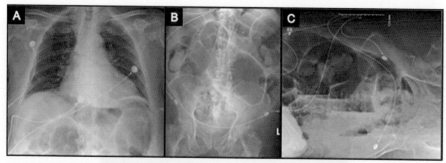

Fig. 4.12 Obstruction series demonstrating a bowel obstruction. (A) Upright chest radiograph demonstrating dilated bowel loops. (B) Supine abdominal radiograph demonstrating dilated bowel loops. (C) Left lateral decubitus abdominal radiograph demonstrating air fluid levels.

uses of fluoroscopy include functional imaging of the gastrointestinal (GI) tract, including upper GI series, small bowel follow through studies, lower gastrointestinal studies (e.g., barium enema), and interventional radiologic procedures. In the operating room, fluoroscopy is used extensively during endovascular procedures for angiography and operative guidance when using catheters and other tools. It is also useful during hepatobiliary procedures to study the biliary tract, commonly referred to as an intraoperative cholangiogram.

Upper GI series: A fluoroscopic study using contrast to evaluate the pharynx, esophagus, stomach, and duodenum (Fig. 4.13). This study can detect ulcers and tumors in these areas, hiatal hernias, and bowel obstructions, among many other pathologic findings. They are also

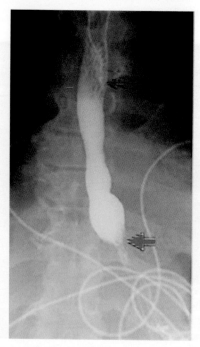

Fig. 4.13 An upper GI study performed with contrast demonstrating a normal esophagus *(red arrow)* and the gastroesophageal junction *(yellow arrow).*

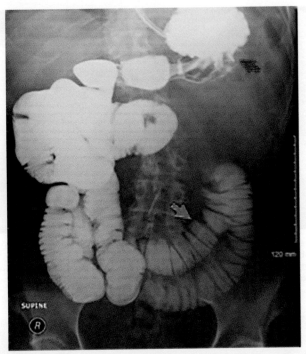

Fig. 4.14 Small bowel follow through study. Contrast demonstrates the stomach *(red arrow)* and small bowel *(yellow arrow)* as it passes through the gastrointestinal tract.

commonly used to evaluate patients postoperatively after esophageal and upper gastrointestinal surgeries, such as esophagectomies or gastrojejunostomies.

Small bowel follow-through study: As its name states, this study evaluates the small bowel from the duodenum to the cecum (Fig. 4.14). Contrast may be followed beyond and into the large bowel if there is an indication to continue the study to this area. Small bowel follow-through studies are helpful in the evaluation of Crohn's disease, small bowel obstruction, and suspected masses. The study can also identify anatomic abnormalities such as strictures, diverticula, and small bowel fistulas.

Lower gastrointestinal study: Commonly referred to as a "barium enema" or "gastrografin enema," this study evaluates the rectum and colon fluoroscopically (Fig. 4.15). Contrast is delivered retrograde via the rectum rather than antegrade. The study can evaluate for diverticular disease, polyps, masses, and ulcerative colitis.

Angiography: Angiography allows for the visualization of the lumen of blood vessels throughout the body by injecting iodinated contrast dye into them under fluoroscopic guidance (Fig. 4.16). Angiography employs the use of catheters to select vessels of interest for the injection of contrast agents to achieve the desired diagnostic images. Arteriography, angiography of the arteries, is commonly used in the diagnosis and treatment of peripheral vascular disease and in the evaluation of traumatic vessel injury. Venography is commonly used to diagnose and treat deep venous thrombosis and pulmonary embolism. Surgeons, interventional radiologists, and cardiologists perform interventions such as angioplasty, stent placement, coil embolization, and many other minimally invasive procedures utilizing angiographic guidance.

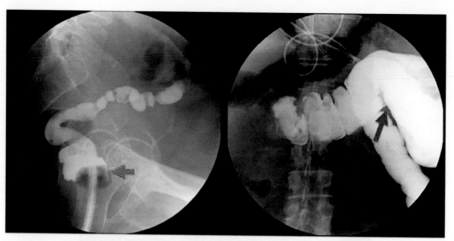

Fig. 4.15 Barium enema. The image on the left shows the rectum and distal sigmoid colon. The yellow arrow demonstrates the balloon catheter that is inserted into the rectum to administer the contrast. The image on the right demonstrates a point later in the study, in which the descending and transverse colon are visualized, including the splenic flexure *(red arrow)*.

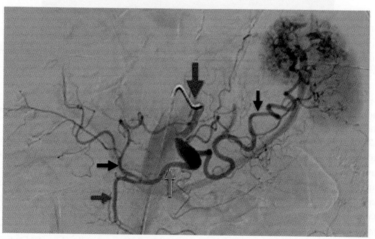

Fig. 4.16 Celiac angiogram. The red arrow indicates the catheter with its tip in the celiac artery. Contrast is administered through this catheter to visualize the common hepatic artery *(yellow arrow)*, gastroduodenal artery *(green arrow)*, proper hepatic artery *(black arrow)*, and splenic artery *(blue arrow)*.

Cross-sectional Imaging: Computed Tomography

The introduction of computed tomography (CT) in the 1970s drastically changed the way in which imaging studies could be used to diagnose and help manage surgical disease. For the first time, one could look into the human body with such great detail that specific diagnoses could often be made based on imaging findings alone. For the surgeon, the CT scan offered a window into the human body that could previously only be achieved by open surgery. CT is one of the most useful diagnostic and operative planning tools available to the surgeon today.

TABLE 4.2 ■ Approximate Hounsfield Units for Various Types of Body Matter

Matter	Hounsfield Units
Air	− 1000
Lung	− 700
Fat	− 100 to − 50
Water	0
Cerebrospinal fluid	+ 15
Blood	+ 30 to + 45
Hematoma	+ 40 to + 90
Spleen	+ 35 to + 55
Liver	+ 40 to + 60
Contrast	+ 100 to + 300
Bone	+ 700 to + 1000

Current CT imaging employs a rotating x-ray beam and multiple arrays of detectors (also rotating around the patient) to obtain images in three different planes (coronal, sagittal, and axial). Computer algorithms are used to piece together the many two-dimensional, slice-like images obtained during the study, allowing for their interpretation. When reading a CT scan in the axial (transverse) plane, one should imagine that they are at the foot of the bed looking up toward the patient's head. The CT image is composed of pixels that are assigned a number from −1000 to 1000 based on the density of tissue represented in that pixel. This unit of measurement is called the Hounsfield unit. The Hounsfield unit represents a measure of how much x-ray energy is absorbed by the tissue represented in each pixel. The various Hounsfield units that represent various tissues in the body are described in Table 4.2. By convention, air is assigned a Hounsfield unit of -1000 HU and is represented as black. Higher-density substances will be white.

Common CT studies include CT examinations of the head, neck, chest (Fig. 4.17), abdomen, pelvis (CT scan of the abdomen and pelvis are often performed together, as seen in Fig. 4.18), and the extremities.

Contrast agents are also employed in CT and help provide additional data that may aid the surgeon in the diagnosis and treatment of a patient. Oral (PO) contrast helps better visualize the bowel and delineate the gastrointestinal tract from surrounding structures. Barium, dilute gastrografin, or other water-soluble contrast may be used as PO contrast when performing CT studies. Iodinated intravenous (IV) contrast enables better evaluation of the vasculature on a CT scan and accentuates abnormalities in solid organs. IV contrast is a necessary component of CT angiography (CTA). CTA is performed with a bolus of IV contrast timed in such a way that images can be obtained during the arterial phase of contrast injection to evaluate vascular anatomy. CTA is an important tool in evaluating the aorta and other major vessels, the pulmonary arteries, and the intra- and extracranial circulation (Fig. 4.19). Computer algorithms also allow for three-dimensional reconstructions of CT images, which can be helpful in operative planning (Fig. 4.20). Arguably, the most common CT scan encountered by the general surgeon is the CT abdomen and pelvis (Fig. 4.21).

The indications for CT scans of different areas of the body, with PO and/or IV contrast, are beyond the scope of this text, but one should always keep in mind what information they hope to gain from a CT scan and how the findings will affect clinical decision making before ordering a study.

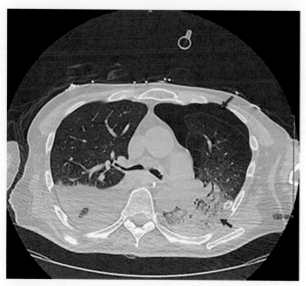

Fig. 4.17 CT of the chest showing a left-sided pneumothorax anteriorly *(red arrow)*, a dense consolidation on the left posteriorly *(blue arrow)*, and a pleural effusion on the right *(yellow arrow)*.

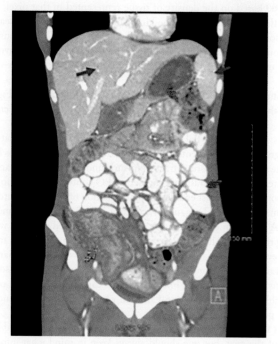

Fig. 4.18 Coronal CT scan of the abdomen and pelvis performed with IV and PO contrast. Note the stomach *(orange arrow)*, spleen *(blue arrow)*, liver *(purple arrow)*, contrast-filled small bowel *(red arrow)*, and a large inflammatory mass in the right lower quadrant *(yellow arrow)*.

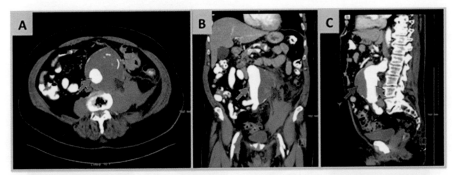

Fig. 4.19 A CT angiogram (CTA) of the abdominal aorta demonstrating a large abdominal aortic aneurysm in three different planes: (A) transverse plane; (B) coronal plane; and (C) sagittal plane. The yellow arrow demonstrates the true aorta filled with contrast and the red arrow demonstrates the thrombosed aneurysmal sac.

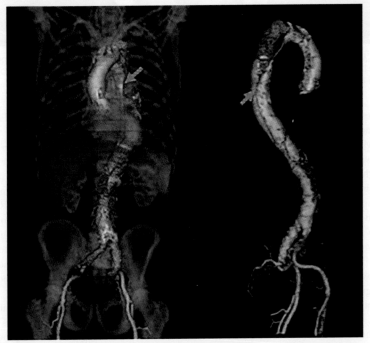

Fig. 4.20 CTA Reconstruction of an aortic dissection. The dissection flap is readily identified (yellow arrows).

Cross-sectional Imaging: Magnetic Resonance Imaging

Magnetic resonance imaging (MRI) utilizes the magnetic spin properties of hydrogen atoms in the water molecules of tissue within the human body to produce images. An MR machine uses a magnet to align these proton spins, which are normally randomly oriented, and then disrupts this alignment using radiofrequency pulses (resonance). After this disruption, the protons return to their resting alignment during a process called relaxation. As relaxation occurs, radiofrequency energy is emitted. This energy can be measured and converted into a grayscale MR image of varying

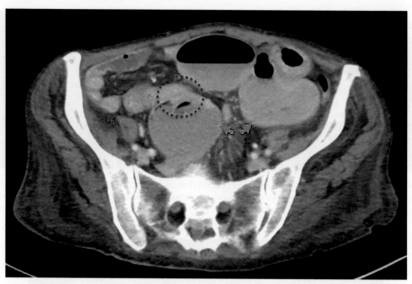

Fig. 4.21 CT of the abdomen/pelvis with evidence of a small bowel obstruction, with a transition point noted within the blue dotted circle. Proximal to the obstruction dilated loops of small bowel are noted *(yellow arrows)* and distal to the obstruction decompressed loops of small bowel are noted *(red arrow)*.

intensities. By varying the sequence of radiofrequency pulses delivered and the time at data is collected, various MR images can be obtained yielding different information.

An MRI sequence is a number of radiofrequency pulses and gradients that result in a set of images with a particular appearance. The main MRI sequences are T1-weighted sequences and T2-weighted sequences. Although the mechanisms behind why and how these different sequences produce images with different characteristics are beyond the scope of this text, the key differences in image appearance are helpful in their interpretation. The shade of gray portrayed in an MR image is described in terms of intensity. A "high-intensity" signal will be white on an MR image, and a "low-intensity" signal will be black. T1-weighted sequences show air and bone as black (low intensity), tissues with high free and/or bound water content as gray (intermediate intensity), proteinaceous tissue as light gray, and fat as white (high intensity). T2-weighted sequences show air and bone as black (low intensity), collagenous and high bound water tissues as gray (intermediate intensity), fat as light gray, and high free water tissues as white (high intensity).

Gadolinium is the main contrast agent used during some MRI examinations. Gadolinium is useful in T1-weighted images and gives them a brighter signal, enhancing MRI's capabilities to detect and delineate focal lesions such as tumors, abscesses, and metastases. Gadolinium improves vessel imaging in MR angiography and allows for characterization of liver lesions. Gadolinium is contraindicated in patients with renal failure due to its association with nephrogenic systemic fibrosis.

MRI is mainly used for neurologic imaging; however, there are many uses for MRI in the general surgery setting. These include magnetic resonance cholangiopancreatography (MRCP), magnetic resonance angiography (MRA), abdominal MRI for hepatic lesions, and MRI for the evaluation of osteomyelitis. MRCP will be briefly covered here.

> *MRCP:* MRCP takes advantage of the relatively stationary nature of bile compared with blood to produce high quality images of the biliary and pancreatic ductal systems, without the use of contrast (Fig. 4.22). MRCP is commonly used to evaluate for cholelithiasis, choledocholithiasis, strictures, neoplasms, and other pancreaticobiliary disease processes. In the general surgery setting, it is most commonly used to evaluate patients with abnormal liver function

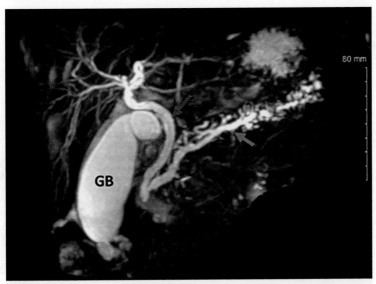

Fig. 4.22 Magnetic resonance cholangiopancreatography (MRCP) exhibiting a patent common bile duct *(red arrow)*, normal gallbladder (GB) and pancreatic duct *(blue arrow)*.

tests, with suspected gallstones or common bile duct obstruction seen on ultrasound. If positive, preoperative endoscopic retrograde cholangiopancreatography with potential stone removal or intraoperative cholangiogram and common bile duct exploration is indicated.

Ultrasound

Ultrasound uses high-frequency sound waves to produce images. Ultrasound takes advantage of the properties of different types of tissue to absorb and reflect acoustic energy. An ultrasound transducer (commonly called an ultrasound probe) is placed against the skin with a thin layer of gel in between to allow for the sound waves to be transmitted to the human body, as these waves do not travel effectively through air. The sound beam enters the tissue and is absorbed and reflected at tissue interfaces. The amplitude of the reflected sound wave is dependent on the type of tissue. This reflected acoustic energy is recorded by the ultrasound probe, and the different amplitudes are assigned different shades of gray to produce an ultrasound image. Strong acoustic signals (bone, gallstones) are near the white end of this spectrum (hyperechoic) and weak acoustic signals (fluid) are near the black end of this spectrum (anechoic or hypoechoic). Depth is determined based on the amount of time it takes for the sound wave to travel and reflect back to the ultrasound probe.

Ultrasound has the advantages of being cheap, portable, noninvasive, and free of ionizing radiation (which makes it well suited for use in pediatrics and in pregnancy). However, it is highly user dependent, and the ability to produce ultrasound images is limited by the inability for sound waves to penetrate gas (commonly encountered in the bowel) and bone. Ultrasound is commonly used to image the heart, abdominal organs (liver, gallbladder (Fig. 4.23), kidneys), reproductive organs, vascular structures, thyroid, and breasts. Doppler ultrasound can be employed to measure flow velocities within vessels and is commonly used in carotid imaging to evaluate for stenoses (Fig. 4.24). Although of great diagnostic importance, ultrasound can also be used to guide invasive procedures such as central line placement and abscess drainage. The use of ultrasound continues to grow and represents an imaging modality that the surgeon-in-training should make a conscious effort to learn and master.

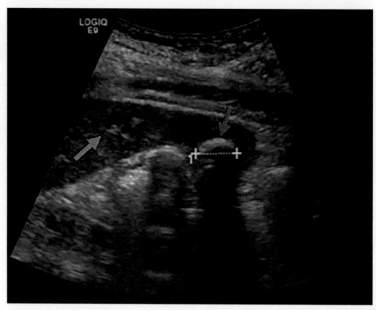

Fig. 4.23 Ultrasound of the gallbladder *(yellow arrow)* showing a gallstone *(red arrow)* at the neck of the gall-bladder.

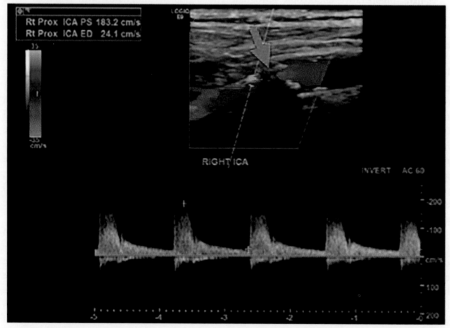

Fig. 4.24 Doppler ultrasound of the right internal carotid artery. The blue and red represent flow toward and away from the ultrasound probe. An atherosclerotic plaque *(yellow arrow)* is seen. The graph on the bottom right shows the change in blood flow velocity with each heartbeat.

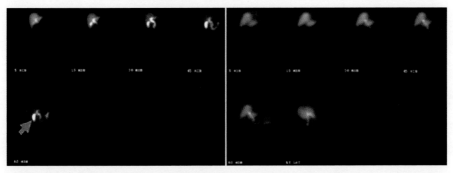

Fig. 4.25   A normal HIDA scan is seen on the left with visualization of the gallbladder *(yellow arrow)*. An abnormal HIDA scan is seen on the right. Note the gallbladder is not observed.

Nuclear Imaging Studies

Nuclear imaging utilizes radiopharmaceuticals that are administered to the patient and selectively uptaken or bound by the tissue or cell type of interest. Radiation is then emitted internally by the radiopharmaceutical, which is detected by special cameras that produce an image, representing the *in vivo* distribution of the radiopharmaceutical. Nuclear imaging is highly sensitive but relatively nonspecific in detecting pathology. Common uses of nuclear studies in the surgical setting include PET scans and bone scans to evaluate for metastatic malignancy, thyroid studies to evaluate thyroid nodules, tagged red blood cell studies to evaluate gastrointestinal bleeding, and hepatobiliary studies to evaluate acute cholecystitis. The hepatobiliary iminodiacetic acid (HIDA) radiotracer is used in a HIDA scan, where it is secreted into the biliary system and its progression through the system is observed and imaged (Fig. 4.25). In a normal study, the gallbladder and duodenum will be visualized as the radiotracer passes through the hepatic ducts, into the common bile duct, through the cystic duct, and into the gallbladder, as well as through the common bile duct into the duodenum. If the cystic duct is occluded, possibly in the setting of a gallstone within the duct, the gallbladder will not be visualized.

Abdominal Pain

Abdominal Pain

CHAPTER 5

Right Lower Quadrant Pain in a 28-Year-Old Female

Murad Karadsheh   ■   Adam Santoro   ■   Amit R.T. Joshi

A 28-year-old female without significant past medical history presents to the emergency department with acute onset of right lower quadrant abdominal pain. The pain was initially periumbilical, then later localized to the right lower quadrant. It is sharp in nature and is accompanied by nausea and vomiting. She also reports an episode of fever.

What Is the Differential Diagnosis for Right Lower Quadrant Abdominal Pain?

Acute abdominal pain is a common complaint causing patients to seek evaluation in emergency departments and often requires evaluation by surgeons. The location of abdominal pain is an important factor that informs the differential diagnosis. There are many conditions that are included in the differential diagnosis of right lower quadrant abdominal pain, especially in females of reproductive age. Bowel related pathologies include appendicitis, mesenteric adenitis, Crohn's disease, gastroenteritis, and Meckel's diverticulitis. Gynecologic pathologies include pelvic inflammatory disease (PID), tuboovarian abscess, ectopic pregnancy, ruptured ovarian cyst, and ovarian torsion. Urologic pathologies include urinary tract infections, renal colic, and epididymitis. The duration, progression, and exact location of abdominal pain and associated symptoms are often helpful at determining the diagnosis.

CLINICAL PEARL (STEP 2/3)

In females of reproductive age, it is important to rule out gynecologic illnesses such as ectopic pregnancy and pelvic inflammatory disease in patients with acute abdominal pain of any location. Bimanual pelvic examination is an important component of the physical exam. Cervical motion tenderness is a hallmark of PID but does not exclude the diagnosis of atypical appendicitis.

Acute appendicitis remains one of the most common causes of an acute abdomen in the United States and worldwide. The rate of acute appendicitis is higher in males, with the highest incidence occurring between the ages of 10 and 19 years (See Chapter 55 for a discussion of appendicits in the pediatric population). Additionally, acute appendicitis is one of the most common indications for an emergent surgical procedure. The classic progression of abdominal pain associated with acute appendicitis is a dull periumbilical pain (visceral pain) that progresses to a sharp pain localized to the right lower quadrant as the peritoneum becomes inflamed. Patients will usually have anorexia and occasionally complain of nausea, vomiting, or loose stools.

CLINICAL PEARL (STEP 2/3)

The classic presentation of migratory pain in acute appendicitis occurs in only 50% to 60% of patients who present with acute appendicitis. Chills, diarrhea, constipation, and dysuria have also been reported in patients with acute appendicitis.

BASIC SCIENCE PEARL (STEP 1)

The appendix is located inferior to the ileocecal junction at the base of the cecum. The location of the appendiceal tip is variable but is most commonly retrocecal. The blood supply to the appendix consists of the appendiceal artery, which arises from the ileocolic artery, the terminal branch of the superior mesenteric artery. The appendiceal artery traverses the mesoappendix, which also contains the lymphatic drainage of the appendix. It is hypothesized that the appendix plays a role in the body's immune system due to lymphoid tissue found in its submucosa. More recent evidence suggests that the appendix is a reservoir of "good" bacteria and may help maintain normal colonic flora or aid in the recolonization of the gut if needed.

CLINICAL PEARL (STEP 2/3)

The appendiceal tip may migrate to pelvic and retroileal locations, which may alter physical examination findings due to inflammation of adjacent structures.

What Is the Pathogenesis of Acute Appendicitis?

Acute appendicitis is an inflammatory process often preceded by an appendiceal obstruction. Obstruction is often due to a fecalith, but other causes include a tumor and lymphoid hyperplasia. The majority of patients with simple acute appendicitis do not have a fecalith or tumor, indicating that an obstructive process may not always be identified in acute appendicitis.

As obstruction occurs, an increase in intraluminal pressure causes occlusion of the small vessels and inflammatory changes. This leads to distension of the appendix and irritation of the visceral afferent nerves of the superior mesenteric ganglion, which produces the broad, periumbilical pain initially experienced. As the inflammation progresses to the parietal surface of the peritoneum, somatic sensory fibers localize the pain to the right lower quadrant of the abdomen. Ischemia, necrosis, and perforation are late findings of this disease process as compromised blood flow to the appendix allows for further bacterial invasion and inflammation.

BASIC SCIENCE PEARL (STEP 1)

Gut-associated lymphoid tissue is found throughout the gastrointestinal tract, though its density and composition vary. The small intestine contains large aggregates of lymphoid tissue referred to as Peyer's patches. The large intestine and appendix contain only small follicular aggregates.

The patient is found lying still in bed. Her temperature is 37.2°C, blood pressure is 120/70 mm Hg, heart rate is 77 bpm, respiration is 18/min, and oxygen saturation is 98% on room air. She is tender to palpation in the lower abdomen, especially in the right lower quadrant. Palpation of the left lower quadrant induces right lower quadrant pain (positive Rovsing sign).

What Are the Physical Examination Findings in Acute Appendicitis?

A thorough physical examination is imperative to diagnose and treat acute appendicitis. The classic patient with appendicitis exhibits right lower quadrant tenderness and rebound tenderness. The patient is often found lying still because any abdominal movement will irritate the inflamed peritoneum, mimicking the rebound tenderness on exam. Slight elevation in temperature and mild leukocytosis are often seen in early, uncomplicated appendicitis. Although the presence of a fever is commonly seen with appendicitis, the absence of a fever does not rule out the diagnosis. Other atypical findings such as diarrhea, dysuria, and upper respiratory tract symptoms are not uncommon.

TABLE 5.1 ■ Named Abdominal Examination Signs in Acute Appendicitis

Sign	Physical Examination Finding
McBurney's Point	The classic point of maximal tenderness, 1/3 the distance from the anterior superior iliac spine to the umbilicus
Rovsing Sign	Right lower quadrant pain with palpation of the left lower quadrant
Obturator Sign	Right lower quadrant pain with passive flexion and external rotation of the right hip
Psoas Sign	Pain with active extension of right hip

Moreover, atypical physical examination findings are often seen due to varying locations of the appendix (Table 5.1). For example, a pelvic appendix often produces suprapubic pain or an obturator sign, whereas a retrocecal appendix may produce flank pain or a psoas sign.

Atypical and complicated appendicitis is often seen in pregnant, immunocompromised, elderly, and pediatric patient populations. In pregnant patients, the location of the pain may vary as the uterus displaces the appendix cephalad throughout the progression of the pregnancy. In addition, nausea and vomiting tend to be more prominent in the pregnant patient, whereas leukocytosis maybe diminished in the immunocompromised patient. Elderly and pediatric patients often present with complicated disease, as presentation may be delayed because symptoms may be more vague.

CLINICAL PEARL (STEP 2/3)

It is critical to identify patients with peritonitis and signs of sepsis, as these are associated with more complicated disease such as perforated appendicitis or periappendiceal abscess.

On laboratory workup, the patient is found to have a negative pregnancy test with a white blood cell count of 9000/mm^3 with 10% bands. Other labs are within normal limits. A computed tomography (CT) scan of the abdomen and pelvis with oral and intravenous contrast demonstrates a thickened appendiceal wall with periappendiceal fat stranding. No oral contrast enters the lumen of the appendix (Fig. 5.1).

What Is the Workup of Acute Appendicitis?

Accurate and early identification of appendicitis is critical in preventing progression of the disease, as perforated appendicitis can lead to significant morbidity and mortality. Ambiguity in the diagnosis can lead to unnecessary surgical exploration, resulting in nontherapeutic appendectomies. However, nontherapeutic appendectomies are arguably justified to decrease the risk of perforated appendicitis. The rate of negative appendectomies has decreased with the advent of preoperative imaging. The Modified Alvarado Scoring System helps predict the need for operative intervention (Table 5.2). The components of the Modified Alvarado Scoring System may be memorized by the mnemonic MANTRELS: Migration to the right lower quadrant, Anorexia, Nausea/vomiting, Tenderness of right lower quadrant, Rebound tenderness, Elevated temperature, Leukocytosis, and Shift of neutrophils to the left. The Pediatric Appendicitis Score (PAS) is discussed in Chapter 55.

After a thorough history and physical, laboratory tests, including a white blood cell count, may aid in the diagnosis. In females of childbearing age, a pregnancy test should be performed to rule out an ectopic pregnancy. Imaging modalities can further aid in the diagnosis of appendicitis when uncertainty exists. CT scan is accepted as one of the most accurate and effective modalities in diagnosing acute appendicitis. Typical findings include an appendiceal wall thickening, periappendiceal fat stranding, phlegmon, appendicoliths, and/or wall enhancement. Ultrasound and MRI can be

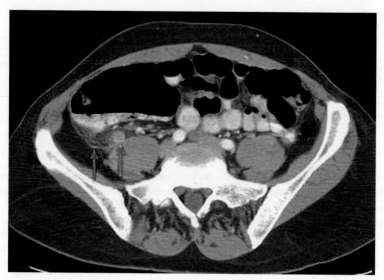

Fig. 5.1   Computer tomography of the abdomen and pelvis with oral and intravenous contrast demonstrates a thickened appendiceal wall *(yellow arrow)* with periappendiceal fat stranding *(green arrow)*.

TABLE 5.2 ■ Modified Alvarado Scoring System

Feature	Score
Symptoms	
Right lower quadrant pain	1
Nausea/vomiting	1
Anorexia	1
Signs	
Right lower quadrant tenderness	2
Fever	1
Rebound tenderness	1
Tests	
WBC ≥ 10,000	2
Left shift of neutrophils	1
Score ≥7	**Surgery is recommended**

particularly advantageous in the pediatric population and pregnant patients, as they produce no ionizing radiation and do not require intravenous contrast. However, the rates of indeterminate examinations of both US and MRI remain higher than CT.

CLINICAL PEARL (STEP 2/3)

The Alvarado Scoring System has not been validated in the setting of pregnancy.

What Is the Management of Acute Nonperforated Appendicitis?

The gold standard treatment of nonperforated appendicitis is appendectomy. Preoperative care should include hydration, electrolyte replacement, bowel rest, and antibiotics. A single dose of a preoperative antibiotic covering both aerobic and anaerobic organisms is recommended. Suggested antibiotics include ampicillin–sulbactam, cefoxitin, and/or cefotetan. Once the necessary preoperative management has been performed, a surgeon needs to decide whether to perform an open appendectomy (OA) or a laparoscopic appendectomy (LA). Regardless of which the surgeon chooses, all patients must be consented for both procedures as well as the complications associated with both.

The decision to perform an open versus laparoscopic appendectomy is based on several factors. LA has gained widespread acceptance and is generally the procedure of choice. Advantages of LA include less postoperative pain, lower rate of wound infection, shorter length of hospital stay, shorter recovery, and improved cosmesis. However, some older studies have found a higher rate of intraabdominal abscesses and increased operative time compared with OA. Certain patients are more suitable for OA: those with significant intestinal dilatation, those with generalized peritonitis, and those that cannot tolerate pneumoperitoneum.

Postoperatively, most patients are able to tolerate a diet immediately with early ambulation and discharge. There is no role for routine postoperative antibiotics in nonperforated appendicitis.

The patient is placed on bowel rest and started on intravenous fluid hydration with normal saline. She receives a dose of ampicillin-sulbactam in preparation for surgery and gives informed consent for appendectomy. She is taken to the operating room for laparoscopic appendectomy. The appendix is easily visualized and found to be hyperemic and enlarged. It is resected without difficulty.

Open Appendectomy

1. Incise either in the right lower quadrant lateral to the rectus muscle or make a lower midline incision.
2. Perform a layer-by-layer dissection into the peritoneal cavity.
3. Identify the appendix by following the *taenia coli* to the base of the cecum; then free it from any adhesions and externalize it.
4. Ligate and divide the appendiceal artery.
5. Suture ligate and divide the base of the appendix.
6. Optional: Bury the appendiceal stump in the cecal wall with a purse string suture.

Laparoscopic Appendectomy

1. Insufflate the abdomen and place three ports: umbilical, suprapubic, left lower quadrant.
2. Inspect the abdomen and identify the appendix by following the *taenia coli* to the base of the cecum.
3. Dissect the appendix and create a window in the mesoappendix at the cecal junction.
4. Divide the appendix at the base with a linear stapler, energy device, or ligature.
5. Divide the mesoappendix with a linear stapler.
6. Deploy a laparoscopic specimen bag and remove the appendix.

CLINICAL PEARL (STEP 2/3)

Laparoscopic appendectomy has the added benefit of complete visualization of the abdominal cavity, allowing diagnosis of concomitant pathology.

CLINICAL PEARL (STEP 2/3)

In the obese patient, laparoscopic appendectomy has been shown to be superior to open appendectomy in several studies. Surgical site infections, length of hospital stay, and operative times were lower in the laparoscopic approach versus the open approach in obese patients.

What Is the Management of Perforated Appendicitis?

Patients with ruptured or complicated appendicitis typically have a delayed or unusual presentation. Deciding on early appendectomy, percutaneous drainage, and/or interval appendectomy remains controversial. However, in all cases, patients are given intravenous hydration and broad-spectrum antibiotics.

In early appendectomy, the patient undergoes urgent appendectomy within 24 hours of hospitalization with any intraabdominal abscesses identified drained intraoperatively. With interval appendectomy, appendectomy is performed 6 to 8 weeks after the initial diagnosis. Presence of a periappendiceal abscess may warrant percutaneous, image-guided drainage. Several nonrandomized trials have suggested that early appendectomy in perforated appendicitis is associated with more complications such as wound infection and bowel obstruction versus patients treated with antibiotics and interval appendectomy. However, other studies have demonstrated that early appendectomy is associated with reduced rate of adverse events and time away from normal activities. In addition, complications such as readmission and abscess formation before the planned interval appendectomy can occur in up to one-third of the patients. Thus recent evidence may be in favor of routine use of early appendectomy in perforated appendicitis. However, no consensus is yet reached between early and interval appendectomy.

If perforated appendicitis is diagnosed intraoperatively, it is acceptable to continue antibiotics postoperatively. Typically, antibiotics are continued until the patient is afebrile with resolution of leukocytosis.

The patient is started on a regular diet postoperatively and antibiotics are stopped. Her symptoms improve, her postoperative pain is well controlled with oral analgesics, and she is able to ambulate without difficulty. She is discharged home that day.

What Are Potential Complications of an Appendectomy?

Although the incidence of major complications of an appendectomy is low, there are some short-term and long-term complications that are important to mention. Short-term complications include ileus or obstruction, urinary retention, pneumonia, bleeding, colonic fistula formation, surgical site infection, and intraabdominal abscess. Long-term complications are secondary to the development of abdominal wall hernia and intraabdominal adhesions, which can cause small bowel obstruction and, in females, tubal infertility. Intraoperative complications, although rare, include vascular injuries and enterotomies.

BEYOND THE PEARLS

- Acute appendicitis is the most common nonobstetric reason for surgery in pregnancy. It has equal distribution in all three trimesters.
- Appendiceal neoplasms have been identified at a higher rate in interval appendectomies than routine appendectomies. Appendiceal neoplasms include carcinoids, adenocarcinoma, and mucinous adenocarcinoma. Age greater than 40 is a risk factor for appendiceal tumors, and a colonoscopy is advised for this patient population.
- Appendicitis in the elderly is less common, and the signs of peritonitis may be blunted. This makes physical examination less reliable. Hence, the role of CT scan and/or diagnostic laparoscopy is crucial.
- If a healthy appendix is visualized, a complete visualization of the abdomen to search for other pathologies must be performed. The appendix should still be removed to avoid confusion.
- Inflammatory bowel disease offers a special challenge. If the appendix appears uninvolved in the inflammatory process, it may be safely removed. However, if involvement of the cecum or appendiceal base is identified, the appendix should be left in place.

Suggested Readings

Addiss, D. G., et al. (1990). The epidemiology of appendicitis and appendectomy in the United States. *American Journal of Epidemiology*, *132*(5), 910–925.

Cameron, J. L., & Cameron, A. M. (2017). *Current surgical therapy*. Elsevier. Philadelphia, PA.

Choi, D., et al. (2003). The most useful findings for diagnosing acute appendicitis on contrast-enhanced helical ct. *Acta Radiologica*, *44*(6), 574–582.

Chung, C. H., Ng, C. P., & Lai, K. K. (2000). Delays by patients, emergency physicians, and surgeons in the management of acute appendicitis: Retrospective study. *Hong Kong Medical Journal*, *6*(3), 254–259.

Di Saverio, S., et al. (2014). The NOTA Study (Non Operative Treatment for Acute Appendicitis): Prospective study on the efficacy and safety of antibiotics (amoxicillin and clavulanic acid) for treating patients with right lower quadrant abdominal pain and long-term follow-up of conservatively treated suspected appendicitis. *Annals of Surgery*, *260*(1), 109–117.

Lee, S. L., Walsh, A. J., & Ho, H. S. (2001). Computed tomography and ultrasonography do not improve and may delay the diagnosis and treatment of acute appendicitis. *Archives of Surgery*, *136*(5), 556–562.

Lu, Y., Friedlander, S., & Lee, S. L. (2016). Negative appendectomy: Clinical and economic implications. *The American Surgeon*, *82*(10), 1018–1022.

Mason, R. J., et al. (2012). Laparoscopic vs open appendectomy in obese patients: Outcomes using the American College of Surgeons National Surgical Quality Improvement Program database. *Journal of the American College of Surgeons*, *215*(1), 88–99.

Nikolaidis, P., et al. (2006). Incidence of visualization of the normal appendix on different MRI sequences. *Emergency Radiology*, *12*(5), 223–226.

Townsend, C. M., Beauchamp, R. D., Evers, B. M., Mattox, K. L., & Sabiston, D. C. (2017). *Sabiston textbook of surgery: The biological basis of modern surgical practice* (20th ed.). Philadelphia, PA: Elsevier.

CHAPTER 6

Right Upper Quadrant Pain in a 44-Year-Old Female

Kristin Sonderman ■ Douglas S. Smink

A 44-year-old female with past medical history significant for obesity presents to clinic with a 6-month history of intermittent abdominal pain. She describes the pain as sharp, located in the right upper quadrant, and typically after eating. Fatty foods seem to trigger the pain. The episodes occur two to three times a week, last for 30 minutes, and then subside. The attacks are associated with nausea but not vomiting. The pain is not associated with movement, and she has not found anything that relieves the pain. She denies any recent weight loss, changes in her diet, acid reflux or regurgitation, epigastric pain, change in bowel habits, hematochezia, or melena. She recalls her mother having similar symptoms. She has no surgical history.

On examination, her temperature is 98.6°F, blood pressure is 130/85 mm Hg, pulse is 87 bpm, respiratory rate is 16/min, and her oxygen saturation is 98% on room air. She appears comfortable and in no acute distress. She has normal heart and lung sounds. Her abdomen is obese, without any tenderness, rebound, or guarding. She has no hepatosplenomegaly and no peripheral edema.

What Is the Differential Diagnosis for Right Upper Quadrant Pain?

The differential for right upper quadrant (RUQ) pain is broad. A thorough history and physical examination can, however, eliminate many disease processes. The differential for RUQ pain includes disease processes of the liver (hepatitis, hepatomegaly), biliary system (uncomplicated biliary disease, sphincter of Oddi dysfunction, cholecystitis, choledocholithiasis, cholangitis), stomach (acid reflux, peptic ulcer disease), pancreas (pancreatitis), duodenum (perforated ulcer), small intestine (obstruction), and urinary system (ureteral stones, pyelonephritis).

This patient's symptoms of episodic, colicky right upper quadrant pain after ingestion of fatty foods with resolution is classic of biliary colic. Her benign physical examination and notable risk factors (female sex, obesity, fertility, and family history) are also convincing. Patients with biliary colic do not always present with such classic symptoms. Atypical symptoms include chest pain, regurgitation, nonspecific abdominal pain, bloating, and early satiety. For these patients, a thorough workup is necessary to avoid missing another cause.

What Is the Workup for This Patient?

A healthy patient who presents with symptoms typical of biliary colic should undergo thorough physical examination, an abdominal ultrasound, and laboratory studies (complete blood count, hepatic panel, and lipase). If the patient presents with atypical symptoms (for example, chest pain), a more thorough workup focusing on those symptoms is required.

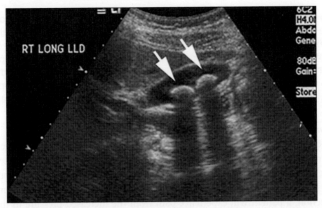

Fig. 6.1 Abdominal ultrasound with cholelithiasis *(arrows)*. (From Gore RM, Levine MS: *High-yield imaging: gastrointestinal,* Philadephia, 2010, Elsevier, pp. 512–514.)

The patient undergoes an abdominal ultrasound, which reveals multiple stones in the gallbladder (Fig. 6.1). There is no gallbladder wall thickening or stranding to suggest cholecystitis. The liver appears normal. The common bile duct is of normal diameter. Her complete blood count, hepatic panel, and lipase are normal. The patient is told she has uncomplicated biliary disease and is scheduled for an elective laparoscopic cholecystectomy. She is instructed to avoid fatty foods until her surgery for symptomatic management.

BASIC SCIENCE PEARL (STEP 1)

Knowing the anatomy of the biliary tree is essential to understanding its pathology and treatment (Fig. 6.2). The gallbladder is a pear-shaped structure attached to the inferior surface of liver in the gallbladder fossa. The gallbladder is divided into the three parts: fundus, body, and neck.

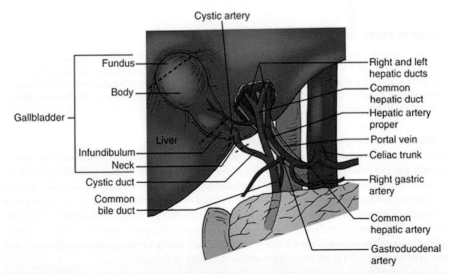

Fig. 6.2 Gallbladder anatomy. (Redrawn from Peterson DR: Gallbladder. In Soni NJ, Arndtfield R, Kory P, editors: *Point-of-care ultrasound,* Philadelphia, 2015, Elsevier, pp. 145–152.e3.)

Bile from the liver drains into either the right or left hepatic ducts, which combine to forming the common bile duct (CBD). The cystic duct joins the common hepatic duct, forming the CBD. Bile enters and exits the gallbladder through the cystic duct. The common bile duct continues to descend posteriorly to the duodenum and joins the pancreatic duct and then empties into the duodenum through the sphincter of Oddi. It is important to recognize that the distal third of the common bile duct traverses the pancreatic perenchyma. The gallbladder is supplied by the cystic artery, which often is a branch of the right hepatic artery, though multiple variants exist.

What Is Uncomplicated Gallbladder Disease and How Is It Treated?

The main functions of the gallbladder are to store and concentrate bile. After ingestion of food, cholecystokinin (CCK) is released, triggering the gallbladder to contract and force bile through the cystic duct. Stasis of concentrated bile in the gallbladder can lead to precipitation of gallstones or sludge. If a gallstone or sludge obstructs the cystic duct (outlet of the gallbladder) during gallbladder contraction, a patient will experience pain from the increased pressure in the gallbladder. When the gallbladder relaxes, the obstruction often resolves, and the pain subsides. Though the prevalence of gallstones is relatively high in the United States, most patients will never develop symptoms. Biliary colic is the name given to the syndrome of intermittent pain related to gallstones in the absence of inflammation in the gall bladder wall. When gallstones are symptomatic, the recommended treatment is elective laparoscopic cholecystectomy to prevent further attacks and to avoid the complications of biliary disease. Avoidance of fatty foods may minimize the frequency of biliary colic but should be considered a temporizing measure until cholecystectomy.

A few weeks later, before she has had a cholecystectomy, the patient develops severe, prolonged right upper quadrant pain, with associated nausea and vomiting. Unlike her previous episodes, the pain does not relent, and she develops a fever. She presents to the emergency department for evaluation.

On physical examination, her temperature is 99.3°F, blood pressure is 125/75 mm Hg, pulse is 110 bpm, respiratory rate is 16/min, and oxygen saturation is 97% on room air. She is diaphoretic and appears uncomfortable. Her abdominal examination is notable for tenderness in the right upper quadrant. The gallbladder is palpable, and he has a positive Murphy's sign.

CLINICAL PEARL (STEP 2/3)

Murphy's sign is a physical examination finding in patients with an inflamed gallbladder. An examiner palpates under the right costal margin while instructing the patient to take a deep breath. As the patient inspires, the gallbladder moves down toward the examiner's hand and, when in contact, causes significant discomfort. A Murphy's sign is present when the patient stops inspiring secondary to the pain.

What Are the Complications of Gallbladder Disease?

Acute cholecystitis, a known complication of gallbladder disease (Table 6.1). Acute cholecystitis is generally due to a gallstone blocking the outlet of the gallbladder or the cystic duct leading to inflammation of the gallbladder wall (Fig. 6.3). The inflammatory process can progress to frank bacterial infection within the gallbladder and, at times, to necrosis of the gallbladder wall. Acute cholecystitis is generally characterized by pain, fever, and tenderness in the RUQ. Ultrasound findings include gallbladder wall thickening, pericholecystic fluid, and a sonographic Murphy's sign (same clinical response to the ultrasound transducer as was elicited by the examiner's hand). Leukocytosis is usually noted, and liver function tests (LFTs) are most often within the limits of normal.

Choledocholithiasis is the presence of gallstones in the common bile duct (CBD). Common duct stones may lead to biliary obstruction, gallstone pancreatitis, and/or cholangitis. Patients

TABLE 6.1 ▪ Signs, Symptoms and Clinical Findings in Biliary Disease

Disease	Characteristic Symptoms	Physical Examination	Typical findings on studies
Biliary Colic	Postprandial RUQ pain, intermittent.	+/- RUQ tenderness.	Ultrasound with stones Normal hepatic panel.
Acute Cholecystitis	Persistent RUQ pain.	RUQ tenderness and guarding, Murphy's sign. Fever.	Gallbladder with stones, wall thickening, peri-cholecystic fluid, leukocytosis.
Choledocholithiasis	Intermittent or persistent pain. Progresses to jaundice, dark urine, and pale stools.	+/- RUQ tenderness, +/- jaundice and scleral icterus	Elevated total bilirubin, direct bilirubin, alkaline phosphatase, and gamma-glutamyl transferase. Ultrasound with cholelithiasis and dilated CBD.
Cholangitis	Persistent RUQ pain. Symptoms of sepsis as disease progresses.	RUQ tenderness, jaundice, fever; may rapidly progress to septic shock.	Elevated total bilirubin, direct bilirubin, alkaline phosphatase, and gamma-glutamyl transferase.

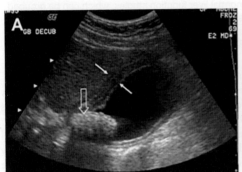 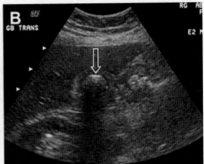

Fig. 6.3   Acute cholecystitis—sonographic findings. Longitudinal (A) and transverse (B) sonograms show a large obstructing stone *(open arrow)* within the gallbladder neck associated with a thick, hypoechoic gallbladder wall *(arrows)*. (From Gore RM, Thakrar KH, Newmark GM, et al: Gallbladder imaging, *Gastroenterol Clin N Am* 39(2):265–287, 2010.)

may present with symptoms of biliary colic or with mild icterus. A completely obstructing stone will lead to progressive jaundice, tea-colored urine, and clay-colored stools. Laboratory findings include abnormal LFT's with an obstructive pattern (elevated bilirubin, alkaline phosphatase, and gamma–glutamyl transferase). Aminotransferases may be mildly elevated. An abdominal ultrasound will usually demonstrate a dilated CBD, but the stones themselves are often difficult to detect by ultrasound. A magnetic resonance cholangiopancreatography (MRCP) can confirm the diagnosis. Endoscopic retrograde cholangiopancreatography (ERCP) allows for imaging as well as stone extraction, and thus can be both diagnostic and therapeutic.

Cholangitis occurs when patients develop a biliary tract bacterial infection secondary to CBD obstruction. Patients with cholangitis classically present with fever, jaundice, and right upper quadrant pain. Patients can quickly develop hypotension, confusion, septic shock, and multiorgan system failure. Laboratory workup will again display an obstructive pattern as well as a significant leukocytosis. Patients must receive prompt IV fluid resuscitation, empiric antibiotic coverage, and urgent biliary drainage. ERCP with sphincterotomy is the procedure of choice; if ERCP cannot be performed, percutaneous transhepatic cholangiography (PTC) should be considered. If endoscopic and percutaneous techniques cannot be performed or are unsuccessful, surgical common bile duct exploration should be performed along with cholecystectomy. After the common duct has been decompressed via ERCP or PTC, most patients should ultimately undergo cholecystectomy.

CLINICAL PEARL (STEP 2/3)

Charcot's Triad describes the classic symptoms of cholangitis (jaundice, fever, RUQ pain). Reynold's Pentad is Charcot's Triad with the addition of hypotension and confusion.

The patient undergoes a repeat gallbladder ultrasound that reveals pericholecystic fluid, gallbladder wall thickening, and a sonographic Murphy's sign. Her labs are notable for leukocyte count of 13,000/mm^3 with normal hepatic panel and lipase. She is diagnosed with acute cholecystitis and started on IV antibiotics. Surgery is consulted for urgent cholecystectomy.

CLINICAL PEARL (STEP 2/3)

There are multiple possible etiologies for abnormal liver function studies, which can be grouped as intrinsic and extrahepatic. These various etiologies present with differences in the elevation of bilirubin, alkaline phosphatase, aspartate aminotransaminase (AST), alanine aminotransferase (ALT) and the ratio of aminotransferases (AST:ALT) which are outlined in Table 6.2.

What Is the Surgical Treatment for Gallbladder disease?

Cholecystectomy is the main surgical treatment for gallbladder disease. Patients who have biliary colic can be scheduled for elective cholecystectomy, whereas those diagnosed with cholecystitis should be admitted to the hospital for urgent cholecystectomy.

Patients with choledocholithiasis can undergo cholecystectomy either after stone removal via ERCP or concurrent intraoperative cholangiogram to identify filling defects in the biliary tree (Fig. 6.4) and common bile duct exploration to remove the stone(s). If CBD stones are detected at the time of cholecystectomy and IOC, a common bile duct exploration can be performed, or the patient can be referred for postoperative ERCP for stone removal.

Patients with cholangitis and those who are medically unfit for urgent surgery should be managed medically with planned interval cholecystectomy. The treatment of choledocholithiasis is removal of the CBD gallstones and subsequent cholecystectomy to prevent further episodes.

TABLE 6.2 ■ Dr Mann's Elsevier volume Surgery: A Competency-Based Companion

	Total Bilirubin	Alkaline Phosphatase	AST	ALT	AST : ALT
Hepatocellular Problem					
Cirrhosis	≥2		90	75	≥1
Alcoholic Liver disease	1–6		200	100	2 : 1
Acute hepatitis	5	270	1,400	1,900	
Extrahepatic/Obstructive Problem					
Choledocholithiasis/cholangitis	6	400	150	150	
Malignant CBD obstruction (pancreatic cancer)	>15	400			

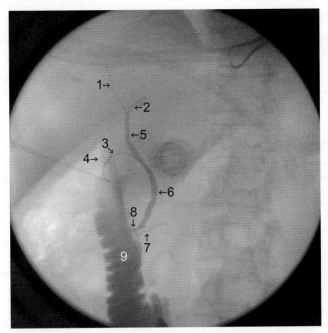

Fig. 6.4 Normal intraoperative cholangiogram. (1) Right hepatic duct; (2) left hepatic duct; (3) cystic duct; (4) two surgical clips holding the cholangiocatheter in the cystic duct; (5) common hepatic duct; (6) common bile duct; (7) pancreatic duct; (8) ampulla of Vater; (9) duodenum. (From Massarweh NN, Flum DR: Role of intraoperative cholangiography in avoiding bile duct injury, *J Am Coll Surg* 204(4): 656–664, 2007.)

Laparoscopic cholecystectomy (rather than open cholecystectomy) is the recommended method for gallbladder removal, given its minimally invasive approach and quick postoperative recovery. If the relevant anatomy cannot be identified laparoscopically, conversion to open may be indicated. The possibility of conversion to open should always be discussed preoperatively with the patient.

Laparoscopic Cholecystectomy

1. Place patient supine, with the surgeon on the left side of the patient.
2. Place a port at the umbilicus for the laparoscope, and place three additional ports in the right upper abdomen and epigastrium.
3. Grasp the fundus of the gallbladder and retract cephalad over the liver exposing the proximal gallbladder (place patient in reverse Trendelenburg for better exposure).
4. Grasp the neck of gallbladder with another grasper to expose the hepatocystic triangle.
5. Dissect out the cystic duct, beginning close to the neck of the gallbladder.
6. Identify the cystic artery running parallel to the cystic duct.
7. Obtain visualization of the *critical view of safety*.
8. Place two hemoclips proximally and one clip distally on both the cystic duct and cystic artery, then divide.
9. Dissect the gallbladder off the gallbladder fossa.
10. Remove gallbladder through umbilical or epigastric incision.

BASIC SCIENCE PEARL (STEP 1)

The cystic artery is typically located within the hepatocystic triangle, formed by the cystic duct, common hepatic duct, and inferior edge of the liver; this triangle is commonly referred to as the Triangle of Calot. Venous drainage occurs either directly into the liver or through a cystic vein draining into the portal vein. A large lymph node is often at the neck of the gallbladder called Lund's node or Calot's node.

CLINICAL PEARL (STEP 2/3)

The critical view of safety (Fig. 6.5) is used to identify the cystic duct and cystic artery and decrease the risk of common bile duct injury. Misidentifying these structures can lead to inadvertent division of the common bile duct, with severe ramifications. Establishing the critical view of safety before division of the cystic duct and artery will minimize this risk. It includes three criteria:

- Clearing of the hepatocystic triangle from fat and fibrous tissue
- Separation of the lower one-third of the gallbladder from the liver to expose the liver bed behind the gallbladder
- Identification of only two structures entering the gallbladder (cystic duct and cystic artery)

Cholangiogram

1. Place a clip on the gallbladder side of the cystic duct.
2. Partially transect the cystic duct and introduce a cholangiocatheter.
3. Inject contrast to visualize the bile ducts (Fig. 6.4).
4. After visualization of CBD stones, flush the catheter and CBD to remove stones.
5. Give 1 to 2mg of IV glucagon to promote relaxation of the sphincter of Oddi and passage of stones.
6. If stones remain, dilate the cystic duct with a forceps or balloon catheter.
7. Extract stones with a grasper, Fogarty catheter, or basket.
8. Repeat cholangiogram to confirm stones are cleared out of the CBD.

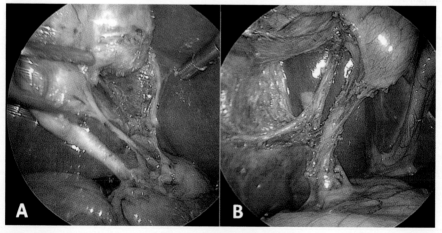

Fig. 6.5   Critical view of safety. (A) Medial view and (B) Lateral view. (From Strasberg SM, Brunt LM: Rationale and use of the critical view of safety in laparoscopic cholecystectomy, *J Am Coll Surg* 211(1):132–138, 2010.)

What Are the Complications of Cholecystectomy?

The most devastating complication of gallbladder surgery is injury to the CBD. Proper exposure of the *critical view of safety* is imperative to minimize risk of this complication. If a CBD injury occurs, these patients are best treated at a referral center with a hepatobiliary surgeon for management and repair of the injury. Additional complications include pancreatitis, bile leak (from either the liver bed or improper clip placement), bleeding, persistent pain, and accidental injury to bowel. Patients may experience loose stool and pain as part of postcholecystectomy syndrome that may be due to sphincter of Oddi dysfunction, postsurgical adhesions, or bile acid diarrhea related to lack of storage of bile. Although rare, long-term medical therapy with bile acid sequestrants, or diet modification with avoidance of large, fatty meals, may be necessary.

Based on the patient's preoperative evaluation, there is no concern for choledocholithiasis. She undergoes an uncomplicated laparoscopic cholecystectomy. Her diet is advanced, and her pain is well controlled postoperatively. She is discharged home on postoperative day 1. At her postoperative visit 2 weeks later, her incisions are well healed, and she is tolerating a regular diet without issue.

BEYOND THE PEARLS:

- The presence of gallstones is common in the U.S. population; however, only patients with symptomatic gallstones need to be treated.
- Abdominal ultrasound is the diagnostic study of choice to evaluate the gallbladder.
- Patients who present with acute cholecystitis should undergo cholecystectomy early during their hospital stay.
- Cholangitis can be a life-threatening emergency; therefore patients should be started on antibiotics immediately with a plan for urgent biliary drainage.
- When performing a laparoscopic cholecystectomy, it is imperative to identify the critical view of safety to prevent bile duct injury.
- If a bile duct injury occurs, patients should be stabilized and treated at a referral center.

Suggested Readings

Gurusamy, K. S. (2010). Surgical treatment of gallstones. *Gastroenterol Clin N Am, 39*(2), 229–244.

Jackson, P. G., & Evans, S. (2017). Biliary system. In C. M. Townsend, Jr., et al. (Ed.), *Sabiston textbook of surgery.* (20th ed., Chapter 54). Philadelphia, PA: Elsevier.

Pham, T. H., & Hunter, J. G. (2015). Gallbladder and the extrahepatic biliary system. In C. F. Brunicardi, et al. (Eds.), *Schwartz's principles of surgery* (10th ed., Chapter 32). New York: McGraw-Hill Education.

Strasberg, S. M., et al. (2010). Rationale and use of the critical view of safety in laparoscopic cholecystectomy. *J Am Col Surg, 211*, 132–138.

Wu, X. D., et al. (2015). Meta-analysis comparing early versus delayed laparoscopic cholecystectomy for acute cholecystitis. *Br J Surg, 102*(11), 1302–1313.

CHAPTER 7

Epigastric Pain in a 47-Year-Old Male

Natasha Leigh ■ Carl Winkler ■ Grace Kim

A 47-year-old male presents to the emergency department complaining of abdominal pain. The pain has lasted 6 hours, has been constant, 8/10 in intensity, and unrelieved by over-the-counter pain medications. The pain is in the center of his abdomen, radiates to his back, and is burning in nature. He is nauseated but has not vomited, and has had subjective fevers at home. He denies any weight change or fatigue and has not noticed any signs of gastrointestinal bleeding. Over the past year he has had similar episodes, approximately monthly, although none this intense. The episodes have no apparent relation to position, activity, or food intake and typically resolve spontaneously in less than 1 hour. He denies any past medical history other than chronic back pain and has never undergone surgery. He takes nonsteroidal antiinflammatory drugs (NSAIDs) for his back pain but no other medications. He denies smoking but admits to drinking three to four glasses of wine nightly. He works as an accountant and has important deadlines in the next 2 weeks.

On physical examination, his temperature is 100.5°F, blood pressure is 110/76 mm Hg, pulse is 105 bpm, respiration rate is 16/min, and oxygen saturation 95% on room air. His body mass index (BMI) is 40. On inspection, he is diaphoretic and in mild distress. He is not jaundiced. His abdomen is soft, nondistended, and tender to deep palpation in the epigastric region without rebound or guarding. Murphy's sign is negative. No organomegaly, masses, scars, or hernias are appreciated. He has dark stool on rectal examination, which is positive for occult blood. There is no cervical, axillary, or inguinal adenopathy.

What Is the Differential Diagnosis for Acute Epigastric Pain?

Though epigastric pain is usually related to foregut pathology, there is a broad differential of causes to consider, which is outlined in Table 7.1. The major distinguishing factors of these diagnoses are in the history (timing of major symptoms, risk factors, associated symptoms) and physical examination (with the abdominal examination being normal in the majority of cases not involving the gastrointestinal tract). There is some overlap between diagnoses, and additional studies may be required to differentiate between them. In this case severe pain radiating to the back and significant alcohol consumption make pancreatitis an important consideration. However, the history of burning pain in the setting of chronic NSAIDs use, recent stress at work, as well as stool positive for occult blood forces the clinician to rule out peptic ulcer disease.

What Diagnostic Studies Should Be Obtained?

Basic laboratory tests including a complete blood count (CBC), basic metabolic panel (BMP), liver functions tests (LFTs), and serum amylase and lipase should be obtained. Table 7.2 summarizes laboratory studies in the investigation of acute epigastric pain. Be aware that the interpretation of many of these findings differs among clinical presentations (e.g., a different location of the abdominal pain).

The need for further imaging will be guided by the differential diagnosis formulated based on the patient's history, physical, and laboratory values. For most patients with acute abdominal pain, an erect chest radiograph (CXR) should be obtained, as this test is fast, noninvasive, and can

TABLE 7.1 ■ Differential Diagnosis for Acute Epigastric Pain

System	Pathology	History Clues	Abdominal Examination
Cardiac	Acute MI	Smoking, dyslipidemia, hypertension	No significant findings
Pulmonary	Lower lobe pneumonia	Productive cough, dyspnea, COPD	No significant findings
Gastrointestinal	Peptic ulcer disease	Burning pain, bloating, relief with antacids	Epigastric tenderness
	GERD	Associated "heartburn" (chest), regurgitation, hoarseness, sour taste	No significant findings
	Small bowel obstruction	Prior surgery, bilious emesis, obstipation	Distention, tympany, hernia/scars, diffuse tenderness
	Acute mesenteric ischemia	Arrhythmia, hematochezia, severe pain	"Pain out of proportion" to physical examination
	Epigastric hernia	Association with straining, bulge at site, prior surgery	Cough impulse, point tenderness over defect, scars
Hepatopancreaticobiliary	Biliary colic / acute cholecystitis	Cholelithiasis, obesity, association with fatty meals	RUQ or epigastric tenderness, Murphy's sign
	Acute pancreatitis	Cholelithiasis, alcohol use, radiation to the back	Epigastric tenderness, diminished bowel sounds
	Pancreatic cancer	Weight loss, jaundice, dull pain, family history	Cachexia, vague epigastric pain
	Hepatitis	HBV/HCV, alcohol use	RUQ tenderness
Genitourinary	Nephrolithiasis	Dysuria, prior renal stones	Flank tenderness
Metabolic	DKA/HHNK	Diabetes mellitus, poor glycemic control, precipitating infection	Diffuse tenderness, no rebound or rigidity, diminished bowel sounds
Infections	Esophagitis, gastritis, enteritis, colitis	Nausea/vomiting, diarrhea, suspect food intake	Diffuse mild tenderness
Vascular	Aortic dissection or aneurysm	Uncontrolled hypertension, tearing pain, known aneurysm	Pulsatile mass, point tenderness
Hematologic	Sickle cell crisis	Personal history of SCD	Splenomegaly (peds)
Neurologic	Opioid withdrawal	Abrupt cessation of opioids, chronic pain	No significant findings

COPD, Chronic obstructive pulmonary disease; *DKA*, diabetic ketoacidosis; *GERD*, gastrointestinal reflux disease; *HBV*, hepatitis B virus; *HCV*, hepatitis C virus; *HHNK*, hyperosmolar hyperglycemic nonketotic; *MI*, myocardial infarction; *RUQ*, right upper quadrant; *SCD*, sickle cell disease

quickly rule out several catastrophic surgical emergencies. The most important sign to exclude is pneumoperitoneum (see Fig. 4.2). In patients who have not undergone a recent operation, free air is pathognomonic of a perforated hollow viscus. An abdominal radiograph may be useful in excluding bowel obstruction or ileus. In gallstone pancreatitis, ultrasonography of the right upper

TABLE 7.2 ■ Useful Laboratory Studies in Workup of Acute Epigastric Pain

Laboratory Test	Derangement	Disease
Complete Blood Count (CBC)	↑ WBC	Nonspecific (infection, inflammation)
	↓ Hb/Hct	Acute upper gastrointestinal bleeding (PUD) Malignancy (chronic anemia)
Basic Metabolic Panel (BMP)	↑ BUN / Creatinine	Nonspecific (volume depletion, primary genitourinary pathology)
	↑ Glucose	DKA, HHNK, infection
Liver Function Tests (LFTs)	↑ AST/ALT	Acute hepatitis (> 1000 IU/L) Gallstone pancreatitis (< 500 IU/L)
	↑ Total/Direct (conjugated) Bilirubin	Gallstone pancreatitis Choledocholithiasis
	↑ ALP	Gallstone pancreatitis Choledocholithiasis
Gamma-Glutamyl Transferase (GGT)	↑ γ-GT	Gallstone pancreatitis
Amylase	↑ Amylase	Pancreatitis (less specific)
Lipase	↑ Lipase > x3 normal	Pancreatitis (more specific)
CA 19–9	↑ CA 19–9	Pancreatic cancer Gallstone pancreatitis
Lactic acid	↑ Lactate	Nonspecific (underresuscitation, ischemia)
Fecal occult blood (FOB)	+ Blood in stool	Peptic ulcer

ALP, Alkaline phosphatase; *ALT*, alanine aminotransferase; *AST*, aspartate aminotransferase; *BUN*, blood urea nitrogen; *DKA*, diabetic ketoacidosis; *Hb*, hemoglobin; *Hct*, hematocrit; *HHNK*, hyperosmolar hyperglycemic nonketotic; *PUD*, peptic ulcer disease; *WBC*, white blood count

quadrant (RUQ) will reveal cholelithiasis and possibly a dilated common bile duct and/or choledocholithiasis. An inflamed pancreas may also sometimes be demonstrated on ultrasound.

Others tests that may be useful depending on clinical suspicion include cross-sectional imaging with a computed tomography (CT) scan, which would be helpful in demonstrating an acute pancreatitis though not required to make this diagnosis. An upper gastrointestinal (UGI) contrast series may reveal a large ulcer crater or extravasation in the case of perforation. Upper endoscopy should be considered to evaluate for peptic ulcer disease; however, its use in the acute setting should be limited to patients with suspected bleeding from gastric or duodenal ulcers. Upper endoscopy is contraindicated in suspected perforation.

CLINICAL PEARL (STEP 2/3)

Free air under the left hemidiaphragm may be obscured by a large, air-filled stomach or "gastric bubble." The clinician should be vigilant to differentiate between air in the stomach and free air under the diaphragm.

SCENARIO 1

On further workup, the patient's complete blood count reveals leukocytes of $11,300/mm^3$ and a hemoglobin of 8.3 g/dL. A basic metabolic panel is significant for blood urea nitrogen of 40 mg/dL and serum creatinine of 1.4 mg/dL. Transaminases and lipase are normal. Fecal occult blood is positive. Upright chest radiograph and an abdominal radiograph do not demonstrate pneumoperitoneum or abnormal bowel gas patterns.

What Is the Most Likely Diagnosis at This Point?

The most likely diagnosis at this point is peptic ulcer disease (PUD) complicated by upper gastrointestinal bleeding. The patient has a mild leukocytosis to indicate the presence of inflammation and anemia, which indicates the presence of bleeding. The patient also shows evidence of acute kidney injury, which may be a result of volume depletion or the effect of NSAIDs.

BASIC SCIENCE PEARL (STEP 1)

The mechanism of action of NSAIDs is in the inhibition of the inflammatory mediator COX-2. The inhibition of COX-2 also leads to an inhibition of prostaglandins, which is responsible for the predominant adverse effects of NSAIDs. Prostaglandins typically serve to aid in the normal physiologic gastric mucosal protection (through mucus and bicarbonate) and to dilate the afferent arterioles in the kidney. NSAIDs, as a result, lead to a decreased protection of the gastric mucosa (leading to ulcer formation) and decreased renal blood flow, especially in those with baseline renal dysfunction (leading to acute and potentially chronic kidney injury).

The patient is admitted to the hospital, started on intravenous fluids, and monitored for bleeding and worsening of his abdominal pain. He undergoes an upper GI endoscopy on the next day, which is significant for a 0.8 cm, clean, nonbleeding ulcer in the first portion of the duodenum. Biopsies of the lesion are taken for pathologic analysis.

What Are the Main Etiologies of PUD?

Gastroduodenal ulceration occurs when the body's natural mucosal defenses are overwhelmed by the acidic (hydrochloric acid) and digestive (pepsin) contents of the bowel. This can occur when the mucosal defenses are diminished, when acid secretion is increased, or both. The majority of cases of peptic ulcer disease can be attributed to *Helicobacter pylori* infection or NSAIDs use. A minority of cases can be attributed to acid hypersecretion exclusively, as in the Zollinger-Ellison syndrome. "Stress ulcers" in critically ill patients represent a related clinical entity brought on by severe physiologic stress. Additionally, smoking and psychological stress have been shown to exacerbate PUD. The data regarding alcohol consumption is mixed. Peptic ulcers are classified according to location, which also typically corresponds to the etiology of the ulcer (Fig. 14.1).

BASIC SCIENCE PEARL (STEP 1)

H. pylori is a gram-negative, urease-positive, rod-shaped bacterium (Fig. 7.1), highly adapted to life in the gastric environment. The exact mechanism by which *H. pylori* predisposes to PUD is not fully understood. However, it is generally accepted that a combination of bacteria-produced toxins, host-inflammatory response to infection, and elevated gastrin levels leading to excess acid production all play a role. This multifactorial pathogenesis is outlined in Fig. 7.2. Through

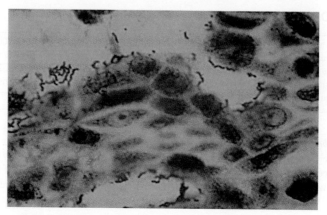

Fig. 7.1 Evidence of *Helicobacter pylori* infection in gastric mucosa.

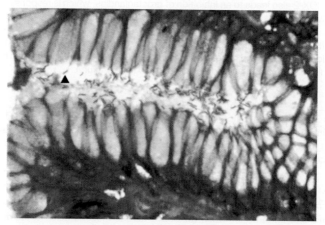

Fig. 7.2 Evidence of Helicobacter pylori infection (arrowhead) in gastric mucosa. (From Klatt EC: The gastrointestinal tract. Ch 7. In: Robbins and Cotran Atlas of Pathology. Philadelphia: Elsevier, 2015, p. 175.)

its production of urease, *H. pylori* is able to hydrolyze gastric urea into ammonia and thereby neutralize the acidity of its immediate environment. This adaptation is critical to protecting the organism from the acidic environment of the stomach.

How Is **H. pylori** *Infection Diagnosed?*

There are several tests used to confirm *H. pylori* infection. Endoscopic methods include biopsy–urease testing, histology, and bacterial culture. These should only be used if the patient requires endoscopy for symptom evaluation, as *H. pylori* testing is not considered a stand-alone indication for endoscopy. Noninvasive tests include urea breath testing, stool antigen assay, and serology. Only the first two are considered tests of active infection, as *H. pylori* serology can remain positive well after eradication.

How Is Duodenal Ulceration Treated?

The first step in treatment of a duodenal ulcer is eradication of *H. pylori* with a 2-week course of "triple therapy," consisting of two antibiotics and a proton pump inhibitor (PPI). One commonly employed regimen includes amoxicillin, clarithromycin, and omeprazole. The treatment can vary based on prior treatment, local antibiotic resistance, and medication allergies. In certain cases, bismuth is added to the regimen and dubbed "quadruple therapy." In 20% of cases, initial therapy fails to eradicate the infection; therefore it is advisable to perform confirmatory testing after treatment. Urea breath testing, fecal antigen assay, and endoscopic biopsy are acceptable methods. Typically, this is performed at least 1 month after completion of the regimen. PPI therapy should be discontinued 1 to 2 weeks prior, as this can produce false-negative results.

The second step in treatment is withdrawal of contributing factors. Patients should be advised to discontinue NSAIDs, quit smoking, limit alcohol consumption, and minimize psychological stress. Foods that induce dyspepsia, although not proven to worsen PUD, may be discontinued for symptom relief.

In complicated ulcer disease, PPI therapy is continued for 4 to 12 weeks depending on the size and location of the ulcer, with longer courses reserved for ulcers larger than 1 cm and gastric ulcers. PPIs are preferred over histamine-2 receptor antagonists because they have been shown to reduce healing time, at least in NSAID-induced ulcers. In some cases, antisecretory therapy is continued until ulcer resolution is confirmed endoscopically. It may also be used indefinitely in refractory cases, or when the ulcerogenic risk factor cannot be eliminated.

The patient's biopsy is positive for urease activity. His hemoglobin remains stable, his abdominal pain resolves, and he is discharged on triple therapy with instructions to try acetaminophen for his back pain instead of NSAIDs, to limit his alcohol intake to one to two drinks per day, and to try to limit his stress at work. He will follow up in 1 month or sooner if his symptoms recur.

What Are the Complications of PUD? How Are These Treated, and When Is Surgery Indicated?

The major acute complications of PUD include penetration, perforation, bleeding, and gastric outlet obstruction. Penetration refers to the ulcer eroding through the bowel wall without free perforation or leakage of luminal contents into the peritoneal cavity. Perforations include leakage of luminal air and/or succus from the ulcer into the abdomen. Notably, many perforations seal spontaneously before presentation. Bleeding is the most common complication necessitating hospitalization, and gastric outlet obstruction is the least common in developed countries. PUD is often clinically silent, making complicated disease the initial presentation. This phenomenon often occurs in elderly patients and those taking NSAIDs. The indications for surgical intervention can be summarized as failure of medical management, whether in the acute or nonacute setting. Additionally, surgery should be offered to all patients with refractory hemodynamic instability and diffuse peritonitis (see Chapter 12).

SCENARIO 2

On further workup, the patient has a white blood cell count of 18,100/mm^3, and the following results on a hepatic panel:
- Aspartate aminotransferase (AST) 350 IU/L
- Alanine aminotransferase (ALT) 300 IU/L
- Alkaline phosphatase (ALP) 400 U/L
- Total bilirubin 4.1 mg/dL
- Direct bilirubin 3.6 mg/dL
- Lipase level 8100 U/L.

A CXR is unremarkable. A RUQ ultrasound demonstrates cholelithiasis and a common bile duct dilated to 6 mm.

What Is the Most Likely Diagnosis at This Point?

The patient is presenting with leukocytosis, elevated transaminases, elevated bilirubin, elevated lipase, and an ultrasound consistent with a stone that has passed from the gallbladder into the biliary system. Without elevated lipase, this patient may be diagnosed with choledocholithiasis (see Chapter 6), but this laboratory pattern is consistent not only with biliary obstruction but also with pancreatic obstruction causing acute gallstone pancreatitis.

What Causes Acute Pancreatitis?

The most common etiologies of pancreatitis in the United States are gallstones and alcohol abuse. Other etiologies include instrumentation of the pancreatic duct (after endoscopic retrograde cholangiopancreatography [ERCP]), trauma, congenital anatomic variations of ductal anatomy, and hypertriglyceridemia. How alcohol consumption leads to pancreatitis is not well established, but it is thought to be due to the increased synthesis of digestive and lysosomal enzymes by pancreatic acinar cells or the oversensitization of pancreatic acinar cells to cholecystokinin (CCK).

Acute biliary pancreatitis occurs when a gallstone becomes lodged at or near the ampulla of Vater and subsequently causes upstream obstruction of both pancreatic and biliary trees. Ultimately, pancreatitis occurs from impaired extrusion of zymogen granules and subsequent activation of proteolytic enzymes in pancreatic acinar cells, initiated by trypsin, which leads to autodigestion of the pancreas.

CLINICAL PEARL (STEP 2/3)

A useful mnemonic to recall the etiologies of acute pancreatitis is I GET SMASHED (Table 7.3).

TABLE 7.3 ■ Etiologies of Acute Pancreatitis

I	IDIOPATHIC
G	GALLSTONES: #1 cause worldwide (35%)
E	ETHANOL: #2 cause in United States (30%)
T	TRAUMA
S	STEROIDS (glucocorticoids)
M	MUMPS (paramyxovirus) and other viruses (EBV, CMV); MALIGNANCY
A	AUTOIMMUNE: IgG4 antibody, SLE, PAN
S	SCORPION STING
H	HYPERTRIGLYCERIDEMIA (>1000), HYPERCALCEMIA, HYPOTHERMIA
E	ERCP: 3rd most common (1%–2%)
D	DRUGS: SAND (steroids & sulfonamides, azathioprine, NSAIDs, diuretics (furosemide, thiazides, didanosine))

CMV, Cytomegalovirus; *EBV*, Epstein-Barr virus; *ERCP*, endoscopic retrograde cholangiopancreatography; *NSAIDs*, nonsteroidal antiinflammatory drugs; *PAN*, polyarteritis nodosa; *SLE*, systemic lupus erythematosus

TABLE 7.4 ■ Ranson Criteria for Acute Gallstone Pancreatitis

On Admission GA LAW*	At 48 hours C HOBBS[a]
Glucose > 200	Calcium < 8
Age > 55 years old	Hematocrit drop > 10%
LDH > 350	PaO$_2$ < 60 on room air
AST > 250	BUN increase > 5
WBC > 16	Base deficit > 4
	Fluid Sequestration > 6 liters

AST, Aspartate aminotransferase; BUN, blood urea nitrogen; LDH, lactate dehydrogenase; PaO$_2$, partial pressure of oxygen in arterial blood; WBC, white blood count
Total points: 0 to 2: 2% mortality; 3 to 4: 15% mortality; 5 to 6: 40% mortality; 7 to 8: 100% mortality
[a]Each criteria scores 1 point

How Is Acute Pancreatitis Managed?

There is a wide disease spectrum in acute pancreatitis from mild to very severe and even death, and the extent of disease informs management. Mild cases have no end organ dysfunction and are usually responsive to conservative management. Severe cases often have organ dysfunction (most commonly acute kidney injury and hypotension from intravascular volume depletion) as well as hemorrhage, infection, and pancreatic necrosis.

The initial management consists largely of supportive care, which includes bowel rest and intravenous fluids. Patients with severe pancreatitis may require large volume resuscitation, and intubation may prove necessary if significant pulmonary edema prevents adequate oxygenation. Pain control, usually with narcotic analgesia, is also essential. Nausea and vomiting, from a local duodenitis, should be managed with a nasogastric tube. Once the nausea has subsided, a clear liquid or low-fat diet should be started. For patients unable to take food orally, a nasojejunal tube may be placed for tube feeding.

In order to risk-stratify patients and to inform how aggressive they should be treated, two common scoring systems are utilized. The Ranson criteria (Table 7.4) can help give physicians an idea of mortality risk, but its positive predictive value is only around 50%. It has largely been replaced with the APACHE II (acute physiology and chronic health evaluation) scoring system. APACHE II is not only a better predictor of outcomes but also has the advantage of being usable at any point in the disease course without time point restrictions, whereas the Ranson criteria are validated for use at the time of patient presentation. Patients with a higher Ranson or APACHE II scores are more likely to do poorly and develop complications. Therefore closer monitoring in a step-down or intensive care unit is often warranted.

Addressing the underlying cause of the pancreatitis is also important. For gallstone pancreatitis, unless contraindicated, the patient should undergo cholecystectomy. Timing is dictated by clinical improvement not on laboratory values alone. For mild cases, a cholecystectomy should be performed before discharge but after resolution of abdominal pain, as 25% of patients will experience recurrent pancreatitis or gallstone-related complications if surgery is delayed more than 6 weeks after diagnosis. For severe pancreatitis, surgery may be delayed until the patient has completely recovered. Alcohol cessation is also critical. If hypertriglyceridemia is causative, apheresis (removal of plasma with reinfusion of blood cells), intravenous insulin (for glucose control if concurrent hyperglycemia), and oral triglyceride-lowering medications should be considered. Autoimmune pancreatitis, when secondary to IgG4 antibodies, is typically responsive to a 4- to 6-week course of glucocorticoids.

CLINICAL PEARL (STEP 2/3)

Early enteral feeding, rather than total parenteral nutrition, within 7 days for patients with severe pancreatitis is associated with decreased infectious complications and a decreased need for surgical intervention and has been shown to improve survival.

The patient is admitted to the hospital, placed on intravenous fluids, and kept nothing by mouth (NPO) for 3 days until symptoms resolved. On day 2 of the hospitalization, transaminases and alkaline phosphatase began to normalize, and the consulting gastroenterologist concluded that the patient has passed the stone and does not require an ERCP. The patient was taken to the operating room on hospital day four and underwent an uncomplicated laparoscopic cholecystectomy. His diet is advanced, which he tolerates, and he is discharged the next day with oral analgesics.

What Are the Possible Complications of Acute Pancreatitis?

Complications related to acute pancreatitis occur both during the hospital admission and in a more delayed fashion.

PANCREATIC NECROSIS

Pancreatic necrosis can occur with severe cases of pancreatitis and can be sterile or infected. Most cases will be sterile (noninfected), asymptomatic, and only discovered on contrast-enhanced CT with areas of hypoenhancement within the pancreatic parenchyma. Areas of necrosis will wall off and spontaneously resolve over the subsequent months to years, but structural loss will persist. A subset of patients will develop infected necrosis, which presents as delayed fever and leukocytosis up to 3 weeks after presentation. CT scan may demonstrate bubbles of gas within an area of necrosis. CT-guided fine-needle aspiration of pancreatic tissue with cultures demonstrating bacterial infection will make the diagnosis and ensure appropriate antibiotic coverage. Imipenem is most frequently used to cover for gram-negative bacilli in such cases. Operative drainage (necrosectomy) may be required if CT-guided drainage and/or antibiotic therapy are unsuccessful.

CLINICAL PEARL (STEP 2/3)

At least 85% to 90% of the pancreatic parenchyma must be destroyed for patients to experience exocrine or endocrine dysfunction. Even with extensive necrosis, it is uncommon for patients to develop diabetes or require enzyme replacement in the long term.

PSEUDOCYST

Disruption of pancreatic ducts, as can be seen in severe pancreatitis, causes leakage of pancreatic enzymes and formation of a walled-off cyst. This cyst lacks an epithelial lining, a so-called "pseudocyst." After 2 months, the wall matures to become thick and fibrotic. Though most remain asymptomatic, larger cysts can cause local compression resulting in abdominal pain or gastrointestinal/biliary obstruction. Pseudocysts are not premalignant, so treatment is only indicated for symptom control. Aspiration alone results in reaccumulation; it has a 54% failure rate and a 63% recurrence rate. Successful drainage can be achieved by forming a permanent connection with the gastrointestinal tract. Cystgastrostomy or cystojejunostomy can be performed endoscopically or surgically depending on the anatomic relationship of the cyst to adjacent organs.

PANCREATIC COLLECTION OR FISTULA

Pancreatic ductal disruption can cause enzyme leakage into the peritoneal cavity and subsequent development of a fistulous tract. The enzymes are inactive, as they have not been in contact with the gastrointestinal tract, and will therefore not cause organ autodigestion. A collection adjacent to the pancreas may be apparent on CT, and, if drained, the fluid will have a high amylase level. Management is largely conservative. A percutaneous drain can be used to manage the output from a pancreatic fistula. With low-output fistulae (less than 200 cc/day), patients may be able to resume a normal diet. Higher-output fistulae may require limiting oral intake (and perhaps nothing by mouth for an extended period of time), total parenteral nutrition (TPN), and octreotide therapy. ERCP with pancreatic stenting may be indicated to divert flow of pancreatic juices in persistent cases.

CHRONIC PANCREATITIS

Repeated episodes of acute pancreatitis may lead to irreversible parenchymal fibrosis with permanent structural changes. Patients will experience chronic epigastric pain and in severe cases may develop malnutrition, secondary to protein and fat malabsorption, and diabetes secondary to pancreatic endocrine dysfunction. The radiographic finding of pancreatic parenchymal calcification with ductal dilation is classic for chronic pancreatitis. Analgesia and supplemental nutrition, to include pancreatic enzyme replacement, are the mainstays of treatment. Surgical management is most commonly indicated for pain refractory to medication and largely consists of ductal drainage.

The patient presents to the surgeon's office 2 weeks after discharge. His abdominal pain has completely resolved, his incisions are healing well, and he is tolerating a regular diet.

BEYOND THE PEARLS

- Both PUD and pancreatitis can present with epigastric pain radiating to the back.
- PUD is typically diagnosed with upper endoscopy.
- The treatment of PUD is acid suppression and antibiotics in patients who are infected with *H. pylori*.
- Surgical management in PUD is reserved for complications of the disease, including perforation, bleeding, and obstruction, as well as in cases that fail to respond to conservative management.
- Acute pancreatitis is initially treated with bowel rest, aggressive hydration, and analgesia.
- Patients with biliary pancreatitis need cholecystectomy after resolution of pancreatitis.
- Complications of severe acute pancreatitis include pancreatic necrosis, pseudocyst, pancreatic fistula, and chronic pancreatitis.

Suggested Readings

Chan, F. K., & Leung, W. K. (2002). Peptic-ulcer disease. *Lancet, 360*(9337), 933–941.
Dudeja, V., Christain, J. D., Jensen, E. H., & Vickers, S. W. (2018). Exocrine pancreas. In C. M. Townsend, Jr., et al. (Eds.), *Sabiston textbook of surgery: The biological basis of modern surgical practice* (p. 1520). Philadelphia: Elsevier.

Malfertheiner, P., et al. (2017). Management of Helicobacter pylori infection—the Maastricht V/Florence consensus report. *Gut*, *66*(1), 6–30.

Podolsky, D., et al. (2015). *Yamada's textbook of gastroenterology* (6th ed., Vol. 1). New York: Wiley-Blackwell.

Swaroop Vege, S. *Clinical manifestations and diagnosis of acute pancreatitis.* https://www-uptodate-com.eresources.mssm.edu/contents/clinical-manifestations-and-diagnosis-of-acute-pancreatitis?source=search_result&search=acute%20pancreatitis&selectedTitle=2~150. Accessed October 31, 2017.

CHAPTER 8

Left Lower Quadrant Pain in a 67-Year-Old Female

Rebecca L. Hoffman ■ Cary B. Aarons

A 67-year-old female with a history of hypertension and noninsulin-dependent diabetes mellitus presents to the emergency department with worsening left lower quadrant pain for the past 24 hours. The pain is constant and does not radiate. She has had several loose stools. Her temperature is 100.7°F, heart rate is 87 bpm, and blood pressure is 132/78 mm Hg. On physical examination, she is tender to light palpation in the left lower quadrant and exhibits voluntary guarding but no rebound tenderness. A bimanual examination is negative for cervical motion or adnexal tenderness. Her laboratory values are notable for a white blood cell count of 14,000/mm^3.

What Is the Differential Diagnosis of Left Lower Quadrant Abdominal Pain?
As with all complaints of abdominal pain, the clinician must formulate a differential diagnosis based on the location of the patient's pain (both historically and on examination) and other associated symptoms. Potential causes of left lower quadrant pain include bowel obstruction, inflammatory bowel disease, gynecologic disease, and nephrolithiasis, among other rarer presentations outlined (Table 8.1). The physical examination is essential at determining the precise location of the pain. For example, some patients will describe left-sided abdominal pain but really have flank pain on examination, making urologic pathology more likely.

This hemodynamically stable patient is presenting with acute, focal left lower quadrant (LLQ) pain without evidence of generalized peritonitis. Her history of loose stools favors a gastrointestinal source of the pain. This is a classic presentation for sigmoid diverticulitis.

CLINICAL PEARL (STEP 2/3)

In a patient presenting with clinical signs and symptoms suggestive of large bowel pathology, obtain a history of prior colonoscopies, as well as a personal and family history of colorectal cancer or other familial malignancies.

What Is the Next Best Step in Diagnosis for Patients With Left Lower Quadrant Abdominal Pain?
History, physical examination, and laboratory analyses often are extremely helpful in narrowing the differential diagnosis of someone with a complaint of abdominal pain, but imaging is typically necessary to precisely determine the diagnosis. The most likely diagnosis will drive the type of imaging test to be ordered. For example, if diverticulitis and a ureteral calculus are both on the differential, a computed tomography (CT) scan without intravenous contrast should be ordered. Despite not defining bowel pathology as readily, a noncontrast scan allows for the detection of calculi in the urinary tract that intravenous contrast would otherwise obscure.

TABLE 8.1 ■ Differential Diagnosis of Left Lower Quadrant Pain

Body System	Diagnosis
Gastrointestinal	Diverticulitis
	Appendicitis
	Bowel Obstruction
	• Small bowel
	• Volvulus (sigmoid > cecal)
	Cancer
	Ischemic Colitis
	Inflammatory Bowel Disease (IBD)
	Irritable Bowel Syndrome (IBS)
	Stercoral Ulcer
	Infectious Colitis
Gynecologic	Endometriosis
	Ovarian Torsion
	Pelvic Inflammatory Disease (PID)
	Tubo-ovarian Abscess
Urologic	Ureteral Calculi
	Pyelonephritis

Given the most likely diagnosis of sigmoid diverticulitis, the next best step to confirm this diagnosis is to obtain cross-sectional imaging in the form a CT scan of the abdomen and pelvis with intravenous contrast. The sensitivity and specificity of CT scans for diverticulitis are both greater than 95%. Plain abdominal radiographs and an upright chest x-ray can also be helpful in quickly diagnosing perforation, obstruction, or volvulus.

The patient undergoes a CT scan of the abdomen and pelvis with IV contrast (Fig. 8.1). There is bowel wall thickening and fat stranding in the area of the mid to proximal sigmoid colon with an associated pelvic abscess measuring 2.4cm x 4.7cm x 6.6 cm.

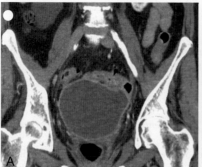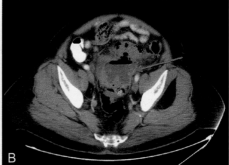

Fig. 8.1   Computed tomography (CT) scan of the abdomen and pelvis with oral and intravenous contrast in the coronal (A) and axial (B) views. Bowel wall thickening and fat stranding are seen in the area of the mid to proximal sigmoid colon with an associated pelvic abscess measuring 2.4cm x 4.7cm x 6.6 cm *(yellow arrow)*. (A, From Sessa B, Galluzzo M, Ianniello, SS, et al: Acute perforated diverticulitis: assessment with multidetector computed tomography. In *Seminars in Ultrasound, CT, and MRI*, 37(1):37–48, 2016. B, From Bodmer, NA, Thakrar, KH: Evaluating the patient with left lower quadrant abdominal pain. *Radiologic Clinics of North America* 53(6):1171–1188, 2015.)

How Is Acute Diverticulitis Classified and How Does the Classification Affect Treatment?
Acute diverticulitis is classified as *uncomplicated* or *complicated* depending on the clinical presentation and CT findings. In general, patients with uncomplicated diverticulitis may present either to their primary care physician or the emergency department with mild to moderate LLQ pain—usually without fever. They may or may not manifest a leukocytosis. Notably, although the CT scan may show thickening of the colon or pericolonic fat stranding, there is no abscess. Such patients can be treated with bowel rest and antibiotics and are often treated in the outpatient setting.

Complicated diverticulitis, however, is defined by the presence of an abscess, perforation, or a fistula on CT scan. The Hinchey classification system is often used to describe the severity of perforation in complicated diverticulitis and ranges from I–IV (Table 8.2).

Patients with complicated diverticulitis should be admitted to the hospital, placed on bowel rest, and started on intravenous fluid and broad-spectrum antibiotics. One of the most important principles in the management of surgical infections is source control. In cases of Hinchey I and II diverticulitis, strong consideration should be given to percutaneous drainage of the abscesses by interventional radiology. Percutaneous drainage is either via a transabdominal, transgluteal, or transrectal approach, with the former being the most preferred route. Successful drainage is achieved in approximately 80% of cases. However, in some cases, the abscess can be in a difficult location that prohibits safe percutaneous drainage. In cases that are not amenable to percutaneous drainage, in which the abscess is less than 4 cm in greatest dimension, antibiotics alone may be sufficient if the patient is otherwise hemodynamically stable. Patients with Hinchey III and IV diverticulitis, on the other hand, generally require operative management consisting of an abdominal washout and typically a Hartmann's procedure (see later in this chapter).

CLINICAL PEARL: USMLE (STEP 1/2/3)

When drained percutaneously, abscess fluid should always be sent for routine gram stain and culture. Bacteria are both aerobic and anaerobic (in 80%–90% of cultures) and include:
- Aerobes
  - Gram-negative bacilli
    - *E. coli*
    - *Enterobacter* sp.
    - *Klebsiella* sp.
  - Gram-positive cocci
    - *Streptococci* sp.
    - *Staphylococci* sp.
    - *Enterococci* sp.
- Anaerobes
  - Gram-negative bacilli
    - *Bacteroides* sp. (especially *B. fragilis*)
  - Gram-positive bacilli
    - *Clostridium* sp. (especially *C. difficile*)

BASIC SCIENCE PEARL: USMLE (STEP 1)

Colonic diverticula are false diverticula, meaning they do not contain all the layers of the colon. Diverticula occur where the vasa recta penetrate the colon wall to provide blood supply to the mucous membrane.

TABLE 8.2 ■ **The Hinchey Classification System**

Hinchey Classification	Description	Typical Clinical Presentation	CT Findings	Image
Stage I	Pericolic or mesenteric abscess	Localized LLQ pain on palpation, mild to moderate leukocytosis, ± fever	Pericolic stranding, segmental bowel wall thickening, pericolic abscess identified by locules of gas and fluid contained within a hyperintense rim.	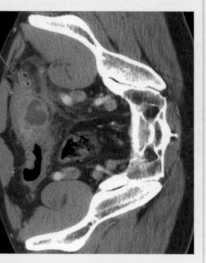
Stage II	Pelvic or retroperitoneal abscess	Localized LLQ pain on palpation, mild to moderate leukocytosis, ± fever	Pericolic stranding, segmental bowel wall thickening, pelvic or retroperitoneal abscess identified by locules of gas and fluid contained within a hyperintense rim.	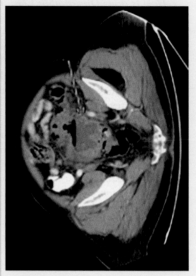

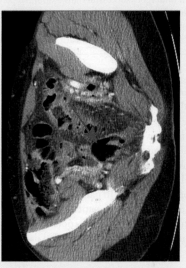

| Stage III | Purulent peritonitis | Peritonitis, leukocytosis, fever, ± hypotension and tachycardia | Free air without definite abscess, and free fluid throughout abdomen (typically less than that seen with IV) |
| Stage IV | Feculent peritonitis | Peritonitis, leukocytosis, fever, ± hypotension and tachycardia | Massive pneumoperitoneum and free fluid |

Stages I, II, and IV from: Sessa, B, Galluzzo, M, Ianniello, SS, et al: Acute perforated diverticulitis: assessment with multidetector computed tomography. *Seminars in Ultrasound, CT, and MRI* 37(1):37–48, 2016.
Stage III from: Hall, J, Hammerich, K, Roberts, P: New Paradigms in the Management of Diverticular Disease, *Current Problems in Surgery* Sep;47(9):680–765, 2010.

The patient undergoes successful transabdominal percutaneous drainage of approximately 25 mL of purulent fluid by interventional radiology, and a drain is left in place. In the first 3 days after drainage, the patient improves. Her white blood cell count drops to 8000/mm^3, and she begins eating a soft diet. She is discharged home with the drain in place, on oral antibiotics.

What Considerations Are Important in the Outpatient Management of Diverticulitis?

If not recently performed, a colonoscopy is recommended for all patients 6 to 8 weeks after an episode of acute diverticulitis to evaluate for malignancy or alternate diagnosis (such as ischemic colitis or inflammatory bowel disease), even though the likelihood of finding a malignancy is extremely low (less than 3%). During the acute phase of the disease, colonoscopy is generally avoided due to the increased risk of perforation.

There is little to no evidence to support a recommendation for a sustained change in diet after an episode of diverticulitis. In particular, nuts, corn, popcorn, and seeds do not cause diverticulitis and need not be avoided in patients who have had a previous attack. Fiber from fruits and vegetables confers the most protection against diverticulitis, and an intake of 20 to 30 g per day is recommended. (This recommended daily intake is independent of a history of diverticular disease).

CLINICAL PEARL: USMLE (STEP 1)

There are several factors which have been identified as contributing to the development of diverticulosis beyond a diet low in fiber (the "Western" diet) and increased pressure in the sigmoid colon. A diet high in red meat confers an increased risk, such that when compared with vegetarians, meat-eaters have a 50-fold increase in diverticular disease. Histologic studies have also noted an increase in collagen deposition and cross-linking in patients with diverticular disease. This leads to a loss of compliance in the colon and increased susceptibility to mucosal tearing in high-pressure areas.

Ten days later you are called to the emergency department to evaluate the same patient. Her percutaneous drain had been removed by interventional radiology since you last saw her, and, despite initially doing well, she developed acute worsening of her abdominal pain, which is now diffuse. On examination, she appears uncomfortable. Her vital signs are notable for a temperature of 101.7°F, a heart rate of 114 bpm, and a blood pressure of 95/66 mm Hg. She has a distended abdomen and exhibits rebound tenderness on abdominal examination. Her white blood cell count is 19,000/mm^3.

What Do You Expect to Find on CT Scan of the Abdomen/Pelvis?

In this clinical scenario, the concern is that the patient has failed more conservative management of her diverticulitis and has now freely perforated her colon. This means she has either Hinchey III (purulent) or Hinchey IV (feculent) peritonitis. In either case, the CT findings would be most impressive for free air and free fluid, in addition to colon wall thickening and adjacent fat stranding. It is often difficult to distinguish Hinchey III from IV based on imaging findings—this is usually a diagnosis made based on intraoperative findings.

What Are the Operative Considerations for Managing Her Hinchey III and IV Complicated Diverticulitis?

The principles behind operative management of any diverticulitis are removing the diseased portion of colon, minimizing concern for intraabdominal infection (washout), and creating a safe exit point for stool. Typically, uncomplicated and Hinchey I and II diverticulitis are managed operatively in an elective fashion, and there is little to no concern for creating a primary anastomosis. However, in the management of Hinchey III and IV diverticulitis, the decision about performing an end colostomy (Hartmann's procedure) versus a primary anastomosis should be individualized in order to mitigate the risk of anastomotic leak. The decision hinges on intraoperative findings, patient comorbidities, hemodynamic stability, and surgeon preference. Although colon resection and creation of an end colostomy remains a common approach, there has been recent evidence that in selected patients, sigmoidectomy with primary anastomosis, with or without a diverting ostomy, may be safe. Some contraindications for primary anastomosis include severe hemodynamic instability, severe malnutrition, immunocompromised state, and significant bowel edema at site of the proposed anastomosis, among others. Alternatively, laparoscopic abdominal lavage, without resection, has been employed in patients with purulent peritonitis (Hinchey III) with low morbidity and mortality. However, results have been mixed regarding this practice, and it is not yet endorsed by the American Society of Colon and Rectal Surgeons clinical practice guidelines.

Hartmann's Procedure

1. Preoperatively mark a site for the colostomy that is lateral to the planned incision, and away from the patient's pant/waist line and any skin folds.
2. Create a midline incision, extending from the umbilicus to the pubic symphysis.
3. Place patient in Trendelenburg position and retract small bowel cranially.
4. Mobilize the sigmoid colon until it can be brought up through the abdominal wall to create a tension-free stoma.
5. Select a proximal area of transection in the descending colon that is not inflamed and divide with a linear cutting stapler.
6. Transect distally at the rectosigmoid junction. The rectum can be identified by noting the loss of discrete tenia coli and epiploic appendages, which usually occurs at about the level to the sacral promontory.
7. Bring the stapled end of the descending colon through the preselected colostomy site in the skin.
8. Close the midline incision before maturation of the ostomy in order to protect the incision from stool contamination.

BASIC SCIENCE PEARL (STEP 1/2/3)

The left ureter crosses anterior to the iliac vessels, usually at the level of the bifurcation of internal and external iliac, and is at risk for injury during left colon surgery. To confirm a structure is the ureter, pinch it gently with a pair of forceps and watch it vermiculate.

CLINICAL PEARL (STEP 2/3)

Ostomies can be grouped in several ways, but the major categorizations define the part of the bowel that is creating the anatomosis (ileum = ileostomy, colon = colostomy) and whether both proximal and distal portions of the bowel are incorporated in the ostomy (i.e., loop) or only the proximal portion (i.e., end). A Hartmann's procedure, by definition, results in an end colostomy.

The patient is found intraoperatively to have feculent peritonitis (Hinchey IV) and undergoes a Hartmann's procedure. Her skin is left open and packed to heal by secondary intention due to concern for fecal contamination. The patient recovers otherwise uneventfully and is discharged home on postoperative day 8 after she resumes a regular diet and her colostomy is functioning normally. She returns to see you in the office in 2 weeks and asks about ostomy reversal.

How Long After a Hartmann's Procedure Do Patients Have to Wait to Have Their Colostomy Reversed?

Although there are no set protocols for the timing of reversal or evaluation of the rectal stump, stoma reversal can generally be attempted 8 to 12 weeks after surgery, barring any postoperative complications. Before proceeding with reversal, most surgeons will evaluate the rectal stump with a gastrografin enema (GGE) for signs of leak or flexible sigmoidoscopy. If the integrity of the rectal stump is intact and the mucosa is healthy, a reversal can be attempted. It is important to discuss the possible inability to reverse a colostomy before any emergent or elective surgery.

BEYOND THE PEARLS

- CT scan of the abdomen and pelvis with IV contrast is the most sensitive and specific way to diagnose diverticulitis.
- The presentation and treatment of diverticulitis varies greatly and ranges from outpatient oral antibiotics to emergency surgery.
- Antibiotics used for the treatment of diverticulitis must cover both aerobic and anaerobic organisms.
- Source control, either by percutaneous abscess drainage or operative washout, is essential in the management of complicated diverticulitis.
- Patients should undergo colonoscopy 6 to 8 weeks after an episode of diverticulitis to assess for malignancy or alternate diagnosis.

Suggested Readings

Durmishi, Y., Gervaz, P., Brandt, D., et al. (2006). Results from percutaneous drainage of Hinchey stage II diverticulitis guided by computed tomography scan. *Surg Endosc, 20,* 1129–1133.

Feingold, D., Steele, S. R., Sang, L., et al. (2014). Practice parameters for the treatment of sigmoid diverticulitis. *Dis Colon Rectum, 57*(3), 284–294.

Hall, J. (2016). Diverticular Disease. In S. R. Steele, T. L. Hull, T. E. Read, et al. (Eds.), *Vol II. The ASCRS textbook of colon and rectal surgery* (ed 3, pp. 645–667). New York: Springer International Publishing.

MsDermott, F. D., Collins, D., Heeney, A., & Winter, D. C. (2013). Minimally invasive and surgical management strategies tailored to the severity of acute diverticulitis. *Br J Surg, 101,* e90–e99.

CHAPTER 9

Groin Mass in a 48-Year-Old Male

Austin D. Williams ■ Jonathan Gefen

A 48-year-old male without significant past medical history presents to the general surgery office with a complaint of left groin pain. The pain is intermittent and seems to worsen with heavy lifting and straining. This has been occurring for approximately 2 years but has recently become more intense. Upon further questioning, he admits to feeling an occasional bulge in his left groin, especially with prolonged standing.

What Is the Differential Diagnosis for Groin Pain?

There are acute and nonacute pathologies that can produce groin pain, and it is imperative to differentiate between them (Table 9.1). Nonacute problems are more common and include hernias (inguinal and femoral), spermatic cord pathology (hydrocele, spermatocele, and varicocele), and lymphadenopathy. Musculoskeletal strains, especially in athletes, and vascular etiologies such as iliac aneurysm and pseudoaneurysm are also in the differential diagnosis. Acute surgical problems include incarcerated and strangulated hernias, testicular torsion, and epididymitis. Details in both history and physical examination are essential in determining the cause of the pain.

What Are the Primary Physical Examination Techniques to Evaluate a Groin Mass?

Most groin pathologies can be diagnosed with a thorough physical examination. It is imperative to examine the patient standing. Both groins should be examined for bulges at rest and with straining (i.e., asking the patient to cough or "bear down"). Most inguinal hernias can be found by directly palpating the inguinal canal. In a male patient, the external and internal inguinal rings can be further examined by invaginating the redundant scrotal skin with the index finger to follow the spermatic cord above the inguinal ligament from the scrotum. Femoral hernias can be palpated inferior to the inguinal ligament, though the distinction is not always clear in obese patients. Palpation of the cord and testes can help differentiate hernias from other pathology.

BASIC SCIENCE PEARL (STEP 1/2/3)

Inguinal anatomy is important in both the evaluation and treatment of hernias of the groin (Fig. 9.1) and in access to the femoral vessels for central venous or arterial access. The inguinal canal is bordered by the external oblique aponeurosis anteriorly (the roof), the conjoined tendon (formed by the inferior edges of the internal oblique and transversus abduminus muscles) superiorly, the inguinal ligament inferiorly, and the transversalis fascia posteriorly (the floor). A direct hernia protrudes through the floor of the inguinal canal medial to the inferior epigastric vessels. An indirect hernia protrudes through the deep inguinal ring lateral to the inferior epigastric vessels. A femoral hernia is found bulging inferior to the inguinal ligament. The femoral hernia defect is bordered by the inguinal ligament anteriorly, Cooper's ligament posteriorly, the lacunar ligament medially, and the common femoral vein laterally.

TABLE 9.1 ■ Differential Diagnosis for Groin Pain and Mass

	Pathology	Physical Examination Finding
Groin	Pseudoaneurysm	Pulsatile mass over femoral or iliac artery
	Inguinal hernia	Bulge in the inguinal canal, cough impulse
	Femoral hernia	Mass palpable inferior to inguinal ligament, cough impulse
	Lymphadenopathy	Painless, firm nodule or cluster of nodules; nonreducible.
Cord	Varicocele	"Bag of worms"; does not transilluminate
	Spermatocele	Can resemble third testis
Scrotum/ Testis	Hydrocele	Smooth, painless, large scrotal swelling; transilluminates
	Testicular torsion	Painful, swollen immobile testis; confirmed by Duplex ultrasound

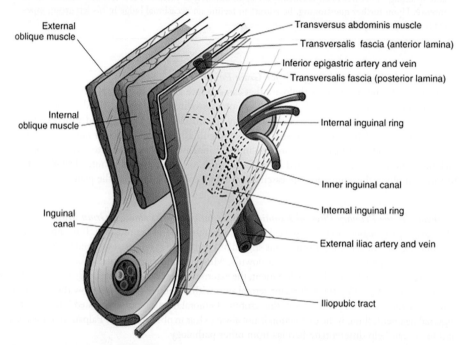

Fig. 9.1 Inguinal anatomy. (From Malangoni MA, Rosen MJ: Hernias. In Townsend CM Jr, Beauchamp D, editors: *Sabiston textbook of surgery,* Philadelphia, 2017, Elsevier, pp 1092–1119.)

On physical examination with the patient standing, there is a bulge in the left groin that is palpable with and without Valsalva maneuver. It is nontender and easily reducible. The right groin and both testes and spermatic cords are otherwise normal.

What Are the Types of Hernias and How Can They Be Distinguished?

A hernia, in general, is the abnormal protrusion of a structure through a defect. Hernias are most commonly found protruding through defects in the abdominal wall and are named based on the location of the defect (Table 9.2). Physical examination is the predominant method of detection.

TABLE 9.2 ■ Types of Abdominal Wall Hernias

Hernia Type	Location of Defect
Inguinal hernias	
Direct	Hesselbach's triangle (bordered by the inferior epigastric vessels laterally, the rectus muscle medially, and the inguinal ligament inferiorly)
Indirect	Internal ring
Pantaloon	Simultaneous ipsilateral direct and indirect hernia
Other abdominal wall hernias	
Femoral	Femoral canal
Umbilical	Umbilicus
Spigelian	Intersection of the semilunar and arcuate lines
Incisional	Any location where a surgical incision has been made

Imaging by computed tomography (CT) scan may be necessary to evaluate hernias through the abdominal wall and their contents, especially if bowel obstruction, incarceration, or strangulation is suspected.

CLINICAL PEARL (STEP 2/3)

Most inguinal and femoral hernias in men can be diagnosed with physical examination only, though the exact type of hernia may not be clear until the time of surgery (see Table 9.2). Radiographic studies, such as ultrasound, CT scan, or MRI, are helpful if the physical examination is equivocal.

CLINICAL PEARL (STEP 2/3)

Although hernias are commonly thought to result from heavy lifting, there is no scientific evidence of this. The activities that put the most pressure on hernias are coughing and jumping rather than lifting. A truss (a strap or undergarment with padding for the inguinal region) can be worn to apply pressure to the hernia and keep it reduced. This can provide comfort but is often cumbersome to wear. Hernias vary widely in size and pain; the size of the hernia does not correlate with the degree of pain.

What Are Some Clinical Findings of Incarceration and Strangulation?

The feared complication of any hernia is that it will become incarcerated (nonreducible) and its contents strangulated (cut off from their blood supply). An incarcerated hernia that is not strangulated may be painless and nontender; this does not require emergent surgery. A strangulated hernia is nonreducible, painful, and tender to palpation. As the hernia contents progress from ischemia to gangrene, the patient can develop local erythema or skin discoloration, generalized abdominal tenderness, peritonitis, fever, tachycardia, and, ultimately, septic shock and death. A strangulated hernia requires emergent surgery. Femoral hernias are more likely than inguinal hernias to present with incarceration and strangulation.

Do All Patients With Abdominal Wall Hernias Require Surgical Repair?

Asymptomatic hernias may be electively repaired or left alone if desired. Patients with a hernia should be instructed to seek immediate attention if signs and symptoms of strangulation occur. Whereas the strangulation risk is low (less than 1 in 500 per year), most hernias will eventually become symptomatic over time. They may become uncomfortable, large, or, painful. At that point, they should be repaired with surgery. Because femoral hernias tend to incarcerate more frequently than inguinal hernias, surgical repair is recommended for even asymptomatic femoral hernias.

The patient is scheduled for an open inguinal hernia repair with mesh. Upon dissection of the hernia sac from the structures of the spermatic cord (see later in this chapter), the hernia sac is seen protruding through the internal ring, consistent with an indirect hernia. The hernia sac is ligated and reduced into the abdomen. A mesh is placed to reconstruct the inguinal floor without tension. His immediate postoperative course is uneventful and he is discharged home the same day.

What Are the Types of Surgery for Inguinal Hernia Repair?

Inguinal hernia repair, or herniorrhaphy, can be broadly classified as open or laparoscopic, with or without mesh. An open repair with mesh is the most common. This approach utilizes an inguinal incision with placement of a permanent prosthetic to cover the hernia defect and buttress the floor of the inguinal canal. An open repair without mesh utilizes sutures and the native tissues of the abdominal wall to create a layered closure of the defect and inguinal canal floor. It is associated with a slightly higher risk of hernia recurrence compared with a mesh repair. A laparoscopic repair, which can only be done with mesh, involves placement of the mesh posterior to the inguinal canal in the preperitoneal space. This approach is more technically challenging, but it has the advantage of less postoperative pain, quicker return to full activity, and less risk of chronic postherniorrhaphy neuralgia. The laparoscopic approach is a good option for recurrent hernias after a previous open repair, and for bilateral hernias, which can be repaired simultaneously through just three small incisions.

BASIC SCIENCE PEARL (STEP 1/2/3)

Three nerves are encountered during an open herniorrhaphy (see Fig. 9.1). The iliohypogastric nerve runs within or superior to the inguinal canal and innervates the skin superior to the pubis. The ilioinguinal nerve runs anterior to the spermatic cord and innervates the pubic region and superior portion of the scrotum or labia majora. The genital branch of the genitofemoral nerve runs within or posterior to the spermatic cord and innervates the scrotum and medial upper thigh. Variation is common, and there is considerable overlap in these distributions. Injury to any of these nerves can cause numbness, paresthesia, or neuralgia. Care must be taken to identify all three nerves and either protect them or resect them prophylactically.

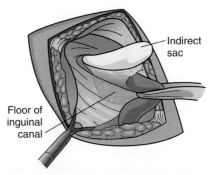

Fig. 9.2 Open inguinal hernia repair. (Redrawn from Mann BD: Operation 9: open inguinal hernia repair. In *Surgery: a competency-based companion,* Philadelphia, 2009, Elsevier, p 685.)

Open Inguinal Hernia Repair

1. Incise along the inguinal canal.
2. Incise the external oblique aponeurosis in the direction of its fibers.
3. Identify the ilioinguinal, iliohypogastric, and genitofemoral nerves.
4. Mobilize the spermatic cord, incise the cremaster muscle, and inspect within the cord for an indirect hernia.
5. Inspect the floor of the inguinal canal for a direct hernia.
6. Reduce or ligate the hernia sac.
7. Reconstruct the floor of the inguinal canal (with or without mesh).
8. Return the cord to its anatomic position and close external oblique.
(Fig. 9.2)

BASIC SCIENCE PEARL (STEP 1/2/3)

The spermatic cord contents are the testicular artery, pampiniform (venous) plexus, genital branch of the genitofemoral nerve, vas deferens, and tunica vaginalis. It is covered by the external spermatic fascia (which arises from the external oblique), the cremaster muscle (fibers from the internal oblique), and the internal spermatic fascia (from the transversalis). Injury to the blood vessels can lead to testicular pain and atrophy. Injury to the vas deferens can contribute to infertility if the contralateral side is also compromised.

Laparoscopic Inguinal Hernia Repair

1. Incise at the umbilicus.
   a. Transabdominal preperitoneal (**TAPP**) approach—Enter and insufflate the peritoneal cavity with CO_2. Place two laparoscopic ports. From within the abdomen, incise the peritoneum to enter the preperitoneal space posterior to the inguinal canal.
   b. Totally extraperitoneal (**TEP**) approach—Incise the anterior rectus sheath on one side of the umbilicus. Retract the rectus muscle laterally to expose the posterior rectus sheath. Insert a balloon dissector along the posterior rectus sheath toward the pubis. Inflate the balloon to develop the preperitoneal space, then remove the balloon and insufflate with CO_2. Place two laparoscopic ports.
2. Dissect the hernia sac from the spermatic cord and reduce the hernia.
3. Mobilize the peritoneum away from the inguinal canal.
4. Position mesh posterior to the inguinal canal and anterior to the peritoneum.
(Fig. 9.3)

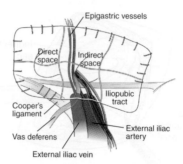

Fig. 9.3 Laparoscopic inguinal hernia repair. (Redrawn from Mann BD: Operation 10: laparoscopic inguinal hernia repair. In *Surgery: a competency-based companion,* Philadelphia, 2009, Elsevier, p 686.)

The patient returns to the office for his postoperative visit 2 weeks later. He is concerned that he still has some pain in his left groin. On examination, there is a well-healing incision in the left groin. There is no erythema, edema, or recurrent hernia.

What Are the Potential Complications of Herniorrhaphy?

Perioperative: Seromas and hematomas are common, especially after repair of large hernias that leave a large, empty space that can fill with fluid. These generally resolve within a few weeks. Postoperative urinary retention, especially after laparoscopic hernia repair, may occur due to a combination of general anesthesia, surgical manipulation of the bladder, and sometimes the presence of an enlarged prostate in older patients. Urinary retention is usually transient but may require overnight placement of a Foley catheter in severe cases.

Long term: The most common long-term complication is chronic postherniorrhaphy pain, reported in up to 30% of cases at 1 year postoperatively. This is thought to be due to irritation or entrapment of the sensory nerves in the inguinal canal. The laparoscopic approach is associated with lower incidence and severity of chronic pain but does not eliminate the possibility. In rare cases, severe neuropathic pain may persist for years and have a very negative effect on quality of life. Treatment options include nerve block injections, oral medication with neurotropic agents such as gabapentin, or reoperation to resect the sensory nerves and revise the hernia repair. The other major long-term complication is hernia recurrence, which is generally reported to occur in less than 2% of cases within 2 years. Hernia recurrence may occur anytime, even decades after surgery.

BEYOND THE PEARLS

- Abdominal wall hernias can present in various locations, most commonly in the groin.
- Patients who have asymptomatic hernias may choose watchful waiting rather than surgical repair, with appropriate counseling on symptoms of incarceration and strangulation.
- Symptomatic hernias should be scheduled for elective repair. Hernias that are incarcerated or strangulated require more urgent repair.
- A wide variety of open and laparoscopic techniques are employed for hernia repair, with the goal of reducing the hernia and repairing the defect in the abdominal wall.
- Postherniorrhaphy chronic pain is a dreaded complication that is difficult to treat.
- Hernia recurrence will occur in a small percentage of cases with any repair technique.

Suggested Readings

Bay-Nielson, M., et al. (2001). Pain and functional impairment 1 year after inguinal herniorrhaphy: A nationwide questionnaire study. *Ann Surg, 233*(1), 1.

Fitzgibbons, R. J., et al. (2006). Watchful waiting vs repair of inguinal hernia in minimally symptomatic men: A randomized clinical trial. *JAMA, 295*(3), 285–292.

Matthews, R. D., et al. (2007). Factors associated with postoperative complications and hernia recurrence for patients undergoing inguinal hernia repair: A report from the VA Cooperative Hernia Study Group. *Am J Surg, 194*(5), 611.

Neumayer, L., et al. (2004). Open mesh versus laparoscopic mesh repair of inguinal hernia. *NEJM, 350*(18), 1819–1927.

CHAPTER 10

Abdominal Pain and Diarrhea in a 43-Year-Old Female

Michael Karon ■ Robert Noone

A 43-year-old female with a past medical history of diabetes mellitus type 2, gastroesophageal reflux disease, and hypertension presents to the emergency department with complaints of generalized abdominal pain and diarrhea for the past 3 weeks. She describes the abdominal pain as crampy in nature, intermittent, and especially associated with bowel movements. Her problem began as small amounts of watery stool occurring four to eight times per day. Over the last 5 days, she has noticed both mucus and blood in her stool. She reports that she has had episodes of diarrhea in the past that have been associated with blood in her stool, but she thought the blood was attributable to hemorrhoids and never reported it to her doctor. She denies vomiting, dysphagia, weight loss, or recent travel.

What Is the Differential Diagnosis of Abdominal Pain and Diarrhea?

When a patient presents to a physician complaining of diarrhea and abdominal pain, it is important to distinguish between infectious and noninfectious causes of diarrhea, as this will ultimately dictate treatment plans. The nature of the diarrhea, as well as its onset and course, will play a large role in determining the etiology. Most acute diarrheal episodes with duration of 14 days or fewer are due to infectious causes of **viral, bacterial,** or **parasitic origin**. **Viruses** that are known to cause diarrhea include rotavirus, norovirus, and adenoviruses. **Bacterial** pathogens such as *Clostridium difficile, Yersinia enterocolitica, Escherichia coli, Salmonella,* and *Yersinia* can all cause infectious diarrhea that is severe at presentation. **Parasitic** diarrheal infections caused by *Giardia* or *Entamoeba histolytica* are less common in the developed world but can present in individuals who have traveled to resource-poor countries.

Noninfectious etiologies of diarrhea include lactose intolerance, celiac disease, irritable bowel syndrome, and inflammatory bowel disease (e.g., Crohn's disease or ulcerative colitis). These syndromes tend to present with diarrhea that is more chronic in nature but may first present as a subacute episode.

BASIC SCIENCE PEARL (STEP 1)

Water is absorbed from ingested material and from fluids secreted by the gastrointestinal tract in both the small and large bowel. Ions, especially sodium, are moved across the bowel mucosa by active cotransport with simple sugars and amino acids. Water follows by osmotic pressure. By the time fecal contents reach the large bowel, 80% of water has been absorbed.

CLINICAL PEARL (STEP 1/2/3)

There are two main mechanisms by which diarrhea occurs: secretory and osmotic. In **secretory** diarrhea the process by which water diffuses from the bowel lumen into the gut epithelium is reversed into an active secretory state, causing transport of ions and fluid *into* the lumen. Toxins and inflammatory reactions are common causes of such active secretion. **Osmotic** diarrhea occurs when a nonabsorbable, osmotically active substrate in the bowel lumen obliterates the normal osmotic gradient that normally draws water out of the bowel lumen into the cells. Under these abnormal circumstances, water remains within the lumen of the bowel and is excreted, resulting in diarrhea.

On physical examination, the patient's temperature is 99.4°F, blood pressure 95/52 mm Hg, pulse 132 bpm, respiratory rate 18 breaths/minute, and oxygen saturation 98% on room air. She is alert and oriented and responds appropriately to questioning but appears in moderate distress. She has decreased skin turgor. There is no jaundice or scleral icterus. Other than tachycardia, she has normal heart and lung sounds. Her abdomen is distended, and she has mild diffuse tenderness throughout. There is no guarding or rebound tenderness.

What Are Important Physical Examination Findings When Evaluating a Patient With Diarrhea?
Because patients may lose a large volume of water when having diarrhea, it is essential to carefully evaluate the patient's volume status. Physical findings associated with low volume include tachycardia, hypotension, decreased skin turgor (ability of skin to regain shape after pinching it for 2–5 seconds), and a dry tongue or gums. Altered mental status can be seen with severe volume depletion, as these patients often have concurrent derangements in their serum electrolyte concentrations.

On abdominal examination of patients presenting with diarrhea, it is extremely important to look for signs of peritonitis, such as tenderness to light percussion, guarding, rebound, and abdominal rigidity. Abdominal distension and the absence of bowel sounds may also be associated with peritonitis. In some instances, these physical examination findings may prompt emergent surgical intervention with or without radiographic imaging (see Chapter 12).

Due to concerns for dehydration, the patient is admitted to the hospital for intravenous fluid resuscitation and further diagnostic workup. Upon further questioning the patient notes that she recently had an upper respiratory infection for which she is being treated with a 2-week course of amoxicillin/clavulanic acid; she is on day 10 of her antibiotic regimen. Due to concern for *Clostridium difficile*-associated colitis, a stool sample is sent for analysis for the *C. difficile* toxin, and cultures are sent for other infectious causes of colitis.

What Are Some of the Other Etiologies of Infectious Diarrhea and How Do They Present?
Common bacterial causes of diarrhea are listed in Table 10.1. Most of these organisms are transmitted via the fecal-oral route or via contaminated food and water. The virulence of the majority of these organisms is via toxin production, which initiates the previously described secretory and/or inflammatory diarrhea. Hand hygiene and proper food preparation are important in preventing the transmission of these illnesses. Although stool culture and analysis for organism-specific toxins will be important for ultimate diagnosis, a patient's history of potential exposures, recent travel, and the quality and quantity of the diarrhea will usually suggest the correct diagnosis and enable the initiation of empiric treatment.

TABLE 10.1 ■ Organisms Responsible for Infectious Colitis

Organism	Signs/ Symptoms	Exposure	Diagnosis	Treatment
Escherichia coli (Several strains dependent on virulence factors)	Watery or bloody diarrhea	Contaminated water/food, fecal-oral	Clinical; Genetic detection methods under development	Dependent on strain: Traveler's diarrhea— doxycycline, trimethoprim/ sulfamethoxazole, fluoroquinolone, or rifaximin Enterohemorrhagic— antibiotics contraindicated
Clostridium difficile	Watery diarrhea in the setting of antibiotic use	Fecal-oral transmission of spores	Stool ELISA for toxins A and B or PCR	IV/oral metronidazole or oral vancomycin
Campylobacter jejuni	Fever, watery diarrhea, abdominal pain (RLQ- terminal ileum and/or cecum)	Uncooked meats (chicken or beef)	Stool culture	Supportive (mild) to macrolides (severe)
Shigella	Dysentery; Watery diarrhea that progresses to bloody diarrhea; assoc. fever/ abdominal pain; affects rectum/ sigmoid colon	Fecal-oral	Fecal WBCs and stool culture	Supportive (mild) to ciprofloxacin(severe)
Vibrio cholerae	Watery "rice- water" diarrhea, vomiting, septic shock	Contaminated water/food	Vibrio serogroup O1 or O139 in stool culture	Supportive care as well as doxycycline

What Is the Pathogenesis of the Development of C. difficile Infectious Colitis?

C. difficile is a Gram-positive, anaerobic organism that can form spores and lie quiescent in the GI tract. Under normal circumstances, gastrointestinal tract microorganisms compete for resources and suppress the growth of C. difficile in the colon. However, when a patient takes an antibiotic that reduces the number of colonic bacteria, normal suppression of C. difficile is reduced. The C. difficile organisms are then able to proliferate and secrete endotoxin. C. difficile toxins A and B cause colitis via damage to the epithelial cell of the colon and cause cell death leading to inflammation. Endoscopic evaluation in patients with C. difficile colitis will find pseudomembranous colitis (Fig. 10.1), characterized by yellowish plaques on the bowel mucosa. These plaques are composed of fibrin and inflammatory cells that can be scraped off; these findings are essentially pathognomonic for C. difficile colitis.

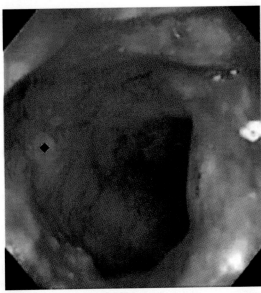

Fig. 10.1 Pseudomembranous Colitis. Colonoscopic view of pseudomembrane colitis in a patient with *C. difficile* infection. These plaques are composed of fibrin and inflammatory cells such as neutrophils and can be scraped of the colonic mucosa during endoscopy. From Klatt ED (ed) (2015). The Gastrointestinal Tract. Chapter 7. In Robbins and Cotran Atlas of Pathology, pp. 175–222.e7, Philadelphia: Elsevier.

CLINICAL PEARL (STEP 2/3)

Almost all antibiotics make patients susceptible to *Clostridium difficile* infection. The most commonly associated antibiotics include clindamycin, cephalosporins, fluoroquinolones, and some penicillins. It is important to note, however, that these antibiotics can also cause diarrhea that is *not* associated with *C. difficile* infection.

CLINICAL PEARL (STEP 2/3)

C. difficile is known to be difficult to culture, so diagnosis is typically based on identification of toxins A and B produced by the organism. The test of choice for diagnosing *C. difficile* is an enzyme-linked immunosorbent assay (ELISA) for the toxins. Polymerase chain reaction (PCR) testing can also be used to identify the organism's DNA in the stool.

What Is the Treatment for C. difficile Colitis?

For mild/moderate disease, the patient should immediately stop previous antibiotic use, begin fluid and electrolyte restoration, and start oral metronidazole, 500 mg three times daily. If the patient does not respond to oral metronidazole, oral vancomycin should be started. However, if the colitis is severe with signs and symptoms of systemic toxicity, IV metronidazole and oral vancomycin would be a more appropriate regimen. A feared complication of *C. difficile* colitis is toxic megacolon that may result in colonic perforation. If the patient has disease severe enough to cause sepsis, toxic megacolon, or perforation, surgery is mandatory. Total abdominal colectomy with end ileostomy and the creation of a rectal stump is the procedure of choice.

The stool ELISA test is negative for the *C. difficile* toxins. Stool cultures finalize without growth of any infectious organism. After 2 days of aggressive fluid resuscitation the patient's symptoms and vital signs improve. She undergoes a colonoscopy to help determine the cause of her diarrhea. Upon entering the rectum with the colonoscope the physician notices circumferential inflammation with extensive edema that continues proximally. There are no "skip lesions" and no true ulcerations. Biopsies of the involved mucosa show pseudopolyps and crypt architecture distortion, but no granulomas are noted.

What Are the Clinical, Endoscopic, and Pathologic Characteristics of Inflammatory Bowel Disease?

Inflammatory bowel disease (IBD) refers to a group of inflammatory diseases that affect the small bowel and colon. The two disease entities that will be discussed here are ulcerative colitis (UC) and Crohn's disease. Patients who initially present with UC tend to describe signs and symptoms such as bloody and/or mucoid stools, tenesmus (sensation to defecate even with an empty rectum), urgency, incontinence, and abdominal pain. The initial presentation of patients with Crohn's may take several forms: protracted diarrhea; abdominal pain, commonly in the right lower quadrant from terminal ileitis (that may mimic appendicitis); and/or perianal fistulas and abscesses. Both UC and Crohn's can present with anemia, weight loss, malaise, lack of appetite, and abdominal pain. If clinically severe, the patient may exhibit signs of SIRS response such as high fevers, tachycardia, hypotension, and leukocytosis.

Most commonly the diagnosis of IBD is made by endoscopic examination with biopsy of the involved tissues. With an acutely ill patient, this may be simple flexible sigmoidoscopy. The characteristic endoscopic appearance of UC is diffuse, symmetric inflammation that does not spare any parts of the colonic mucosa and tends to extend from the rectum and continue proximally. The severity of inflammation often decreases as the colon is examined more proximally. The inflammation can range from mild edema to frank ulcerations of the colonic mucosa. Full colonoscopy should be performed when the acute phase has subsided, in order to determine the full extent of the disease. Understanding that patients with UC are at risk for developing malignancy, a stricture in the setting of UC should be considered possibly malignant in nature until proven otherwise. Crohn's disease looks different from UC on endoscopic examination. When Crohn's is considered, a colonoscopy that includes examination of the terminal ileum should be performed with biopsies of the ileum, as the ileum is one of the most common sites involved in Crohn's. On colonoscopy the hallmark finding is patchy inflammatory changes with "skip lesions" that represent areas of spared mucosa; ulcerations may be found in Crohn's that are linear ("bear claw") in appearance, giving a characteristic "cobblestone" appearance. Of note, whereas UC almost always involves the rectum, Crohn's disease more commonly has rectal sparing.

A diagnosis cannot be made solely on physical appearance of the mucosa and requires tissue biopsies harvested as part of the endoscopic examination. Pathologic characteristics of ulcerative colitis include pseudopolyps, crypt distortion, and the absence of granulomas. Noncaseating granulomas are pathognomonic findings for Crohn's disease, but are found in only 15% of cases. Remember that it is easier to make a diagnosis of Crohn's disease in a surgical resection specimen than endoscopic biopsy because specimen examination is full thickness, and transmural inflammation and granulomas can more easily be identified.

CLINICAL PEARL (STEP 2/3)

In patients who present with moderate to severe disease, the benefits of colonoscopy in providing an accurate diagnosis must be weighed against the risks of perforation. Flexible sigmoidoscopy may be a safer alternative and should be considered.

What Are the Options for Medical Management of Ulcerative Colitis and Crohn's Disease?

Treatment options for ulcerative colitis can be viewed in two categories: (1) management of active acute colitis to induce remission, and (2) maintenance therapy to remain in remission. The severity of the inflammation in ulcerative colitis determines the initial therapy. For mild to moderate severity the mainstay of medical therapy is 5-ASA or mesalamine, in both the topical (suppository or enema) and oral forms. If the patient does not respond adequately to these medications, then oral corticosteroids (e.g., prednisone, beclomethasone, or budesonide) should be used to induce remission. When disease activity is severe, it is best to admit the patient to the hospital for intravenous corticosteroids, usually methylprednisolone or hydrocortisone. Patients for whom corticosteroids are contraindicated (e.g., poorly controlled diabetes or previous steroid-induced psychosis) and patients not responding to IV steroid therapy within 3 days should be treated with cyclosporine. Tacrolimus or infliximab may be used to induce remission. Once the patient with severe colitis is in remission, the use of TNF-alpha inhibitors (infliximab or adalimumab) or azathioprine should be used as maintenance medications. In the patient with toxic colitis or megacolon who does not respond quickly to supportive treatment and steroids, abdominal colectomy should be performed.

Surgical management of Crohn's disease is unlikely to be curative, thus medical management plays a large part in patient care. Similar to UC, the medical management of Crohn's is based on disease severity and on considerations of both induction of remission and maintenance therapy. Treatment depends on the location of the disease. In mild to moderate disease involving the colon the first-line agent is predominantly sulfasalazine. A patient whose symptoms are unresponsive to this therapy should be considered to have more severe disease and should be treated with oral corticosteroids such as prednisone or prednisolone. For patients resistant to corticosteroids, the use of anti-TNF agents such as infliximab is indicated. The SONIC trial (2010) concluded that the use of infliximab monotherapy or infliximab in combination with azathioprine was more effective at inducing and maintaining steroid-free remission than azathioprine alone. As a result of this study, infliximab is commonly used to induce remission and for maintenance therapy for patients who either do not respond to corticosteroids or who have had severe side effects from corticosteroids. If medical management does not provide adequate remission and maintenance, then surgery may be indicated to remove the involved portion of the intestine.

The patient is diagnosed with ulcerative colitis, achieves remission with 5 days of in-hospital medical therapy, and is discharged and referred to a gastroenterologist for follow-up. Despite attempts over the next several months to manage her ulcerative colitis with medical therapies, she continues with persistent abdominal cramping, fecal incontinence, and tenesmus. She is referred to a surgeon for discussion of surgical management.

What Are the Indications for Surgical Management of Ulcerative Colitis?

The options for surgical management of patients with UC depend on whether surgical intervention is urgent or elective. The most common reason to perform an urgent operation in UC is fulminant colitis or toxic megacolon that does not improve within 2 to 3 days of medical therapy. The procedure of choice is a total abdominal colectomy with end ileostomy. This procedure avoids a time-consuming, complex dissection of the rectum and leaves the rectum in place to facilitate reconstructive surgery in the future.

Surgery for UC patients who have disease intractable to medical therapy or who develop malignancy can be performed on an elective basis and includes the following options:

- The most common elective procedure performed for UC is total proctocolectomy with ileo-anal pouch reconstruction. In this procedure the surgeon removes the colon and rectum with preservation of the anal sphincter complex. A reservoir, or "pouch," is created using a portion of the distal ileum (Fig. 10.2). The pouch is then connected to the anus via a stapler or by

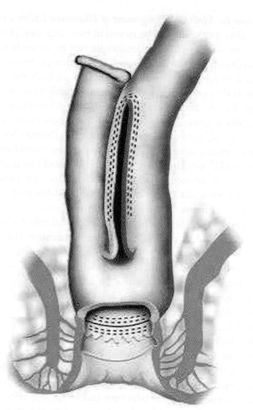

Fig. 10.2   J-pouch. Created by a portion of the distal ileum and connected to the preserved anal sphincter complex after total proctocolectomy. (From Araghizadeh F: Ileostomy, Colostomy, and Pouches. Ch 117. In: Sleisenger and Fordtran's Gastrointestinal and Liver Disease, Philadelphia: Elsevier, 2016, pp. 2062–2075.e4).

handsewn anastomosis. A major long-term problem is "pouchitis," a chronic inflammation of the pouch that may be related to the change in intestinal microflora.

- Total proctocolectomy with end ileostomy involves resecting the entire colon, including the rectum, and leaving the patient with a permanent ileostomy. This should be considered in a patient for whom an ileo-anal pouch might be high risk, such as an older patient with multiple comorbidities or a patient with lax anal sphincters who would be expected to have poor bowel control.
- Total proctocolectomy with continent ileostomy involves resection of the colon and rectum but is unique in that the surgeon uses the ileum to create an ileostomy with a reservoir for stool with a valve that the patient can periodically catheterize with a tube to evacuate the stool.

As UC is confined to the colon, surgical resection should be curative.

What Are the Indications for Surgical Management of Crohn's Disease?

Similar to the surgical treatment of UC the indications for surgical intervention in Crohn's disease include medical intractability, fulminant colitis/toxic megacolon, and concern for malignancy. However, in Crohn's disease, surgical intervention is commonly required for obstruction, fistulous disease, and the presence of intraabdominal abscesses. The general principle of operative management in Crohn's is to resect the involved bowel segment, preserving as much small intestine as possible. Multiple resections, which may be required over the course of a patient's lifetime, run the risk of the development of short bowel syndrome.

Options for surgical management include:

- Ileocecal resection for localized inflammation usually involves removing the terminal ileum and cecum and then anastomosing the remaining portion of the ileum to the ascending colon.
- Total proctocolectomy with end ileostomy is used mainly for patients with extensive colonic involvement including the rectum.
- Total abdominal colectomy with ileorectal anastomosis is used in patients who do not have rectal involvement and who wish to remain in-continuity.
- Localized colonic/small intestinal resection is segmental resection that may be used in patients who have localized Crohn's complications such as fistulas, strictures, or obstructions.
- Stricturoplasty is used to treat strictures without resection in patients at risk for short gut, particularly in diffuse jejunoileitis.

After meeting with a colorectal surgeon and discussing her surgical options, the patient decides to proceed with a total proctocolectomy with ileo-anal pouch. She does well postoperatively, her major complaint being anal skin irritation due to multiple bowel movements. When seen by her surgeon 1 month later, she has no abdominal pain, the number of her bowel movements has decreased to 3 to 5 per day, and her skin irritation has resolved.

BEYOND THE PEARLS

- Diarrhea is a common complaint and can be caused by infectious or inflammatory problems in the small bowel or the colon.
- Stool culture, examination for ova and parasites, and specialized testing for *Clostridium difficile* toxin are important steps in the workup of diarrhea, but empiric treatment of suspected infectious etiologies can usually be initiated based on history and physical examination.
- Minimizing intestinal inflammation is the goal of the medical treatment of inflammatory bowel disease. Surgical management is indicated for failures of medical management and for the management of disease complications.

Suggested Readings

Colombel, J. F., Sandborn, W. J., Reinisch, W., Mantzaris, G. J., & Kornbluth, A. (2010). Infliximab, azathioprine, or combination therapy for Crohn's disease. *New England Journal of Medicine, 363*(11), 1086–1088. https://doi.org/10.1056/nejmc1005805.

Fordtran, J. S. (2006). Colitis due to *Clostridium difficile* toxins: Underdiagnosed, highly virulent, and nosocomial. *Baylor University Medical Center Proceedings, 19*(1), 3–12. https://doi.org/10.1080/08998280.2006.11928114.

Gomollón, F., Dignass, A., Annese, V., Tilg, H., Assche, G. V., Lindsay, J. O., et al. (2016). 3rd European evidence-based consensus on the diagnosis and management of Crohn's disease 2016: Part 1: Diagnosis and Medical Management. *Journal of Crohns and Colitis, 11*(1), 3–25. https://doi.org/10.1093/ecco-jcc/jjw168.

Mahmoud, N. N., Bleier, J. I., Aarons, C. B., Paulson, E. C., Shanmugan, S., & Fry, R. D. (2017). Colon and rectum. In *Sabiston textbook of surgery: The biological basis of modern surgical practice* (20th ed.). Philadelphia, PA: Elsevier.

Vavricka, S. R., Schoepfer, A., Scharl, M., Lakatos, P. L., Navarini, A., & Rogler, G. (2015). Extraintestinal manifestations of inflammatory bowel disease. *Inflammatory Bowel Diseases, 21*(8), 1982–1992. https://doi.org/10.1097/MIB.0000000000000392.

CHAPTER 11

Abdominal Pain and Distention in a 63-Year-Old Male

Derek Freitas ■ Mary Ann Hopkins

A 63-year-old male with a past surgical history of an open appendectomy when he was 25 years old presents to the emergency department with abdominal pain and distention. The pain started approximately 1 day ago and has gotten progressively worse. He reports it feels crampy and comes in waves, but it is now becoming more constant. He also feels that his abdomen is more bloated than usual. On further questioning, he reports one episode of green emesis and denies ever having a colonoscopy.

What Is the Differential Diagnosis for Abdominal Pain and Distention?

Evaluations of patients with abdominal pain and distention are some of the most common consults for general surgeons. The differential diagnoses include a few possible emergencies as well as other less critical etiologies. Potentially emergent and urgent diagnoses include large bowel obstruction (LBO), small bowel obstruction (SBO), or severe colonic dilation from an ileus or colitis. Other diagnoses to consider include constipation, ascites, gastroenteritis, tumors, and even pregnancy. Table 11.1 provides a shortened list for the differential diagnosis of abdominal pain and distension.

Why Are the History and Physical Examination So Important for Diagnosing the Cause of Abdominal Pain and Distention?

Although a patient's history is always important, it is perhaps even more so in helping differentiate potential causes of abdominal pain and distention (see Table 11.1). A history of any abdominal surgery predisposes to adhesions that can be lead points for obstruction. Patients with hernias are also at a higher risk of bowel obstruction. Similarly, a patient's recent colonoscopy history is important to know, as colon cancer is a common cause of LBO. Patients with diverticulitis, sigmoid or cecal volvulus, and Crohn's disease are also at risk for LBOs. Patients with severe *Clostridium difficile* colitis or ulcerative colitis can be at risk for toxic megacolon.

Associated symptoms are also important to elucidate—mainly whether the patient has continued to have bowel movements, has flatus, and has been vomiting. SBO is almost always associated with obstipation (complete failure to pass any stool or flatus). Fevers, an elevated white blood cell count, and tenderness on palpation may be indicative of an infectious colitis. Conversely, if the patient has had no nausea or vomiting, is afebrile and without significant pain, and continues to pass flatus, the differential tends to go toward more benign causes such as gaseous distention or constipation. The timing of vomiting relative to pain can also be somewhat indicative of the cause. If the distention and pain started first and then vomiting followed several hours or days later, then obstruction is more likely. However, if the patient started vomiting immediately and distention and pain developed subsequently, an obstruction might be less likely.

TABLE 11.1 ■ **Examination and Laboratory Findings for Possible Causes of Abdominal Pain and Distention**

Possible Diagnosis	History, Examination, and Laboratory Findings
Small bowel obstruction	No flatus, hyperactive bowel sounds, distended tympanitic abdomen, ± tenderness, vomiting
Large bowel obstruction	No flatus, hyperactive bowel sounds, distended tympanitic abdomen, ± tenderness, vomiting
Infectious colitis/ toxic megacolon	Distended, tender, fevers, leukocytosis
Severe constipation	Distended but potentially soft, hard stool in rectal vault, + flatus,
Severe ileus/Ogilvie syndrome	Distended tympanitic abdomen, ± tenderness
Ascites	Distended nontympanitic abdomen, fluid wave, ± tenderness
Tumor	Possible distended abdomen secondary to palpable mass, ± ascites, ± pain
Gastroenteritis	Pain, possible distention, mild pain, vomiting, diarrhea
Pregnancy	+ bHCG, distended abdomen with palpable uterus

CLINICAL PEARL (STEP 2/3)

Do not let the presence of bowel movements rule out a diagnosis of intestinal obstruction. Depending on where the obstruction is and how recently the patient became obstructed, there may still be stool past the obstruction that will continue to pass. Absence of flatus (obstipation) is more sensitive for diagnosing a full obstruction.

What Are the Primary Physical Examination Techniques to Evaluate Abdominal Pain and Distention?

The physical examination is essential in helping to begin to narrow the differential diagnosis and to further determine whether the patient is presenting with a surgical emergency. Key examination maneuvers include palpation of the abdomen, percussion, and auscultation. Auscultation should be performed initially to determine the presence of hyperactive bowel sounds, which have a predicative value in diagnosing SBO (but are not as useful in other diagnoses). Absence of bowel sounds would suggest ileus. Percussion can elicit tympany, which is indicative of dilated, air-filled bowel. Palpation is vital to determine whether the abdomen is: distention is elicited via observation, not palpation; 2) soft or firm; and 3) tender. The location of abdominal tenderness is especially important, though many patients with an obstructive process will have diffuse abdominal tenderness. The presence of signs of peritonitis—extreme diffuse tenderness, rebound tenderness, involuntary guarding—indicate that the patient has presented with a problem that may need immediate surgical intervention. Many patients may have a distended abdomen but may not have obstruction. Patients with a complete obstruction or severe ileus tend to be very distended with a firm, tympanic abdomen, almost like an overinflated beach ball. Conversely, someone suffering from chronic constipation may appear very distended, but the abdomen will tend to be softer and you may be able to feel a dilated colon with appreciable masses of stool. The presence of copious hard stool on rectal examination may point you toward this diagnosis as well. However, patients with early obstructions or ileus may present mildly distended with a soft abdomen. A pregnant patient may complain of abdominal distention, but a palpable uterus may easily be appreciated. Similarly, a patient presenting with ascites may have a very distended abdomen, but it will not be tympanic and may have a fluid wave. Examining the patient for hernias in the abdominal wall and the groin is an important part of this examination to assess for bowel incarceration or strangulation as a cause of the patient's symptoms.

What Imaging Modalities Are Indicated to Assess a Patient With Abdominal Pain and Distension?

Imaging adds important adjunct information to the history and physical examination in the evaluation of patients who present with abdominal pain and distension. The initial radiographic assessment can be performed with abdominal radiographs that are fast and readily available. Findings may include distended bowel—small or large—the pattern of which helps define a potential obstruction. For example, dilated small loops of bowel throughout the abdomen with a decompressed terminal ileum and colon indicates a point of obstruction in the distal small bowel.

Computed tomography (CT) of the abdomen and pelvis is more specific than abdominal radiography. Contrast enhancement with both oral and intravenous contrast aids in the detection of intraabdominal pathology, though intravenous contrast should not be used in patients with renal impairment. Findings include bowel wall thickening to suggest inflammation or edema, the presence of dilated and decompressed bowel with a transition point between the two which suggests a bowel obstruction, a transition point related to a hernia not appreciated on physical examination, and the presence of any other process in the abdomen that could cause pain or distension by external compression of the bowel.

CLINICAL PEARL (STEP 2/3)

In cases of a suspected bowel obstruction the American College of Radiology Appropriateness Criteria recommend a computerized tomography (CT) scan of the abdomen and pelvis with intravenous (IV) contrast. If there is a concern for a high-grade SBO, the guidelines recommend against the use of oral contrast. The IV contrast assists in identifying any possible bowel ischemia or mesenteric edema that could be indicative of a surgical emergency. If the patient cannot get IV contrast, the Appropriateness Criteria recommend a noncontrast CT of the abdomen and pelvis.

On physical examination there are bowel sounds and the abdomen is very distended, firm to palpation, and tympanic. The patient's abdomen is only very minimally tender to palpation. Laboratory analyses including a complete blood count and basic metabolic panel are normal. CT scan of the abdomen and pelvis reveals dilated proximal small bowel and decompressed distal small bowel, with a transition point in the right lower quadrant (Fig. 11.1).

How Is a Small Bowel Obstruction Managed? What Determines If a Patient Needs Surgery?

Patients for whom there is concern for a small bowel obstruction should be made nothing by mouth (NPO), have a nasogastric (NG) tube inserted and placed on suction, and have IV crystalloid fluids initiated. Laboratory analyses should include a complete blood count (CBC), basic metabolic panel (BMP), and venous lactate. Oftentimes, these patients will have electrolyte abnormalities that should be corrected.

Whether to pursue additional surgical management depends on several factors. Patients who have undergone abdominal surgery previously are most likely to have a bowel obstruction due to intraabdominal adhesions. These patients can frequently be treated nonoperatively with hydration, NG tube decompression, and serial abdominal examinations until resumption of bowel activity. Indications for surgical intervention in adhesive small bowel obstruction are closed loop obstruction (in which the bowel twists on itself causing a blind loop with both inflow and outflow obstructed), and a physical examination (severe abdominal pain, tenderness, rebound, or guarding) or imaging (poor perfusion of the bowel and/or mesenteric edema on contrast-enhanced CT imaging) that suggests small bowel ischemia. Ischemia may evolve over the course of treatment, so serial abdominal examination and laboratory analyses (including white blood cell counts and lactate) should be performed.

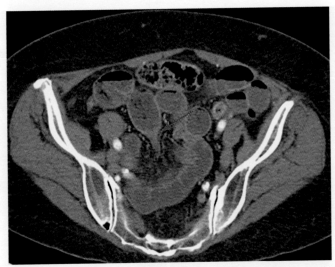

Fig. 11.1 CT scan of the abdomen demonstrating dilated small bowel loops proximal to a transition point in the lower abdomen (yellow arrow) to decompressed small bowel. There is also fecalization of the small bowel proximal to the transition point. (From Rubesin SE, Gore RM: Small bowel obstruction. In Gore RM, Levine MS, editors: *Textbook of Gastrointestinal Radiology,* ed 4, Philadelphia, 2015, Elsevier, pp 806–826.)

If patients do not have a history compatible with an adhesive bowel obstruction (no previous abdominal surgery; i.e., a "virgin abdomen,"), the cause of the obstruction must be elucidated, and they will often require surgery. An obstruction secondary to a hernia (whether it is an irreducible ventral or inguinal hernia or an internal hernia) is a clear indication for surgery. Small bowel volvulus in adults or children or malrotation pediatric patients is an indication for operative intervention (see Chapters 54 and 55 for a discussion of abdominal pain in children). Mass effect due to an intraabdominal tumor or intraluminal tumor is also an indication for surgery.

CLINICAL PEARL (STEP 2/3)

The vast majority of small bowel obstructions secondary to adhesions in the absence of closed loop etiology or ischemia can be managed nonoperatively with hydration, making the patient NPO, and placing a nasogastric tube. Adhesions are the most common cause of SBOs in the United States, and with proper management will frequently resolve with return of bowel function within 3 days. Those that do not resolve within 3 to 5 days require surgery. It is critical to monitor for signs and symptoms (fever, worsening pain, worsening abdominal examination) that require more urgent surgical intervention.

How Is a Large Bowel Obstruction Managed? How Does It Differ Depending on the Etiology and Status of the Ileocecal Valve?

The etiology of a LBO largely determines how it is managed, but most LBOs will need some intervention either emergently or on a more elective basis, as the original cause of the obstruction is unlikely to resolve on its own. Common etiologies include an obstructing mass, stricture, and volvulus.

A volvulus is treated based on clinical findings and the location of the volvulized portion of bowel. For a sigmoid volvulus (Fig. 11.2A), endoscopic decompression to untwist the sigmoid colon is an option in patients who are stable and without signs or symptoms of bowel ischemia. The patient will still need an eventual surgical intervention, as the sigmoid is prone to volvulize

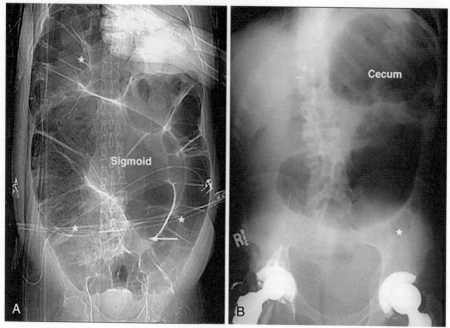

Fig. 11.2   Abdominal radiographs demonstrating large bowel obstructions due to sigmoid volvulus (A) and cecal volvulus (B). Note that the sigmoid becomes displaced into the right upper quadrant and the remainder of the colon becomes distended (*) proximal to the sigmoid obstruction (arrow). (From Mizell JS, Turnage RH: Intestinal obstruction. In Feldman M, Friedman LS, Brandt LJ, editors: *Sleisenger and Fordtran's Gastrointestinal and Liver Disease,* ed 9, Philadelphia, 2010, Elsevier, pp 2154–2170.e3.)

again. For cecal volvulus (see Fig. 11.2B), endoscopic decompression is difficult and unlikely to be effective, and therefore a surgical intervention of some form is needed at the time of diagnosis (cecal pexy versus resection, depending on the patient's clinical status and comorbidities).

One important point in the pathophysiology of a LBO is the competence of the ileocecal valve. If the valve is incompetent, the obstruction will back up into the small bowel and can be treated similarly to a small bowel obstruction initially. If the valve is competent, however, this becomes a surgical emergency as the nondecompressed bowel creates a situation similar to a closed loop obstruction without the ability to decompress passed the cecum. A cecal diameter of 9 to 12 cm on imaging is concerning for impending perforation and should prompt operative intervention. Commonly, a diverting transverse or sigmoid loop colostomy is performed to decompress the large bowel both proximally and distally. An end colostomy may be inadequate, as the colon left behind just proximal to the obstruction would still be unable to be decompressed.

CLINICAL PEARL

As with any surgery, electively planned surgery or urgent surgery is likely to lead to better outcomes than emergent surgery. This gives the surgeon the ability to optimize a patient medically and reduce risks related to any comorbidities as well as allowing the surgeon to have proper planning for the operation. Therefore temporizing interventions, such as endoscopic decompression of a sigmoid volvulus or diverting colostomy for an obstructing colon cancer before definitive resection, can reduce perioperative and postoperative complications.

What Are Other Causes of Abdominal Pain and Distention Aside From Obstructions and How Are They Treated?

Patients with severe **constipation** are usually easily identifiable. They will report chronic difficulty passing stool, will likely continue to pass flatus, and typically will not report any nausea or vomiting. Imaging studies will typically show a significant stool burden. First-line management for this patient is a proper diet and laxative regimen and minimizing any medications that promote constipation (narcotics, anticholinergics). Rarely, very severe constipation can lead to colonic inflammation (stercoral colitis) and possibly even ischemia simply from the pressure and dilation of the colon caused by the hard stool. Unchecked, this could lead to **stercoral perforation,** which is a surgical emergency. Therefore worsening abdominal pain in a patient with severe constipation should not be ignored.

An **ileus** may be another common cause of the previously mentioned symptoms. Ileus is common in postoperative patients and can arise from a combination of factors, including lack of patient mobility and the use of narcotics. Imaging typically demonstrates diffusely dilated bowel with air extending all the way into the distal colon and rectum. Mild to moderate ileus can be treated by encouraging ambulation and minimizing narcotics and anticholinergics. Progressive ileus may require the patient to be made NPO to prevent the risk of vomiting, and severe ileus may require nasogastric tube decompression until the patient has the return of bowel function.

Ogilvie syndrome or **colonic pseudoobstruction** is another diagnosis to consider. These patients present very similarly to a large bowel obstruction, but imaging shows a diffusely dilated colon without any clear point of obstruction. Treatment is similar to treating an ileus. Severe Ogilvie syndrome may lead to massive colonic dilation. In these cases, intravenous neostigmine or endoscopic decompression may be indicated. Refractory cases potentially require operative intervention to prevent perforation. The risk for perforation increases significantly when the cecum approaches 10 cm in diameter, as the cecum is the thinnest portion of the colon.

Toxic megacolon may be another cause of abdominal distention and pain. This may be a dreaded sequela of severe ulcerative colitis (UC) or *Clostridium difficile* (CD) colitis. Patients presenting with severe UC or CD should be placed in a highly monitored setting, be made NPO and have a nasogastric tube placed, and receive aggressive steroid or antibiotic therapy as appropriate. Additionally, they should receive repeated abdominal examinations and their white blood cell count and electrolytes trended. If there is progression of their colitis, worsening dilation, or frank perforation, then these patients should be operated on immediately.

A few other diagnoses to consider include **ascites, tumors,** and **pregnancy.** Patients with ascites secondary to any number of causes can present with significant abdominal distention. Examination and imaging are likely to demonstrate a large volume of intraabdominal fluid. Management of these patients depends on the underlying cause of the ascites. Importantly, do not let a finding of ascites mislead you if the patient is also presenting with clear signs of an obstruction. It is not infrequent to find a patient with large-volume ascites and a malignant obstruction of the bowel. Similarly, patients with intraabdominal tumors may present with abdominal pain and distention. You may be able to appreciate a palpable mass or masses representing the tumor. The pain in these patients may be more long-standing, but as with a patient presenting with ascites, you must perform a thorough history and physical, as malignant obstruction and/or perforation is not uncommon. Last but not least, it is not completely unheard of for a patient to present with a distended abdomen and vomiting and be found to be pregnant. Therefore a beta HCG should be checked for women of childbearing age. However, pregnancy does not exclude any of the previously mentioned diagnoses, and therefore they should be ruled out before attributing any symptoms and signs solely to pregnancy.

The patient is admitted to the surgery service with a nasogastric tube in place and is resuscitated with intravenous fluids. He undergoes serial abdominal examination and laboratory analyses, and his electrolytes are repleted as needed. On his second hospital day, he begins to pass flatus, and his NG tube is removed. The following day his abdomen is much less distended, he has a bowel movement, and his diet is advanced at first to liquids and then to solid food. He is discharged home the next day. He is counseled about the potential recurrence of his obstruction and that he requires no dietary modifications to prevent this.

BEYOND THE PEARLS

- The most common cause of a small bowel obstruction is adhesions from prior surgery or a hernia. Other etiologies include malrotation with volvulus, malignant obstructions, and impaction from bezoars.
- Many small bowel obstructions without concern for ischemia or closed loop obstruction can be managed medically with hydration, NPO, and nasogastric tube decompression.
- A common cause of large bowel obstructions is obstructing colorectal cancers. Other etiologies include inflammatory strictures from Crohn's or diverticulitis, large bowel volvulus, or hernia (including ventral and inguinal).
- Large bowel obstructions with a competent ileocecal valve require emergent intervention due to the presence of a closed loop obstruction.
- Nonobstructive etiologies can also cause abdominal pain and distention including toxic megacolon, severe constipation, ileus, Ogilvie syndrome, ascites, tumors, and pregnancy.

Suggested Readings

American College of Radiology ACR Appropriateness Criteria: *Suspected Small-Bowel Obstruction.* https://acsearch.acr.org/docs/69476/Narrative. Accessed October 9, 2017.

Brothers, T., Strodel, W., & Echkauser, F. (1987). Endoscopy in colonic volvulus. *Ann Surg, 206*(1), 1.

Danese, S., & Fiocchi, C. (2011). Ulcerative Colitis. *N Engl J Med, 365,* 1713–1725.

McGee, S. (2007). *Evidence-Based Physical Diagnosis* (Vol. 2). Philadelphia, PA: Saunders/Elsevier.

Ponec, J., Saunders, M., & Kimmey, M. (1999). Neostigmine for the treatment of acute colonic pseudo-obstruction. *N Engl J Med, 341,* 137–141.

Sheth, S., & LaMont, T. (1998). Toxic megacolon. *Lancet, 351,* 509–513.

CHAPTER 12

"Free Air" in a 72-Year-Old Female

Kevin L. Grimes ■ Christopher P. Brandt

A 72-year-old female presented to the emergency department after awaking this morning with sudden-onset, severe epigastric abdominal pain. Initial laboratory data include serum amylase and lipase levels, which are normal. The ED physician obtained an upright chest radiograph (CXR), which demonstrates "free air" under the diaphragm (Fig. 12.1). The surgical service is consulted for further evaluation and management.

What Is the Differential Diagnosis for Free Air?

Free air under the diaphragm is also called pneumoperitoneum. The most concerning cause of free air is a perforated viscus, which can include stomach, small intestine, or colon. The two most frequent causes in developed countries are gastroduodenal perforation secondary to ulcer disease and perforated diverticulitis. Perforations due to cancer, bowel obstruction, intestinal ischemia, inflammatory bowel disease, foreign body, or endoscopic procedures are also possible but less common. In developing countries, small bowel perforations due to typhoid or *Salmonella* enteritis may occur.

Patients who have had recent surgery, either open or laparoscopic, may have free air in the post-operative period, which usually resolves within 5 to 6 days. However, any post-operative patient, whether open or laparoscopic, who has free air associated with peritoneal findings, must be considered to have an anastomotic leak or an inadvertent enterotomy until proven otherwise.

BASIC SCIENCE PEARL (STEP 1/2/3)

Perforation of retroperitoneal structures may result in pneumoretroperitoneum rather than pneumoperitoneum, and air would not be found freely mobile under the diaphragm. Instead, air may be seen tracking along the kidneys on cross-sectional imaging. Retroperitoneal structures include the second, third, and fourth portions of the duodenum, the ascending and descending colon, and the rectum and anus.

What Are the Key Components of the Physical Examination in Patients for Whom There Is a Concern for Free Air?

In a patient presenting with free air, the most important components of the initial examination are the vital signs, general appearance, and abdominal findings. Patients with perforated viscus may present with signs of sepsis, such as fever, tachycardia, or hypotension, and may require immediate resuscitation. Patients will often look acutely uncomfortable, and the general appearance may also reveal signs of malignancy, such as pallor or cachexia.

The abdominal examination may demonstrate surgical scars, distention, or masses; the patient may have localized or generalized tenderness or signs of frank peritonitis, including diffuse rigidity, involuntary guarding, and rebound tenderness. If the patient does not have frank peritonitis with diffuse abdominal tenderness, the maximum point of tenderness on abdominal examination may

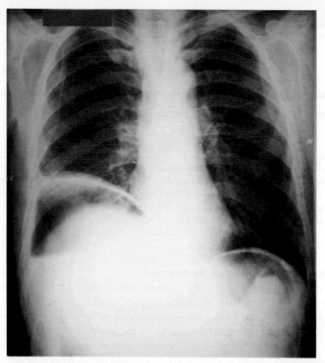

Fig. 12.1 Upright chest x-ray demonstrating pneumoperitoneum consistent with perforated viscus. (From Squires RA, Postier RG: Acute abdomen. In Townsend CM, Beauchamp D, Evers MB, editors: *Sabiston textbook of surgery,* ed 19, Philadelphia, 2012, Elsevier, p 1141.)

TABLE 12.1 ■ Differential Diagnosis and Key Examination Findings

Diagnosis	Key Examination Findings
Perforated gastroduodenal ulcer	Epigastric tenderness; guarding
Perforated diverticulitis	Left lower quadrant tenderness; guarding
Perforated small bowel obstruction	Abdominal distention and tenderness; guarding
Perforated large bowel obstruction (cancer, volvulus)	Abdominal distention or mass; tenderness; guarding
Perforated small bowel lymphoma or colon cancer	Cachexia, abdominal mass, tenderness

offer additional information as to the underlying etiology of the pain. Key physical examination findings for the major differential diagnoses are outlined in Table 12.1. Bowel sounds will often be diminished or absent due to associated intestinal ileus.

On physical examination, the patient is alert, mildly overweight, and appears uncomfortable. Her blood pressure is 155/85 mm Hg, and her pulse is 102 bpm. She has cool extremities. Her abdomen is nondistended, and there are no palpable masses. She has generalized tenderness, particularly in the epigastric region, and she demonstrates voluntary guarding.

What Imaging Studies Are Indicated in This Patient?

An upright chest x-ray is the quickest and most cost-effective study and may be diagnostic. Free air can be seen between the liver and the right hemidiaphragm and, less commonly, under the left hemidiaphragm, though this can be obscured by gas in the stomach—the so-called gastric bubble. If the patient cannot sit or stand upright, an abdominal radiograph with the patient in the left lateral decubitus position (left side down) can also reveal free air between the right lobe of the liver and the abdominal wall. An abdominal radiograph in the right lateral decubitus position (right side down) would be nondiagnostic because of the gastric bubble. Plain radiographs have a sensitivity of only 75%, however, and often do not reveal the underlying cause of pneumoperitoneum.

The decision may be made to proceed directly to operative exploration in a patient with free air on a radiograph without additional imaging. However, in a stable patient, a computed tomography (CT) scan of the abdomen and pelvis may be obtained, especially if there is any question about the presence of free air on radiographs. The sensitivity of CT scan in detecting free air is 98%, and it may also reveal additional information regarding etiology, which may help inform treatment decisions.

CLINICAL PEARL (STEP 2/3)

Sepsis is common in patients presenting with a perforated peptic ulcer; it is present in approximately one-third of patients and accounts for up to 50% of mortalities. Preoperative fluid resuscitation, initiation of broad-spectrum antibiotics, and rapid surgical source control are keys to reducing morbidity and mortality.

The patient undergoes CT of the abdomen and pelvis, which reveals a moderate amount of free air under the diaphragm as well as inflammation and fluid in the vicinity of the pylorus (Fig. 12.2). The surgeon explains that, based on these findings, a perforated peptic ulcer is the most likely etiology for the patient's abdominal pain and free air.

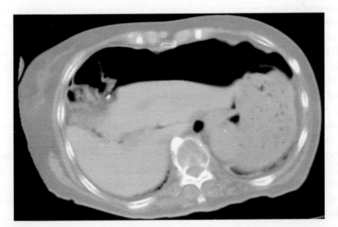

Fig. 12.2 Computed tomography scan demonstrating pneumoperitoneum consistent with perforated viscus. (From Tanaka R, Kameyama H, Nagahashi M, Kanda T, Ichikawa H, Hanyu T, et al: Conservative treatment of idiopathic spontaneous pneumoperitoneum in a bedridden patient: a case report, *Surgical Case Reports* 1(1):69, 2015.)

TABLE 12.2 ■ Types of Peptic Ulcer

Type	Location	Acid Hypersecretion
Duodenal	Duodenal bulb	Yes
Gastric—Type I	Lesser curve	No
—Type II	2 ulcers: gastric & duodenal	Yes
—Type III	Prepyloric	Yes
—Type IV	Cardia	No
—Type V	Any, related to NSAIDs	No

What Are the Types of Ulcers?

There are six types of peptic ulcers: duodenal and five different gastric ulcers (Table 12.2). Duodenal ulcers and gastric ulcers type II and III are related to acid hypersecretion. The other ulcers are related to a decreased mucosal defense.

BASIC SCIENCE PEARL (STEP 1/2/3)

Parietal cells, which are located in the fundus and cardia of the stomach, are responsible for secreting hydrochloric acid and intrinsic factor. A hydrogen-potassium ATPase on the apical surface of the cells pumps hydrogen ions into the gastric lumen. Acid secretion is stimulated by histamine (the most significant contribution), acetylcholine (from the parasympathetic nervous system), and gastrin (secreted by gastric enterochromaffin-like cells).

What Are the Risk Factors for Ulcer Disease?

The main risk factors for development of erosive ulcers fall into two categories: injury to the mucosal barrier and increased acid production.

Mucosal Injury:

- **Helicobacter pylori** is present in approximately 50% of the global population and is primarily associated with duodenal ulcers. H. pylori is found in more than 90% of patients with duodenal ulcers and 60% to 70% of patients with acute perforation.
- **NSAIDs** disrupt the mucosal barrier and expose the mucosa to acid. The mechanism is thought to be related to decreased prostaglandin production due to COX-1 inhibition. Selective COX-2 inhibitors are associated with a lower risk of ulcer disease.
- **Alcohol** directly damages the gastric mucosa.

Increased Acid:

- **Smoking** is believed to inhibit pancreatic bicarbonate secretion, leading to increased acidity in the duodenum. Tobacco also inhibits healing of duodenal ulcers.
- Oversecretion of gastrin due to **a gastrinoma** (also known as **Zollinger-Ellison syndrome (ZES)**) stimulates the parietal cells of the stomach to increase acid production. Over 90% of patients with ZES will develop peptic ulcers. **Alcohol** also increases gastrin production.
- **Fasting,** especially for extended periods of time for religious holidays such as Ramadan or Yom Kippur, may increase acid release and exposure.

Do All Patients With a Perforated Peptic Ulcer Require Surgery?

The majority of patients with perforated peptic ulcers are best managed with urgent surgical exploration. However, in some series, up to half of perforated peptic ulcers seal spontaneously, and a subset of patients may be initially managed nonoperatively. Patients in good clinical condition with minimal symptoms may be appropriate for a trial of nonoperative management, which should include prompt intravenous antibiotics, a proton pump inhibitor (PPI), nothing by mouth, and a water-soluble contrast study demonstrating that the leak has sealed.

Patients should be carefully chosen for attempted nonoperative management, because the risk of mortality increases with each hour that surgery, if needed, is delayed. In particular, there is a higher rate of failure of nonoperative management in patients older than 70 years.

For patients who require an operation, exploration is the first step in order to determine the cause of the pneumoperitoneum seen on imaging and, specifically, the type of perforated ulcer. Duodenal ulcers can simply be patched, whereas gastric ulcers should always be biopsied because of the risk of cancer. If the patient is known to be *H. pylori* negative, has been treated previously for *H. pylori*, or has clinically intractable ulcer disease, consideration should be given to more definitive antiulcer surgery, such as vagotomy and pyloroplasty or partial gastrectomy.

The patient is taken directly to the operating room for exploratory laparotomy. Bilious fluid is encountered in the upper abdomen, and a 1-cm perforation is identified on the anterior duodenum just distal to the pylorus. A modified Graham patch is performed (Fig. 12.3), and her immediate postoperative course is uneventful.

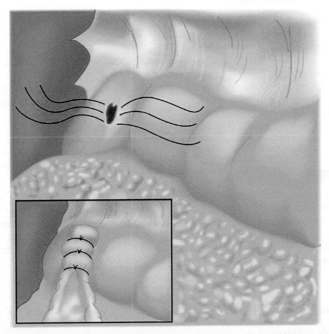

Fig. 12.3 Closure of perforated duodenal ulcer with Graham patch. (From Turnage RH, Badgwell B: Abdominal wall, umbilicus, peritoneum, mesenteries, omentum, and retroperitoneum. In Townsend CM, Beauchamp D, Evers MB, editors: *Sabiston textbook of surgery,* ed 19, Philadelphia, 2012, Elsevier, p 1088.)

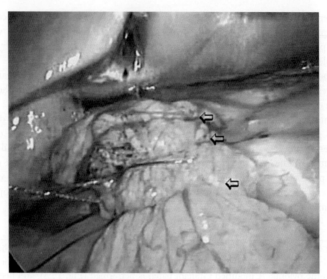

Fig. 12.4 Laparoscopic Graham patch *(sutures marked by arrows)*. (From Lam PW, Lam MC, Hui EK, Sun YW, Mok FP: Laparoscopic repair of perforated duodenal ulcers: the "three-stitch" Graham patch technique, *Surg Endosc* 19(12):1627–1630, 2005.)

Open Modified Graham Patch

1. Perform an upper midline incision.
2. Identify the stomach, pylorus, and first portion of the duodenum.
3. Mobilize a tongue of greater omentum.
4. Place sutures into healthy tissue on the proximal and distal sides of the ulcer, leaving the tails long.
5. Cover the ulcer with the omentum and loosely tie the sutures to hold the patch in place.

Modified Graham patch can be performed laparoscopically by placing ports at the umbilicus and in the right and left midabdomen. A tongue of greater omentum can be mobilized and sutured laparoscopically to form a patch (Fig. 12.4), similar to the open procedure.

CLINICAL PEARL (STEP 2/3)

The classic Graham patch simply stuffed omentum into the ulcer to plug the hole. The modified Graham patch includes the addition of sutures on either side of the ulcer to hold the omentum in place. The ulcer can be closed primarily before application of the patch, although sometimes the ulcer may be too large (greater than 2 cm) or the surrounding tissue may be too inflamed for closure to be performed safely. There is no difference in clinical outcomes if the patch is applied without ulcer closure.

What Is the Postoperative Management of Patients Undergoing Repair of a Perforated Peptic Ulcer?

Immediate postoperative care is tailored to the age, physiologic status, and degree of inflammation. Although there is no standardized time course, care includes correction of fluid and electrolyte abnormalities, initiation of PPI, continuation of antibiotics until signs of sepsis resolve, and reintroduction of enteral nutrition. There is no advantage to routine use of a contrast study after omental patch.

Patients should be advised to quit smoking, discontinue NSAIDs, and limit alcohol intake. In patients who are *H. pylori* positive (see Chapter 7), eradication of the infection reduces the incidence of ulcer recurrence. A standard course of treatment consists of a 14-day course of triple therapy (PPI + clarithromycin + amoxicillin), though other treatment regimens are also effective.

For perforated gastric ulcers (or if the exact location of an ulcer relative to the pylorus is unclear), upper endoscopy should be performed approximately 6 weeks after surgery to rule out malignancy, particularly if an intraoperative biopsy was not performed. Approximately 13% of gastric perforations are due to cancer.

> The patient is found to be *H. pylori* negative. She is discharged from the hospital on postoperative day 3 with a proton pump inhibitor. She returns to the office in 2 weeks for follow-up. Her incision is well healed and she has no complaints.

BEYOND THE PEARLS

- Patients with perforated peptic ulcer classically present with sudden onset of severe epigastric pain.
- Risk factors for ulcer disease include *H. pylori* infection, NSAID use, and smoking.
- Sepsis is common and is the main cause of mortality.
- Surgical repair is the gold standard treatment for perforated peptic ulcer; each hour that surgery is delayed results in increased risk of mortality.
- Gastric ulcers should always be biopsied due to the high incidence of gastric cancer.
- Postoperative *H. pylori* eradication and use of PPIs reduce the risk of ulcer recurrence.

Suggested Readings

Chung, K. T., & Shelat, V. G. (2017). Perforated peptic ulcer—an update. *World J of Gastrointest Surg, 9*(1), 1–12.

Lam, P. W., Lam, M. C., Hui, E. K., Sun, Y. W., & Mok, F. P. (2005). Laparoscopic repair of perforated duodenal ulcers: the "three-stitch" Graham patch technique. *Surg Endosc, 19*(12), 1627–1630.

Poris, S., Fontaine, A., Glener, J., Kubovec, S., Veldhuis, P., Du, Y., et al. (2018). Routine versus selective upper gastrointestinal contrast series after omental patch repair for gastric or duodenal perforation. *Surg Endosc, 32*(1), 400–404.

Soreide, K., Thorsen, K., Harrison, E. M., Bingener, J., Moller, M. H., Ohene-Yeboah, M., et al. (2015). Perforated peptic ulcer. *Lancet, 386*(10000), 1288–1298.

Tanaka, R., Kameyama, H., Nagahashi, M., Kanda, T., Ichikawa, H., Hanyu, T., et al. (2015). Conservative treatment of idiopathic spontaneous pneumoperitoneum in a bedridden patient: a case report. *Surg Case Rep, 1*(1), 69.

Townsend, C. M., Beauchamp, D., & Evers, M. B. (Eds.) (2012). *Sabiston textbook of surgery: The biological basis of modern surgical practice* (19th ed.). Philadelphia: Elsevier Saunders.

Gastrointestinal Surgery

Gastrointestinal Surgery

CHAPTER 13

Reflux in a 67-Year-Old Male

Rebecca Evangelista

A 67-year-old male with a long history of heartburn and reflux is referred to the surgery clinic by his primary physician for evaluation after the development of postprandial regurgitation. His symptoms were initially well treated with proton pump inhibitor therapy but have gotten progressively worse with weekly episodes of regurgitation. He has maximized the dose of his initial PPI and added others without significant improvement. A review of his other medical history is significant only for hypertension and prediabetes, both of which have been diet controlled.

What Is the Differential Diagnosis for Reflux and Regurgitation?
There are a variety of problems that can present with differing degrees and elements of reflux and dysphagia. Table 13.1 lists the differential diagnosis to consider for the symptoms of reflux and dysphagia. The pathophysiology of each disease process differs, and they present with a history that is unique, including the chronicity, timing related to eating, and associated symptoms. Chapter 21 discusses the presentation of esophageal carcinoma, which will not be discussed here.

What Are the Primary Studies That Will Distinguish Between These Diagnoses?
Although history and physical examination are the first step in evaluating any patient, the treatments for the disease processes resulting in reflux and regurgitation are varied and, in some cases, potentially harmful if an incorrect diagnosis is made. Therefore, several studies are indicated to help understand the patient's pathophysiology. With common things being common, the diagnostic workup should start with looking for evidence of the most likely issues, such as a right upper quadrant ultrasound to look for gallstones and an esophagogastroduodenoscopy (EGD) to visualize esophageal pathology. Using these two studies the medical team is likely to distinguish among most of the potential diagnoses. If these studies both appear normal, esophageal manometry is indicated to study the motility of the esophagus as is an upper gastrointestinal study with oral contrast (typically barium) to evaluate for anatomic abnormalities that may be missed. Computed tomography (CT) scan is rarely useful to help distinguish between potential causes of reflux and regurgitation, but one may be necessary for surgical planning if achalasia, large hiatal hernia, or Zenker's diverticulum is found.

CLINICAL PEARL (STEPS 2/3)

The information taken during the history is the key to guide the workup of dysphagia. Asking for details about the timing of symptoms, whether and how the symptoms are related to food and liquid consumption, and details of any associated pain can guide subsequent workup. For example, if solid food is being regurgitated shortly after a meal, Zenker's diverticulum may be at the top of the differential. In contrast, a feeling that food is not completely "going down" after swallow puts esophageal motility disorders and achalasia at the top of the differential.

TABLE 13.1 ■ Differential Diagnosis for Reflux and Regurgitation

Disease	Pathophysiology
Gastroesophageal reflux disease (GERD)	Acidic contents from the stomach into the esophagus due to lack of closure of the distal esophagus
Achalasia	Neurodegenerative changes to the distal esophagus resulting in failure of LES relaxation and progressive aperistalsis of the esophageal body
Hiatal hernia	Displacement of the GE junction above the diaphragm
Zenker's diverticulum	False diverticulum from herniation of the esophageal mucosa posteriorly between the CP muscle and inferior pharyngeal constrictor muscle
Esophagitis	Inflammation of the esophageal mucosa related to food allergies, acid exposure, infections, and direct medication exposure
Esophageal stricture	Narrowing of the esophagus from intrinsic or extrinsic disease
Gallstones	Biliary colic can mimic symptoms of reflux

The patient undergoes a workup that consists of esophagogastroduodenoscopy (EGD) and a barium swallow (upper GI series), which is shown in Fig. 13.1. He is diagnosed with a paraesophageal hernia and is referred to a surgeon to discuss potential treatment options. The surgeon recommends surgery but describes several other studies that need to be completed before he can undergo surgical repair.

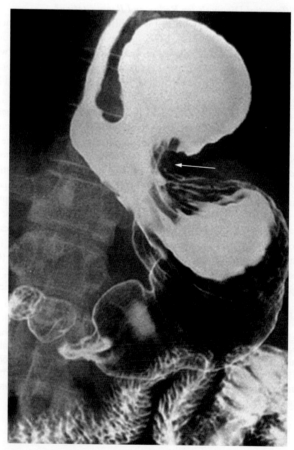

Fig. 13.1 Barium swallow showing the gastroesophageal junction and a portion of the stomach herniated above the diaphragm *(arrow)*. (From Hardwick R: The esophagus, stomach and duodenum. In Garden J, Parks RW, editors: *Principles and practice of surgery*, ed 7, London, 2018, Elsevier, pp 179–205.)

What Are the Indications for Surgical Treatment of a Hiatal Hernia?

The mere presence of a hiatal hernia is not an indication for surgery. Only hiatal hernias that are symptomatic are considered for surgical correction. Reflux symptoms that are refractory to PPIs are the most common. Whereas ordinary heartburn will usually respond to acid suppression, the regurgitation of large amounts of gastric contents will not improve with medical therapy alone. An inability to sleep in the supine position due to regurgitation is a common complaint. Other symptoms, such as cough from chronic aspiration of refluxed gastric contents, asthma or asthma-like symptoms, persistent clearing of the throat, and chronic hoarseness, are less common but important indications for surgical treatment. Massive hiatal hernias leading to chest pain, nausea, or pulmonary symptoms from lung displacement are also an indication for surgery.

How Are Hiatal Hernias Categorized?

There are four types of hiatal hernias, and they are categorized based on the abnormal presence (herniation) of the gastroesophageal (GE) junction, the stomach, and other abdominal organs into the chest (Fig. 13.2):

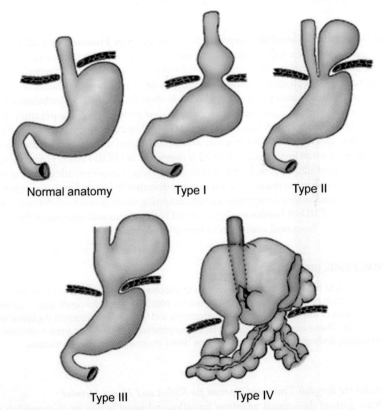

Normal anatomy   Type I   Type II

Type III   Type IV

Fig. 13.2 Normal gastroesophageal anatomy and four types of hiatal hernias. (From Vega JA, Velanovich V: Paraesophageal hernia: etiology, presentation, and indications for repair. In Yeo CJ, editor: *Shackelford's surgery of the alimentary tract*, ed 8, Philadelphia, 2019, Elsevier, pp 279–283. Modified from Duranceau A, Jamieson GG: Hiatal hernia and gastroesophageal reflux. In Sabiston DC Jr, editor: *Textbook of surgery and the biological basis of modern surgical practice*, ed 15, Philadelphia, 1997, Saunders, p 775.)

- Type I: This is a "sliding hernia," with only the GE junction displaced above the diaphragm.
- Type II: The GE junction remains below the diaphragm, with herniation of the gastric fundus above the diaphragm.
- Type III: Both the GE junction and the proximal stomach are herniated above the diaphragm.
- Type IV: There is herniation of the GE junction and proximal stomach along with herniation of other abdominal structures such as the duodenum, colon, pancreas, or omentum.

BASIC SCIENCE PEARL (STEPS 1/2/3)

There are sphincters at both the upper and lower esophagus, but the anatomy and physiology of each differs significantly. The upper esophageal sphincter separates the pharynx from the esophagus, and its anatomic composition includes the cricopharyngeus and inferior pharyngeal constrictor muscles. Muscle relaxation permits passage of food boluses from the pharynx into the esophagus. The lower esophageal sphincter anatomically does not have extrinsic muscular components; instead, it represents a specialized portion of the circular muscle of the esophagus. Relaxation permits food boluses to travel from the esophagus to the stomach. The anatomic position of the sphincter within the abdomen also adds to the tonicity of the sphincter, given the pressure differential between the chest and the abdomen.

What Other Studies Should Be Completed Before the Surgical Treatment of Reflux Disease?

Although gastroesophageal reflux disease is the most likely cause of the vast majority of patients' reflux symptoms, the surgeon must complete a full workup to assess for other underlying diseases such as alterations in esophageal motility. Therefore, a complete assessment should be undertaken before surgical treatment even when a hiatal hernia is identified. A 48-hour ambulatory pH evaluation of the esophagus is the gold standard for diagnosis of gastric reflux. The pH study quantifies the degree of acid reflux and correlates it with the patient's subjective symptoms. This study utilizes a scoring system, called the DeMeester score, which is calculated using data related to esophageal pH and a patient's symptoms. A value of 14.72 is diagnostic of GERD and is predictive of symptomatic improvement after surgery. Esophageal manometry, or pressure recordings during the swallow phase, is also required to evaluate for any motility disorders before undertaking surgery. When there is clinical suspicion for gastroparesis, a gastric emptying study should be performed to rule this out as a cause for GERD. A barium swallow is useful both for anatomic imaging of the esophagus and stomach and for functional evaluation of motility and reflux.

CLINICAL PEARL (STEPS 2/3)

Achalasia is one of the most common disorders of esophageal motility. The etiology of achalasia is the degeneration of ganglion cells in the myenteric plexus in the esophageal wall. This leads to lack of peristalsis of the esophagus and the accompanied failure of relaxation of the lower esophageal sphincter. These classic findings can be demonstrated both on esophageal manometry and with the classic finding of a "bird's beak" in the distal esophagus on barium swallow.

What Are the Surgical Treatment Options for Reflux and Hiatal Hernia?

The primary goals of the surgical treatment for reflux and hiatal hernia are to reestablish normal anatomy through reduction and closure of the hiatal hernia defect (by narrowing the esophageal hiatus) and to affix the GE junction in the abdomen to restore normal pressure dynamics. The second goal is achieved by performing a fundoplication in which a portion of the gastric fundus is wrapped around the GE junction and secured. A **Nissen** fundoplication is a complete, 360-degree

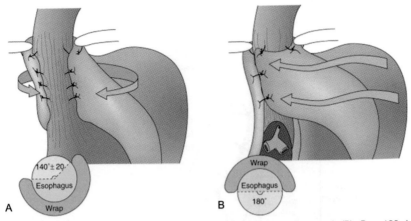

Fig. 13.3 Partial fundoplications. (A) Toupet 270-degree posterior wrap and (B) Dor 180-degree anterior wrap. (Redrawn from Oelschlager BK, Eubanks TR, Pellegrini CA: Hiatal hernias and gastroesophageal reflux disease. In Townsend CM, Beauchamp RD, Evers MN, et al, editors: *Sabiston textbook of surgery*, ed 19, Philadelphia, 2012, Elsevier.

wrap of the fundus around the distal esophagus. It is the most effective technique for preventing reflux. However, in cases of esophageal dysmotility or large hernias without reflux symptoms, a partial wrap may be undertaken. The **Toupet** fundoplication, the most common example of a partial fundoplication, is a 270-degree posterior wrap, whereas a **Dor** fundoplication is a 180-degree anterior wrap (Fig. 13.3). A partial wrap, while still effective in preventing reflux, may minimize the risk of postoperative dysphagia. Again, the goal of a wrap is not to narrow the GE junction, but rather to affix it within the abdomen.

Paraesophageal Hernia Repair and Nissen Fundoplication

1. Access the abdomen laparoscopically.
2. Mobilize the hernia sac from the mediastinum and reduce it into the abdomen, assuring that the GE junction and at least 2 cm of distal esophagus are below the diaphragm.
3. Divide the gastrohepatic, gastrosplenic, and the phrenoesophageal ligaments to mobilize the gastric cardia.
4. Place a bougie (flexible solid tube) through the mouth and esophagus into the stomach to maintain an adequate diameter of the esophageal lumen.
5. Suture the right and left diaphragmatic crura posterior to the esophagus to close the hernia defect. Mesh can be used if needed.
6. Pull the anterior wall of the gastric fundus to the patient's right and anterior to the distal esophagus, and the posterior wall of the gastric fundus to meet the anterior wall of the fundus at the 10 o'clock position on the distal esophagus. The fundus should be mobile enough to stay in the wrapped position without undue tension or compression of the esophagus.
7. Place three interrupted permanent sutures between the anterior and posterior walls to secure the wrap (Fig. 13.4).
8. Remove the bougie and close the incisions.

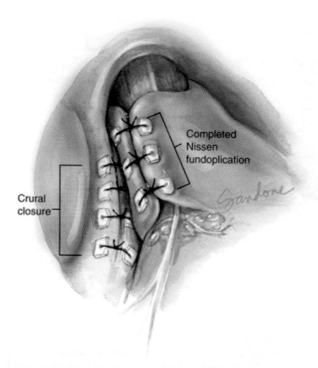

Fig. 13.4   Posterior crural repair and Nissen fundoplication. (Redrawn from Boyett D, Lidor A: Laparoscopic 360-degree fundoplication. In Cameron JL, Cameron AM, editors: *Current surgical therapy*, ed 12, Philadelphia, 2017, Elsevier, pp 1477–1480.)

CLINICAL PEARL (STEPS 2/3)

Hiatal hernia patients with morbid obesity may be better suited for a bariatric operation, with or without a concurrent hiatal hernia repair. Correcting the obesity will improve reflux symptoms and will lower the chances of hiatal hernia recurrence.

BASIC SCIENCE PEARL (STEPS 1/2/3)

An important anatomic consideration when performing operations on the esophagus is the path of the vagus nerves along the distal esophagus. The left vagus nerve transitions to an anterior position, and the right vagus nerve transitions posteriorly. The anterior vagus lies very close to the esophagus and must be identified where it lies on its longitudinal muscle fibers. The posterior vagus is positioned slightly more separate from the esophagus and is identified as a band in the soft tissue between the distal esophagus and the diaphragmatic crura.

What Are the Important Postoperative Complications Related to a Nissen Fundoplication?
- Dysphagia
  Dysphagia is normal for the first few days or weeks after surgery due to edema and transient dysfunction of the distal esophagus. If the fundoplication is too tight, dysphagia can persist, and may require reoperation or endoscopic dilatation.

- Anatomic wrap disruption
  Wrap disruption could include slippage of the wrap higher onto the esophagus, slippage of the wrap too low onto the stomach, or herniation of the entire wrap into the mediastinum. If the patient becomes significantly symptomatic, any form of wrap disruption will require surgical repair.
- Recurrence of gerd
  After 10 years following Nissen fundoplication, 5% to 25% of patients will again require medical therapy for GERD despite adequate wrap position.
- Gastroparesis
  Gastroparesis may result from injury to the left vagus nerve and may respond to medical therapy. Pyloroplasty is a more invasive option for refractory symptoms.
- Gas bloat syndrome
  Thought to be secondary to the inability to belch due to a tight wrap, symptoms include epigastric pain, distension, and early satiety. This is usually self-limited but sometimes requires endoscopic dilatation if persistent.

CLINICAL PEARL (STEPS 2/3)

There are a number of endoscopic procedures that have been devised as a treatment for reflux. The Stretta procedure, which applies radiofrequency energy to the wall of the distal esophagus, showed early promise but has fallen out of favor. The LINX procedure involves laparoscopically placing a ring of magnets around the distal esophagus. The TIF procedure is an endoscopic technique for placing sutures that mimic the effects of a fundoplication. Some of these procedures have shown early promise and are gaining popularity, but long-term results are still being collected. None of these techniques is indicated for a large hiatal hernia.

The patient undergoes pH monitoring with a DeMeester score of 16 and a manometry is performed that reveals no abnormalities in esophageal motility. After informed consent is obtained, the patient is taken to the operating room for a laparoscopic paraesophageal hernia repair with Nissen fundoplication. He tolerates the procedure well, though he complains of trouble swallowing on the first postoperative day. His symptoms improves over the next 2 days, and he is discharged on a diet of soft foods. On his 2-week postoperative visit, he has no complaints; he is tolerating soft foods without dysphagia, and his incisions are healing well. He is advanced to a regular diet and is asked to call as needed with any issues.

BEYOND THE PEARLS

- Gastrointestinal reflux is a very common complaint and is most commonly managed medically with proton pump inhibitors and H2-blockers.
- Asymptomatic hiatal hernias, usually those found incidentally on imaging, do not require surgical repair.
- A complete workup for esophageal dysmotility and other causes of dysphagia needs to be completed before performing a paraesophageal hernia repair or fundoplication.
- Repair of paraesophageal hernia may be performed open or laparoscopically; this decision is based on the severity of the hernia, patient factors, and the comfort of the surgeon.
- Fundoplications can be complete (360-degree—Nissen), or partial (270-degree posterior—Toupet; 180-degree anterior—Dor).
- Some dysphagia in the first postoperative days and weeks is expected due to edema. If the patient is unable to tolerate their own secretions postoperatively, however, concern is that the wrap is too tight and may need to be revised.

References

El-Sayed Abbas, A., Cameron, J. L., & Cameron, A. M. (2017). The management of gastroesophageal reflux disease. In *Current surgical therapy* (12th ed., pp. 10–19). Philadelphia: Elsevier.

Evans, S. R. T., Jackson, P. G., Czerniach, D. R., Kalan, M. M., & Iglesias, A. R. (2000). A stepwise approach to laparoscopic Nissen fundoplication. *Arch Surg, 135*, 723–728.

Lebenthal, A., Waterford, S. D., & Fisichella, P. M. (2015). Treatment and controversies in paraesophageal hernia repair. *Front Surg, 20*(13). April.

CHAPTER 14

Upper Gastrointestinal Bleeding in a 58-Year-Old Female

Heather Lillemoe ■ Kyla Terhune

A 58-year-old female with a past medical history of hypothyroidism and osteoarthritis presents to the emergency department with melena. She endorses a 2-day history of tarry black stools and light-headedness. On review of systems, she reports intermittent epigastric discomfort that she has had "for years" and chronic joint pain in her knees and hips. Her past surgical history includes an open appendectomy in childhood. She is an active smoker (20 pack-year history) and drinks approximately 2 to 3 glasses of wine every night. She takes only levothyroxine daily and ibuprofen as needed for joint pain.

On physical examination, her pulse is 108 bpm, blood pressure is 98/52 mm Hg, respiration rate is 18/min, temperature is 97.2°F, and oxygen saturation is 98% on room air. Her body mass index (BMI) is 26. On appearance, she is thin and slightly anxious. She has no evidence of jaundice but has slight pallor, and her extremities are cool to touch. Her abdomen is soft, not tender or distended, without guarding. She has a small, well-healed incision in her right lower quadrant.

What Is the Differential Diagnosis for Upper Black Tarry Stools?

Bleeding from the upper gastrointestinal (GI) tract (esophagus, stomach, and duodenum) typically presents as hematemesis (vomiting blood) or melena (black tarry stools). Bleeding from the lower gastrointestinal tract (colon, rectum, and anus) typically presents as hematochezia (red blood mixed with stool) or bright red blood per rectum. It is important to recognize that patients with proximal colonic bleeds may also present with melena. Lower GI bleeds are discussed in Chapter 15.

The most common cause of upper GI bleeding is peptic ulcer disease, which includes ulcers of both the stomach and duodenum (Fig. 14.1). Variceal disease secondary to portal hypertension is another common etiology of upper GI bleeding and must be considered in a patient with a history of cirrhosis or known risk factors for liver disease. Mallory-Weiss syndrome, or mucosal tears due to forceful retching, must also be on the differential in a patient with the appropriate history. Erosive disease, including esophagitis, gastritis, and duodenitis, are other diagnoses that lead to upper GI bleeding.

Less common etiologies include: angiodysplasia, neoplasm (polyp or mass), Dieulafoy's lesion (a large tortuous vessel in the stomach wall), aortoenteric fistula, Cameron ulcers (an erosion typically seen in conjunction with hiatal hernias), hemobilia, and iatrogenic bleeding. A complete list of differential diagnoses for upper GI bleeding can be found in Table 14.1.

The patient's initial laboratory values are within normal limits except for hemoglobin of 8.3 g/dL, BUN 36 (mg/dL), and creatinine 1.32 (mg/dL). Repeat vital signs demonstrate persistent tachycardia (112 bpm) and hypotension (92/48).

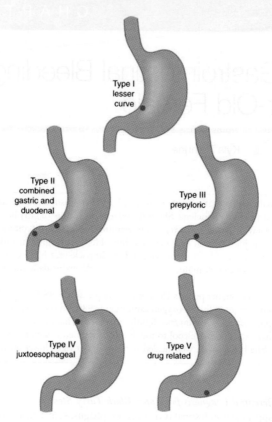

Fig. 14.1 Anatomic location of the types of peptic ulcers. (Redrawn from Ali A, Ahmed BH, Nussbaum MS: Surgery for peptic ulcer disease. In Yeo CJ, editor: *Shackelford's surgery of the alimentary tract*, ed 8, Philadelphia, 2019, Elsevier***.)

TABLE 14.1 ■ **Causes of Upper GI Bleeding**

Common		Uncommon	
	Peptic ulcer disease		Angiodysplasia
	Mallory-Weiss syndrome		Neoplasm (benign or malignant polyp or mass)
	Esophagogastric varices		Dieulafoy's lesion
	Erosive disease (esophagitis, gastritis, duodenitis)		Aortoenteric fistula
			Cameron ulcers
			Hemobilia
			Iatrogenic

What Is the Appropriate Next Step in Management for Unstable Patients With Melena?
The most important thing to remember when evaluating a patient with upper GI bleeding is, as in any emergency scenario, the "ABCs": airway, breathing, and circulation. Once it is established that the patient has a secure airway, adequate oxygenation, and is hemodynamically stable, further diagnostic and therapeutic interventions can be initiated.

In this case scenario the patient has symptoms and signs that are concerning for hypovolemic shock, including hypotension, tachycardia, cool extremities, and elevated BUN/creatinine ratio. She is also anemic with hemoglobin of 8.3 g/dL, which is concerning given her history of dark stools. She requires close monitoring and resuscitation before intervention.

There are several studies that can be used to assess the area of bleeding, which are reviewed in detail in Chapter 15. In summary, a computed tomography (CT) angiogram can be utilized in patients with normal kidney function. A nuclear, tagged red blood cell scan is another radiographic option for assessing the area of bleeding. Both require that the patient still be bleeding and at a sufficient rate to detect extravasation of contrast or tagged red blood cells. Endoscopy is both diagnostic and therapeutic, but requires sedation.

The patient receives a 1-liter bolus of crystalloid, and her vital signs improve. She is started on intravenous proton-pump inhibitor (PPI) therapy. The gastroenterology service is asked to evaluate the patient and proceeds with esophagogastroduodenoscopy (EGD), which reveals ulceration in the first portion of the duodenum and an actively bleeding vessel. This is managed successfully with clipping and epinephrine injection. The proceduralist feels confident that the vessel was controlled.

CLINICAL PEARL (STEP 2/3)

Fig. 14.2 depicts the characteristic endoscopic findings for a few of the common causes of upper GI bleeding. Fig. 14.2 A shows an example of a duodenal ulcer, the pathology found in this patient. Certain EGD findings are associated with a higher risk of rebleeding, thus requiring repeat intervention. In this patient, the visualization of an actively bleeding vessel has a very high likelihood of recurrent bleeding without further management; thus a definitive intervention must take place during endoscopy, followed by medical management and close monitoring (Table 14.2).

What Are the Most Commonly Encountered Complications of Duodenal Ulcers?
Perforation, bleeding, and obstruction are the most common serious complications seen from duodenal ulcers. The majority of patients who require operative intervention suffer from either perforation or bleeding. Obstruction is usually a late complication, presenting as gastric outlet obstruction. In recent years the rates of surgical intervention for PUD have declined as endoscopic and medical therapies continue to improve. See Chapter 12 for a full discussion of peptic ulcer disease.

The patient's symptoms improve after initial intervention, and she is slowly normalized. On hospital day 4, she is able to tolerate a regular diet and has normal laboratory values. Her melena has resolved. That evening, she decides to go for a walk in the hall because she cannot sleep. She begins feeling lightheaded after one lap and attempts to call for her nurse but suddenly falls to the ground.

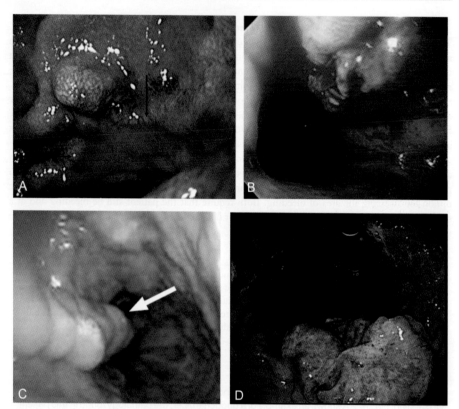

Fig. 14.2   Relative endoscopic images in upper GI bleeding. (A) Duodenal ulcer. (B) Mallory-Weiss syndrome. (C) Varices. (D) Neoplasm. (A, from Zimmermann L, Dudeck O, Schmitt J, et al: Duodenal ulcer due to yttrium microspheres used for selective internal radiation therapy of hepatocellular cancer, *Gastrointest Endosc* 69(4):977–978, 2009. B, from Kim HM, Lee S, Cho JH, et al: Sa1626 A pilot study of single-use endoscopy (ez scan) in patients suspicious of GI bleeding, *Gastrointest Endosc* 75(4) Suppl:AB225–AB226, 2012. C, from Cansu A, Ahmetoglu A, Kul S, et al: Diagnostic performance of using effervescent powder for detection and grading of esophageal varices by multidetector computed tomography, *Eur J Radiol* 83(3):497–502, 2014. D, from Dent B, Griffin SM: Gastric tumors, *Surgery (Oxford)* 32 (11):608–613, 2014.)

TABLE 14.2 ■ **Stigmata of Ulcer-Related GI Bleeding and Associated Risk of Rebleeding**

Stigmata	Risk of Recurrent Bleeding Without Therapy
Active arterial bleeding (spurting)	Approaches 100%
Nonbleeding visible vessel	Up to 50%
Nonbleeding adherent clot	8%–35%
Ulcer oozing (without other stigmata)	10%–27%
Flat spots	<8%
Clean-based ulcers	<3%

Adapted from Hwang, JH, et al: The role of endoscopy in the management of acute nonvariceal upper GI bleeding, *Gastrointest Endosc* 75(6):1132–1138, 2011.

What Is the Most Appropriate Next Step in Management?

This patient may have had a medical event (such as myocardial infarction), but one must also consider a recurrent bleed from her duodenal ulcer leading to hypotension and the subsequent loss of consciousness. She had a very high risk of rebleeding given her findings on endoscopy. She should be immediately evaluated by a rapid-response team and resuscitated. Electrocardiogram, laboratory evaluation, and appropriate radiographs should be obtained to rule out medical causes for her loss of consciousness. The gastroenterology team should be immediately contacted for potential endoscopic intervention, and a surgical team should be consulted. Often in the setting of acute rebleeding, a patient will have large-volume melena or bleeding per rectum to suggest a GI source for the event and help eliminate other possible etiologies. Although this patient did not demonstrate obvious bleeding, it must be high on the list of causes for her change in status.

The patient is quickly moved to the intensive care unit where she is resuscitated with packed red blood cells. The surgical team is consulted. She requires intubation given her unresponsiveness, and the gastroenterology team performs an emergent EGD. The endoscopist is unable to successfully find or treat the source of bleeding as her view is completely obstructed by blood.

CLINICAL PEARL (STEP 2/3)

In the setting of recurrent bleeding after endoscopy, repeat endoscopy is the intervention of choice. It is typically recommended to pursue endoscopic measures up to three times before other surgical intervention takes place as endoscopy reduces the need for an operation and has fewer associated complications. Another technique to consider in the event of rebleeding is interventional radiology coil embolization, particularly with patients who are poor surgical candidates. If all else fails, surgical exploration and management should occur.

The surgical team is called to the bedside given the failure of endoscopic management. The patient has now required transfusion of six units of packed red blood cells. Interventional radiology is contacted, but the team cannot mobilize fast enough in the middle of the night. The decision is made to take the patient to the operating room.

Exploratory Laparotomy and Oversewing of Bleeding Duodenal Ulcer

1. Create a midline or upper midline incision.
2. Mobilize the duodenum by dividing its lateral peritoneal attachment (Kocher maneuver).
3. Create a lateral longitudinal duodenotomy distal to the pyloric ring.
4. Use digital pressure to control or temporize bleeding to allow for resuscitation by the anesthesia team. Perform adequate ligation of the gastroduodenal artery (which has been eroded by the posterior duodenal ulceration) as depicted in Fig. 14.3. Use permanent sutures placed in a figure-8 fashion.
5. Close the duodenotomy with a two-layer technique.

CLINICAL PEARL (STEP 2/3)

Traditionally, the operation of choice for a bleeding duodenal ulcer consisted of a truncal vagotomy with pyloric drainage (via pyloroplasty). This can still be performed in the setting of a patient with acid hypersecretion who is unable (or unwilling) to continue long-term medical acid suppression therapy. However, such an operation is not an ideal choice in a hemodynamically unstable or high-risk patient. This patient was hemodynamically unstable, and her etiology is most likely from excessive NSAID use; thus vagotomy and pyloroplasty is not indicated. Operations for acid suppression must be carefully tailored to the patient, and their associated morbidity must be weighed against the effectiveness of medical management.

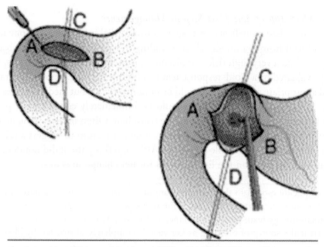

Fig. 14.3   Oversewing of a bleeding duodenal ulcer. (Redrawn from Mann BD, et al: *Surgery: a competency-based companion,* Philadelphia, 2009, Elsevier.)

What Are Some Important Aspects in the Postoperative Management of Patients After Surgical Management of a Bleeding Ulcer?

Patients who have had significant bleeding and a lengthy operative procedure are likely to have fluid and electrolyte imbalances that require close monitoring. After the operation, the patient should be maintained on an intravenous proton-pump inhibitor until tolerating a regular diet and then an oral agent can be initiated. Cessation of NSAIDs is imperative in the prevention of further mucosal injury. Follow-up EGD should be scheduled with the gastroenterologist after several weeks to assure proper tissue healing.

> The patient requires several blood transfusions postoperatively but is ultimately discharged on post-operative day 6 with a normal hemoglobin. She returns for a follow-up visit 3-week postoperatively and has no complaints. Repeat endoscopy 6 weeks postoperatively reveals no evidence of gastritis, duodenitis, or ulceration. She is maintained on oral proton pump inhibitor therapy.

BEYOND THE PEARLS

- The differential for upper GI bleeding is broad, but the most common causes include peptic ulcer disease, esophagogastric varices, Mallory-Weiss syndrome, and erosive disease.
- There are key EGD findings that are associated with a high risk of rebleeding. Such stigmata must be closely monitored and repeat endoscopy performed if there is any suspicion for incomplete endoscopic treatment at the initial procedure.
- Peptic ulcer disease is almost always caused by either infection with *H. pylori* or overuse of NSAIDs. Tissue biopsy should be performed at the time of endoscopic intervention, and if positive, subsequent eradication of *H. pylori* with triple therapy should follow.
- There are five types of peptic ulcers, designated by anatomic location, with the goal of guiding surgical therapy. This classification is important to know and is often a popular test question.
- For recurrent bleeding after endoscopic management of a nonvariceal upper GI bleed, repeat endoscopy is the initial intervention of choice. Other, less invasive means include coil embolization by interventional radiology.
- The key to surgical management of a bleeding duodenal ulcer is adequate ligation of the gastroduodenal artery without inadvertent injury to other vital structures.

Suggested Readings

Beaulieu, R. J., et al. (2016). The management of duodenal ulcers. In J. L. Cameron & A. M. Cameron (Eds.), *Current surgical therapy* (11th ed., pp. 76–80). Philadelphia: Saunders/Elsevier.

Clancy, T. E., et al. (2006). Procedures for benign and malignant gastric and duodenal disease. In W. W. Souba & M. P. Fink (Eds.), *ACS surgery: principles and practice*: WebMD, Inc. Accessed October 30, 2017.

Hwang J. H., et al. (2012). The role of endoscopy in the management of acute non-variceal upper GI bleeding, *Gastrointest Endosc* 75(6):1132–1138.

Lau, J. Y. W., et al. (1999). Endoscopic retreatment compared with surgery in patients with recurrent bleeding after initial endoscopic control of bleeding ulcers. *N Engl J of Med, 340*(10), 751–756.

CHAPTER 15

Lower Gastrointestinal Bleeding in a 71-Year-Old Male

Anna Spivak ■ John H. Marks

A 71-year-old male presents to the emergency department with painless, bright-red blood bleeding per rectum. He describes it as large volume, and states that it has occured eight times over the past 24 hours. His vital signs are temperature 98.8°F, blood pressure 105/65 mm Hg, and heart rate 95 per minute. His medical history is significant for hypertension, hyperlipidemia, and back pain and he takes daily aspirin, lisinopril, atorvastatin, and ibuprofen. He has never had a colonoscopy and is not aware of any colon cancer or inflammatory bowel disease history in his family.

What Is the Differential Diagnosis for Bright Red Blood Per Rectum?

As discussed in Chapter 14, patients with bright red blood per rectum (hematochezia) are differentiated from those with tarry black stools (melena) as they are likely to have bleeding from the lower gastrointestinal (GI) tract. Bleeding originating from any source distal to the ligament of Treitz is considered a lower GI bleed. Bright red blood per rectum typically originates in the colon or rectum. However, it must be kept in mind that hematochezia could also represent brisk bleeding from an upper gastrointestinal source. Bleeding can be acute or chronic and can vary in amount. Chronic bleeding presents with anemia, fecal occult positive stools, and intermittent hematochezia or melena. Acute bleeding, however, often presents with mutiple episodes of hematochezia or melena over a short period of time.

There are numerous pathologic conditions that can present as a lower GI bleed. Diverticular hemorrhage is the most common source of lower GI bleeding in adults. Other causes include neoplasm, infectious or ischemic colitis, inflammatory bowel disease, hemorrhoids, arteriovenous malformation, colonic angiodysplasia, stercoral ulceration, and radiation colitis or proctitis.

GI bleeds are no exception to the rule that the patient's history is key in narrowing the differential diagnosis and focusing the workup and treatment. A patient's history of previous colonoscopy and its findings are key to recognizing preexisting pathologies that may predispose to a GI bleed. Other important historical elements are the use of anticoagulants, aspirin, or NSAIDs; a history of inflammatory bowel disease; alcohol abuse; and personal or family history of colon cancer.

What Are the Steps in Workup of a Patient With Bright Red Blood Per Rectum?

The ABCs (airway, breathing, and circulation) are always first in the assessment of any patient, but especially in a bleeding patient, as acute blood loss can lead to shock. Due to the high likelihood that transfusion will be necessary, good intravenous (IV) access is important. Laboratory analysis should include a complete blood count (CBC), a coagulation panel, and a blood type and crossmatch. Note that if the patient's bleeding is very acute, a drop in the hemoglobin may not yet manifest, despite significant blood loss. The use of anticoagulants, including novel medications for which there may be no reversal agent, is very common; therefore, both medication history and review of labs are important to identify appropriate therapy for reversal of anticoagulation.

Physical examination may give clues to the identification of the source of bleeding. Abdominal tenderness may suggest an area of inflamed bowel. Rectal examination can help identify hemorrhoidal bleeding, and bedside anoscopy should be utilized to evaluate the anus and proximal rectum for sources of bleeding.

CLINICAL PEARL (STEP 2/3)

In the setting of a lower GI bleed, be sure to rule out upper GI bleeding as a source. A bloody aspirate on nasogastric tube lavage will confirm an upper GI source; the presence of bilious output, which attests to the presence of duodenal contents, will rule out an upper GI source. A clear aspirate, on the other hand, is an equivocal result and does not exclude an upper GI source. In equivocal situations in which the suspicion for an upper GI source is high (e.g. peptic ulcer disease, cirrhosis, chronic NSAIDs use), upper endoscopy is needed.

The patient's labs are drawn. His hemoglobin is 6.8 g/dL and a blood transfusion is initiated. He has normal coagulation studies, but his creatinine is 1.8 mg/dL. A nasogastric tube is inserted, and its output is bilious. His abdominal examination is normal. Internal and external hemorrhoids are appreciated on digital rectal examination, and there is a significant amount of blood that passes per rectum. Anoscopy demonstrates several small nonbleeding hemorrhoids.

What Imaging Studies Are Available to Localize the Source of a Lower GI Bleed?

There are several modalities of imaging to localize the source of a lower GI bleed. It is important to note that these studies rely on extravasation of a contrast agent at the site of bleeding, so they must be performed while the patient is actively bleeding.

A computed tomography (CT) angiogram (CTA) is a radiographic study that utilizes intravenous contrast that is timed with the CT scanner to visualize arterial flow in the body location being scanned. This is the most rapid and easiest way to attempt to localize a bleed and has high sensitivity and accuracy for localizing or excluding bleeding. This modality should not be used in patients with renal impairment, given the potential for exacerbation of the impairment by the intravenous contrast.

A tagged red blood cell bleeding scan is a nuclear medicine study that utilizes Tc-99m-tagged erythrocytes given intravenously. Subsequent scintigraphy allows the area of intraluminal extravasation to be visualized. This study is most appropriate for small, intermittent bleeding, the rate of which must be at least 0.1 mL/min in order to be detected. Although the scintographic localization is not precise, the study allows for source identification in 25% to 60% of cases.

Angiography, typically performed by interventional radiology, is a real-time fluoroscopic evaluation of bleeding using intravenous contrast (which again should be avoided in patients with renal impairment). Angiography is the best test for massive bleeding. It detects bleeding at a rate of 0.5 ml/min, and provides precise localization. If the rate of bleeding is too slow to be localized, an infusion of vasodilators, heparin, or thrombolytic agents may increase the sensitivity and accuracy of the study (a so-called "provocative angiogram"). Angiography can be diagnostic as well as therapeutic because interventional radiologists are able to coil embolize or thrombose the source of the bleed once localized. At times, technical difficulty or concern for bowel ischemia may preclude safe intervention even when the source of bleeding is identified.

Colonoscopy is the modality of choice for slow or chronic bleeding. Similar to angiography, it can be both diagnostic and therapeutic, but the patient needs to undergo bowel preparation prior to the procedure in order to ensure adequate visualization. Bowel preparation may not be necessary in the setting of an acute bleed, however, because blood acts as cathartic, emptying the bowel of stool. Blood in large, however, can obscure thorough visulization of bleeding sites. Via colonoscopy, hemoclips, epinephrine injection, cauterization, and thermal coagulation can be used to control the source of bleed if identified during endoscopy. Importantly, colonoscopy is contraindicated in the unstable patient and in the setting of suspected acute inflammation due to the risk of colonic perforation.

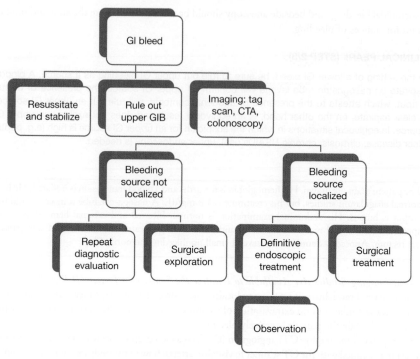

Fig. 15.1   Algorithm for workup and treatment of GI bleeding.

When Is Surgical Intervention Indicated in a Lower GI Bleed?

Because endoscopic and radiographic interventions are available in the treatment of lower GI bleeds, surgery is reserved for when these methods are either unsafe or unsuccessful. An algorithm for workup and treatment (Fig. 15.1) demonstrates that these less invasive methods are preferable over surgery. It is easier to identify the bleeding source with these direct imaging modalities, and non-surgical treatment limits morbidity and mortality. Surgery is indicated for patients exhibiting hemodynamic instability, a transfusion requirement of greater than 6 units of packed red blood cells, or recurrent episodes of bleeding which cannot be controlled by other means. While the location of a bleed generally dictates the operative approach and the extend of the operation, a total abdominal colectomy should be performed if the source of bleeding cannot be definitively identified on tagged red blood cell scan, CTA or colonoscopy.

The patient is admitted to the intensive care unit (ICU) and undergoes fluid resuscitation and surgical consultation. Given his renal impairment, a tagged red blood cell scan is performed but does not reveal the location of bleeding. During the course of the next several hours the frequency of his bloody bowel movements significantly decreases and ultimately stops. During his first 24 hours in the ICU, he undergoes transfusion of three units of packed red blood cells and bowel preparation. On colonoscopy he is found to have a large mass in his descending colon with some adherent as well as extensive (but non-bleeding) diverticulosis throughout the descending and sigmoid colon. A biopsy of the mass is taken and pathologic analysis reveals colon adenocarcinoma.

What Is the Staging Workup for Colon Cancer?

Colon cancer is the fourth most common cancer among both sexes. When colon cancer is diagnosed early, 5-year survival approximates 90%. Because colorectal cancer screening with colonoscopy is

TABLE 15.1 ■ **American Joint Committee on Cancer Staging for Colon Cancer**

AJCC Stage	Tumor Stage	Nodal Stage	Metastasis
0	Tis (intramucosal)	N0	M0
1	T1 (into submucosa) or T2 (into muscularis propria)	N0	M0
2	T3 (into entire wall but not through) or T4 (through wall with local extension)	N0	M0
3	Any T	N1 (1–3 nearby lymph nodes) or N2 (>3 lymph nodes)	M0
4	Any T	Any N	Positive metastasis

recommended to start at age 45, nearly 40% of colorectal cancer will be diagnosed in early stages and will have an excellent prognosis.

When a colon cancer is diagnosed, it is important to stage it appropriately to determine prognosis and to direct therapy. Distant metastases must be ruled out with cross-sectional imaging. A CT of the chest assesses for lung metastases and a CT of the abdomen and pelvis assesses the extension of the primary tumor, whether any lymph nodes appear prominent, and whether there are any metastases to the liver. The staging of colon cancer can be found in Table 15.1.

A carcinoembryonic antigen (CEA) should also be ordered. It is important to note that a CEA is not diagnostic for colon cancer; however, it is used postresection to monitor for recurrence.

What Are the Treatment Options for Colon Cancer?

Surgery is used to treat most localized colon cancer (stages I–III). The extent of the surgery depends on the location of the tumor. It is important to note that a colectomy for malignancy includes the mesentery of the resected portion of the colon in order to remove the mesenteric lymph nodes for evaluation. Adjuvant chemotherapy may be recommended depending upon the stage of the tumor.

Patients with stage IV colon cancer, whose liver metastases are amenable to surgical resection, may undergo synchronous or subsequent metastasectomy (i.e., removing the metastatic lesion(s) in addition to the primary tumor). These patients will also require adjuvant and/or neoadjuvant chemotherapy.

CLINICAL PEARL (STEPS 2/3)

It is always important to discuss the possibility of an ostomy with patients undergoing colorectal surgery, even when the surgical intent is to avoid an ostomy.

CLINICAL PEARL (STEPS 2/3)

Squamous cell anal carcinoma of the anus is recognized as a common entity which is treated differently from adenocarcinoma of the rectum. Patients with squamous carcinoma of the anus undergo neoadjuvant treatment with 5-fluorouracil and mitomycin, and radiation. They may or may not then undergo surgical resection depending on their response to neoadjuvant therapy. This is termed the Nigro protocol and, with some modification, has been the standard of treatment for squamous cell carcinoma of the anus since the 1970s.

The patient's creatinine improves, and he undergoes CT scan of the chest, abdomen and pelvis, which reveals no local extension beyond the colon and no metastatic lesions. His CEA is elevated at 14 ng/mL. After discussion regarding treatment, he elects to undergo a laparoscopic left colectomy.

Laparoscopic Left Colectomy

1. Place laparoscopic ports.
2. Mobilize splenic flexure of the colon.
3. Identify and transect the inferior mesenteric artery and vein.
4. Mobilize the lateral attachments of the descending colon.
5. Transect the rectum (distal margin) and transverse colon (proximal margin) with linear staplers and remove the specimen via an extraction site (enlarged right lower quadrant port site).
6. Perform a coloanal anastomosis* with an EEA stapler. The anastomosis must not be on tension and must have good blood supply.

---

*Indocyanine green (ICG) florescent technology may be used to evaluate tissue perfusion before making anastomosis. The fluorescent dye shows that the tissue is well preserved (green) (Fig. 15.2).

CLINICAL PEARL (STEPS 2/3)

An oncologic resection requires 5 cm margins proximal and distal to the mass and must include the associated mesentery which contains regional lymph nodes, which are subsequently evaluated for regional metastasis. After neoadjuvant therapy, in an effort to avoid a permanent colostomy, margins as small as 5 mm are acceptable. However, a larger margin should always be obtained whenever possible.

BASIC SCIENCE PEARL (STEPS 1/2/3)

The blood supply to the colon comes from the superior mesenteric (SMA) and inferior mesenteric (IMA) arteries (Fig. 15.3). The SMA gives off the middle, right, and ileocolic arteries that supply the ascending and transverse colon. The IMA supplies the descending and sigmoid colon as well as rectosigmoid junction. Watershed areas (overlapping flow from distal endpoints of two vessels) are Griffith's point (between the ascending left colic and marginal artery of Drummond, collateral between SMA and IMA supplying splenic flexure) and Sudeck's point (between the IMA and superior rectal arteries). These two areas are vulnerable.

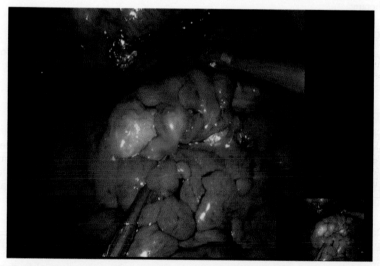

Fig. 15.2 Tissue perfusion may be evaluated before making the anastomosis using indocyanine green (ICG) fluorescent technology. The fluorescent dye shows that the tissue's blood supply is well preserved (green).

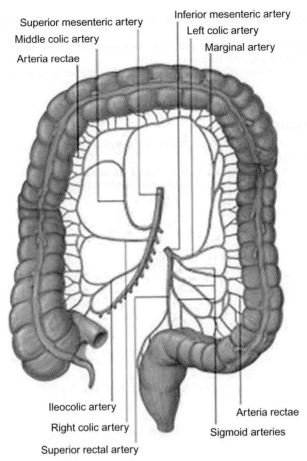

Superior mesenteric artery

Middle colic artery

Arteria rectae

Inferior mesenteric artery

Left colic artery

Marginal artery

Ileocolic artery

Right colic artery

Superior rectal artery

Arteria rectae

Sigmoid arteries

Fig. 15.3 Blood supply to the colon. The superior mesenteric and inferior mesenteric arteries are direct branches of the abdominal aorta.

CLINICAL PEARL (STEPS 2/3)

Potential surgical pitfalls are the failure to identify an inadvertent enterotomy, ureteral and duodenal injuries, splenic capsule laceration, and hypogastric nerve injury.

The patient undergoes laparoscopic left colectomy. Postoperatively, he is started on clear liquid diet; with evidence of progressive bowel activity, is advanced to a regular diet. Postoperatively, his hemoglobin remains stable, and he requires no further blood transfusions. He discharged on post-operative day five and is given instructions to follow up with the surgeon and medical oncologist in approximately 2 weeks.

BEYOND THE PEARLS

- When a patient presents with bright red blood per rectum (hematochezia), it is vital that a brisk upper GI bleed be ruled out.
- Localization of a bleed is important for its ultimate treatment.

- Most imaging studies used to evaluate GI bleeding require that, the patient has active bleeding.
- Angiography and colonoscopy and their associated treatment modalities can be both diagnostic and therapeutic for lower GI bleeds.
- Segmental colectomies are the primary treatment for localized (stages I–III) colon cancer.

Suggested Reading

Beck, D. E., Wexner, S. D., Hull, T. L., et al. (2014). *The ASCRS manual for colon and rectal surgery* (2nd ed.). New York: Springer.

Ghassemi, K. A., & Jensen, D. M. (2013). Lower GI bleeding: Epidemiology and management. *Curr Gastroenterol Rep Jul, 15*(7), 333. https://doi.org/10.1007/s11894-013-0333-5.

CHAPTER 16

Morbid Obesity in a 29-Year-Old Female

Jean F. Salem ■ Richard D. Ing

A 29-year-old female with morbid obesity and prediabetes presents to the bariatric surgery office to discuss the surgical treatment options. She has failed all attempts to lose weight, including diet and physical exercise.

On physical examination, her temperature is 99.1°F, blood pressure is 133/86 mm Hg, pulse is 88/min, respiration rate is 16/min, and oxygen saturation is 98% on room air. Her height is 5'3" and weight is 237 pounds, making her body mass index (BMI) 42 kg/m². She is a nonjaundiced, well-developed, obese woman. Her abdomen is soft and nontender and has no scars.

What Is the Definition of Morbid Obesity?

Obesity is classified according to body mass index (BMI). BMI is a function of a patient's height and weight and is calculated by dividing a patient's weight in kilograms by the square of his or her height in meters. Table 16.1 shows the categorization of underweight through morbid obesity according to BMI.

BASIC SCIENCE PEARL (STEP 1)

Much of the research aimed at understanding obesity has focused on the hormonal regulation of appetite, metabolism, and body fat distribution. Studies have identified that leptin, ghrelin, insulin, androgens, and estrogens all contribute to the regulation of these processes. Ghrelin is a hormone produced by the gastrointestinal tract that is responsible for hunger. It has also been shown to regulate reward perception in central dopaminergic tracts. Gastric bypass has been shown to dramatically lower ghrelin levels, enhancing the restrictive aspect of the procedure.

What Are the Treatments for Obesity?

Obesity was recognized as a disease by the American Medical Association in 2013. It is associated with increased risk for type 2 diabetes, hypertension, dyslipidemia, coronary artery disease, stroke, gallbladder disease, and sleep apnea. Bariatric and metabolic surgery is a proven, effective, and enduring treatment for obese patients, with resultant morbidity and mortality reduction.

Although many over-the-counter therapies exist that claim to help patients lose weight, most are not backed by good scientific evidence that they cause weight loss, and some can be unsafe. Diet and exercise have been shown to help patients lose weight and improve their cardiovascular and musculoskeletal health. However, conflicting evidence exists as to what type of diet is best at providing necessary micro- and macronutrients while promoting weight loss. There are several surgical procedures (grouped together as bariatric surgery) that can help patients lose weight also.

TABLE 16.1 ■ Classification of BMI

BMI (kg/m^2)	Classification
< 18.5	Underweight
18.5–24.9	Normal
25–29.9	Overweight
30–34.9	Obese (class 1)
35–39.9	Obese (class 2)
40	Morbidly obese

What Are the Indications and Contraindications for Bariatric Surgery?

The surgical treatment of obesity is reserved for patients with a body mass index (BMI) greater than 40 kg/m^2 or with BMI greater than 35 kg/m^2 and one or more major obesity-associated comorbid conditions (Box 16.1) when less invasive methods of weight loss have failed.

Recent clinical practice guidelines set forth by the American Association of Clinical Endocrinologists, the Obesity Society, and the Society for Metabolic and Bariatric Surgery have stated that surgery may be appropriate for patients with a BMI of 30 kg/m^2 or greater for cardiovascular disease risk reduction and glycemic control with type 2 diabetes.

Contraindications to bariatric surgery include uncontrolled psychiatric conditions, untreated eating disorders, drug and alcohol abuse, advanced neoplasia, current pregnancy, and high medical risk. Relative contraindications observed by many surgeons are lack of family support, unrealistic expectations, and refusal to commit to postoperative diet recommendations and follow-up.

What Is Included in the Preoperative Evaluation and Workup for Bariatric Surgery?

The preoperative evaluation of patients seeking weight loss surgery must include a comprehensive medical history, psychosocial history, physical examination, and appropriate laboratory testing to assess surgical risk. All patients should undergo an evaluation for obesity-related comorbidities and causes for obesity. A preoperative checklist was proposed by the American Society for Metabolic and Bariatric Surgery (Box 16.2).

A multidisciplinary approach is essential in the preoperative evaluation of the bariatric patient. Many of the items suggested in the checklist assure that patients' medical comorbidities are being thoroughly assessed and treated preoperatively in order to optimize surgical outcomes. This evaluation includes the medical management of comorbidities, dietary modifications, exercise training, and psychological assistance as needed. Preoperative glycemic control should be optimized using a diabetes comprehensive care plan, including healthy dietary patterns, medical nutrition therapy, physical therapy, and pharmacotherapy if needed.

BOX 16.1 ■ Obesity-related Comorbidities

- Type 2 diabetes
- Hypertension
- Sleep apnea
- Nonalcoholic fatty liver disease
- Osteoarthritis
- Dyslipidemia
- GI disorders
- Coronary artery disease

BOX 16.2 ■ Preoperative Checklist for Bariatric Surgery

- Complete history and physical examination (obesity-related comorbidities, causes of obesity, weight loss history)
- Routine labs (including complete blood count, electrolytes, fasting blood glucose, lipid panel, kidney function, liver profile, urine analysis)
- Nutrient screening with iron studies, B_{12}, folic acid, and vitamin D
- Cardiopulmonary evaluation with sleep apnea screening (electrocardiogram, chest radiograph, echocardiography when indicated)
- Gastrointestinal evaluation (Helicobacter pylori screening in high-prevalence areas; gall bladder evaluation and upper endoscopy if clinically indicated)
- Endocrine evaluation (Hb A_{1c} with suspected or diagnosed diabetes; thyroid stimulating hormone with symptoms of thyroid disease; androgens with polycystic ovary syndrome suspicion; screening for Cushing's syndrome if clinically suspected)
- Clinical nutrition evaluation by registered dietician
- Psychosocial-behavioral evaluation
- Document medical necessity for bariatric surgery
- Informed consent
- Continue efforts for preoperative weight loss
- Optimize glycemic control
- Pregnancy counseling
- Smoking cessation counseling
- Verify cancer screening by primary care physician

The patient undergoes a thorough preoperative workup, including a sleep study for obstructive sleep apnea; laboratory evaluation for endocrine disorders such as diabetes and hypothyroidism; gastroenterology evaluation for reflux and H. pylori; psychosocial, nutritional, and exercise counseling; and enrollment in a support group. She is able to lose approximately 12 pounds. She and the bariatric surgeon discuss the different surgical options and their respective risks and benefits.

What Types of Bariatric Surgery Are Available, and to Which Patients Should Each Be Offered?
Several different bariatric and metabolic procedures are available: laparoscopic adjustable gastric banding (LAGB), laparoscopic sleeve gastrectomy (LSG), laparoscopic Roux-en-Y gastric bypass (LRYGB), and laparoscopic biliopancreatic diversion (BPD), BPD/duodenal switch (BPD-DS) (Fig. 16.1). Although most commonly performed laparoscopically, these procedures can be performed in an open fashion as well. LSG has become the most common bariatric procedure performed, followed by LRYGB. LAGB was once popular but is now rarely used because of inferior long-term outcomes.

Gastric plication is an investigational procedure that is designed to create gastric restriction without placement of a device or resection of tissue. Laparoscopic mini gastric bypass has recently gained popularity because it is technically less demanding than LRYGB, and it offers comparable benefits; however, it has not yet been recognized by national societies as a valid bariatric procedure.

LRYGB was for years the most common bariatric procedure. LSG, however, is a much more straightforward operation, with lower risk of long-term complications. Several studies have shown that LRYGB and LSG are equally effective regarding weight loss, quality-of-life improvement, and control of obesity-related conditions such as diabetes. However, some studies have demonstrated that LRYGB is more effective than LSG for control of type 2 diabetes, metabolic syndrome, and gastroesophageal reflux disease. The best choice for any bariatric procedure depends on the

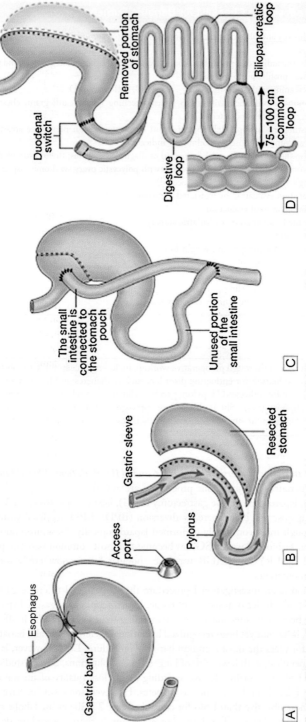

Fig. 16.1 Different validated bariatric procedures. (A) Adjustable gastric band. (B) Sleeve gastrectomy. (C) Roux-en-Y gastric bypass. (D) Biliopancreatic diversion/duodenal switch.

individualized goals of therapy (e.g., weight loss and/or metabolic control), available expertise, patient preferences, and personalized risk stratification.

Laparoscopic Sleeve Gastrectomy

1. Induce pneumoperitoneum and insert laparoscopic trocars in the upper abdomen.
2. Divide all the vessels along the greater curvature of the stomach to the angle of His.
3. Lift the stomach and divide all posterior attachments to the pancreas.
4. Alongside an orogastric tube, staple and divide the stomach in a vertical fashion toward the angle of His.
5. Test the staple line by filling the "sleeved" stomach with methylene blue through an orogastric tube to be sure there is no leak.

BASIC SCIENCE PEARL (STEP 1)

The short gastric arteries, arising from the splenic artery, supply the greater curvature of the stomach.

What Are the Potential Early Complications of Laparoscopic Sleeve Gastrectomy?

Bleeding following LSG occurs in 1% to 6% of cases. The source of bleeding can be intra- or extraluminal. The most common site of bleeding is the staple line. Similar to the RYGB, early recognition and management is essential. Gastric leak is one of the most serious and dreaded complications of LSG. It occurs in up to 5% of patients. The most common site is at the angle of His. Depending on the timing of presentation, the clinical condition, and the amount of leak, several therapeutic strategies exist: conservative monitoring, percutaneous drainage, or operative treatment. Surgical treatment usually entails an abdominal washout, attempt at surgical repair of the leak, and establishment of a feeding jejunostomy.

CLINICAL PEARL (STEP 2/3)

Tachycardia in the early postoperative course is worrisome. It is one of the earliest signs of an anastomotic leak. It warrants laparoscopic exploration even if radiographic studies are negative.

Laparoscopic Roux-en-Y Gastric Bypass

1. Induce pneumoperitoneum and insert laparoscopic trocars in the upper abdomen.
2. Divide the jejunum with a linear cutting stapler approximately 30 cm from the ligament of Treitz.
3. Measure 150 cm distally and align the bowel at this point with the proximal end of the transected jejunum. Create the jejuno-jejunostomy with an endoscopic stapler.
4. Create the gastric pouch by dividing the proximal stomach with a stapler near the top of the lesser curve.
5. Create the gastrojejunostomy by anastomosing the proximal end of the Roux limb to the gastric pouch.
6. Close the "Petersen defect" (the gap between the mesentery of the Roux limb and the mesentery of the transverse colon) with running nonabsorbable suture. This will help prevent an internal hernia in the future.

CLINICAL PEARL (STEP 2/3)

A Roux limb refers to a transected loop of distal jejunum that is brought up and connected to a visceral organ that requires enteric drainage. This could be a gastric pouch in bariatric surgery, the esophagus in gastric resection, the pancreas in chronic pancreatitis, or the liver when portions of the biliary tree are resected. The Roux limb is accompanied by a distal jejunostomy, which connects the proximal jejunum to the Roux limb and drains the foregut structures.

CLINICAL PEARL (STEP 2/3)

Patients who undergo LRYGB typically experience 60% to 70% excess body weight loss, with more than 75% control of comorbidities.

What Are the Potential Complications of Laparoscopic Roux-en-Y Gastric Bypass?

Anastomotic leak remains one of the most common causes of morbidity and mortality after LRYGB. The incidence of postoperative leak ranges from 0% to 5.6%, and leak-associated mortality can be up to 37% to 50%. Together with pulmonary embolism, this represents more than 50% of the causes of death in patients undergoing bariatric surgery. The most frequent site of leak is the gastrojejunostomy. Early recognition and management is the key. Depending on the patient's clinical condition and the magnitude of the leak, different treatment options can be offered ranging from conservative management to percutaneous drainage to reoperation. Bleeding is another major complication and can occur in up to 4.4% of cases. The most frequent site is from the gastric remnant staple line. Early recognition is essential. Usually, early postoperative bleeding is an indication for urgent surgical intervention. Late presentation (longer than 48 hours) can be managed conservatively in most cases.

Late complications can be a significant source of morbidity after a LRYGB. Bowel obstruction secondary to internal hernias occurs in 3% to 4.5% of cases. Surgical exploration should be performed without delay to prevent bowel ischemia. Other late complications include cholelithiasis (22%–70%), dumping syndrome (24%–50%), anastomotic stricture (6%–20%), marginal ulcers (0.6%–16%), gastrogastric fistula (1%–2%), gastric remnant distension, weight regain, and nutritional deficiencies. Altered absorption puts patients at higher risk of deficiencies of iron, calcium, vitamin B_{12}, thiamine, and folate. Lifelong compliance with appropriate dietary choices and vitamin supplementation is imperative.

> The patient elects to undergo a laparoscopic sleeve gastrectomy. Her immediate postoperative course is uneventful, and she is discharged home 2 days later on a full liquid diet. She is given appropriate nutritional counseling and supplements in order to avoid nutritional deficiencies. She is seen in the office for a postoperative follow up 2 weeks later. She is healing well, has lost 8 pounds, and has no complaints.

What Are the Long-term Outcomes of Bariatric Surgery?

RYGB is associated with 70% to 90% excess weight loss (EWL) at 2 years and 60% to 70% EWL at 10 years. Remission of type 2 diabetes mellitus (T2DM) has been reported to be 75% at 2 years and 51% at 12 years. Remission of hypertension is 71% at 5 years.

LSG is associated with 63% to 76% EWL at 3 years and 52% to 67% EWL at 8 years. Remission of T2DM at 3 years has been reported to be 38% and 20% at 5 years. Remission of hypertension is 65% at 5 years.

> Over the next year, your patient loses nearly 80% of her excess body weight. She later regains some of that weight but is maintaining a BMI of 30 at 5 years postoperatively. On follow-up, she complains of a new onset of heartburn. She is prescribed a proton pump inhibitor.

What Are the Late Complications of Sleeve Gastrectomy?

LSG has been implicated with gastroesophageal reflux disease, but the relationship has not been fully elucidated. The first-line treatment is medical therapy with proton pump inhibitors. Refractory cases may require conversion to RYGB. Stricture is a rare complication that occurs usually at the level of the incisura angularis. It can present early after surgery or, more commonly, in a delayed fashion. Early strictures can usually be treated conservatively, whereas chronic strictures usually require either endoscopic dilation or surgical treatment (seromyotomy or conversion to RYGB).

BEYOND THE PEARLS

- Weight loss surgery is the most effective treatment for morbid obesity, producing durable weight loss, improvement or remission of comorbid conditions, and longer life expectancy. When combined with medical therapy, bariatric surgery is more effective than medical therapy alone in decreasing or, in some cases, resolving hyperglycemia.
- LSG and LRYGB are equivalent in weight loss, quality of life, and complications up to 3 years postsurgery. There is a lack of prospective randomized-controlled trials comparing long-term metabolic outcomes of these two procedures.
- Metabolic and nutritional derangements are common after bariatric surgery, making postoperative lifelong compliance with appropriate dietary choices and vitamin supplementation imperative. Altered absorption, especially in LRYGB, puts patients at higher risk of micronutrient deficiencies, particularly iron, calcium, vitamin B_{12}, thiamine, and folate.

Suggested Readings

Courcoulas, A. P., Yanovski, S. Z., Bonds, D., et al. (2014). Long-term outcomes of bariatric surgery: A national institutes of health symposium. *JAMA Surg, 149*(12), 1323–1329.

Mechanick, J. I., Youdim, A., Jones, D. B., et al. (2013). Clinical practice guidelines for the perioperative nutritional, metabolic, and nonsurgical support of the bariatric surgery patient—2013 update: Cosponsored by American Association of Clinical Endocrinologists, the Obesity Society for Metabolic & Bariatric Surgery. *Surg Obes Relat Dis, 9*(2), 159–191.

Peterli, R., Wolnerhanssen, B. K., Vetter, D., et al. (2017). Laparoscopic sleeve gastrectomy versus Roux-Y-gastric bypass for morbid obesity—3-year outcomes of the prospective randomized Swiss multicenter bypass or sleeve study (SM-BOSS). *Ann Surg, 265*(3), 466–473.

CHAPTER 17

Anorectal Pain in a 45-Year-Old Male

Emily Kunkel ■ Henry Schoonyoung

A 45-year-old male without significant past medical history presents to the general surgery office with a complaint of rectal pain. He states that the pain has been present for 2 to 3 months and has been getting progressively worse. He states that the pain is aggravated by bowel movements and that he has noticed some blood on the toilet paper when he wipes. The patient also reports noting a rectal bulge that is tender to palpation.

What Is the Differential Diagnosis for Anorectal Pain?

There are many pathologies that can produce anorectal pain, and it is important to be able to distinguish between these different causes, as the therapies used to treat them can vary greatly. As is typical, the patient's history of the pain, including its onset, duration, and characteristics, can help distinguish between causes of anorectal pain. Key physical examination findings are also useful in differentiating between these causes. For example, hemorrhoids, abscesses, and prolapse can all be associated with an anorectal mass, whereas fissures, fistulas, and squamous cell carcinoma can cause a tender cut or tear around the anorectal region. Table 17.1 lists the most common causes of anorectal pain, their causes, and the key presenting symptoms that can aid in diagnosis.

What Are the Important Aspects of the History and Physical Examination in the Evaluation of a Patient With Anorectal Pain?

In addition to eliciting the duration, quality, and location of the pain and its association with bowel movements, the patient should be asked about any changes in bowel habits (constipation, changes in stool caliber) and if there is any discharge or bleeding from the rectum. Associated symptoms such as fevers, chills, discharge, and prolapsing tissue are among the important details to elicit in the patient's history.

Physical examination provides further details for differentiating between the causes of anorectal pain. A rectal examination must be performed for all complaints of anorectal pain. A good rectal examination starts with the positioning of the patient in either a prone-jackknife position, knee-chest position, or left lateral decubitus position. A visual inspection is performed first, noting any bulges, fissures, or lesions on the perianal skin and anal opening. Having the patient perform a valsalva maneuver may aid in visualization and diagnosis of various pathologies and can lead to protrusion of tissue not appreciated on initial examination. Taking note of any ulcers, lesions, or rashes that are visible around the anus or in the anal canal is also important.

A digital rectal examination should be performed using a gloved index finger and water-soluble lubricant to examine rectal tone and contractility and to assess for rectal masses. Anal fissures are associated with increased rectal tone and spasticity of the anal sphincter. Deep anal abscesses can be further characterized by a rectal examination to examine the perirectal spaces, ischioanal fossa, and deep postanal space for areas of maximal tenderness and fluctuance. Hemorrhoids can be

TABLE 17.1 ■ **Common Presenting Symptoms for Anorectal Pain**

	Pathology	Presenting Symptoms
Fissure	Tear in anal mucosa	Sharp pain associated with bowel movements that lasts after the movement is finished for minutes to hours
Abscess	Localized infection caused by plugging of anal ducts	Painful fullness in the anorectal region, associated with fevers and/or chills
Fistula	Abnormal communication between anal crypts and perianal skin	Swelling, pain, mucus, or fowl-smelling discharge; often associated with history of anorectal abscess or inflammatory process; may be an intermittent drainage with waxing and waning cycle of drainage and healing
Prolapse	Weakness in muscles and ligamentous structures	Pain, constipation, fecal incontinence, rectal mass protruding from anus
Proctitis	Inflammation of the rectal mucosa	Mild diarrhea, tenesmus, itching, burning, pain, rectal bleeding (rarely severe)
Hemorrhoids	Abnormal dilation of veins in the submucosal vascular plexus	Internal: Painless bleeding, itching External: Pain when thrombosed, itching, difficultly with hygiene

characterized by a digital rectal examination by identifying the presence of a thrombosis within the hemorrhoidal bulge or by the reducibility of the mass.

Anoscopy or proctosigmoidoscopy can aid in visualization of hemorrhoids or other deep lesions that are unable to be fully characterized on digital examination.

CLINICAL PEARL (STEPS 2/3)

Fecal impaction can also present with a painful rectal mass. This arises in the setting of chronic constipation and is identified by physical exam as a large mass of dry stool in the rectum. The patient may report some rectal drainage produced from watery stool that may leak around the mass and result in incontinence.

What Are the Important Pathophysiological and Pathologic Differences Between the Causes for Perianal Pain?

FISSURE

A fissure will most commonly be located in the anterior or posterior midline, where the musculature and blood supply to the anoderm is the weakest. Anal fissures are very tender, and patients will often not tolerate a rectal examination. Chronic fissures, defined as fissures that are present for 3 months or longer, often have a sentinel skin tag that will not undergo dynamic protrusion upon a valsalva maneuver (compared with a hemorrhoid).

CLINICAL PEARL (STEPS 2/3)

Anal fissures are most frequently located in the posterior midline (90%–99%). Fissures located off the posterior midline, especially in male patients, should raise the concern for etiologies other than constipation and hypertonicity of the sphincter, such as Crohn's disease, cancer, and sexually transmitted infections.

BASIC SCIENCE PEARL (STEPS 1/2/3)

The anal sphincter complex is made up of an internal sphincter, which is a layer of circular smooth muscle under involuntary control, and an external sphincter, which is made of several layers of striated muscle under voluntary control. Cooperative relaxation allows for defecation, and sphincter dysfunction can lead to either incontinence or sphincter hypertonicity.

ABSCESS

A perirectal abscess will present as a firm area of swelling that is fluctuant on palpation. The area may express pus upon palpation but will usually be too tender to express any exudate. Abscesses can occur in four locations: perianal, ischiorectal, supralevator, and intersphincteric (Fig. 17.1). Supralevator and intersphincteric locations may not have external signs. An infected anal crypt gland usually causes these very painful infections. These crypt glands, though they empty into the dentate line, are situated in different locations. The location of the gland itself dictates the location of the peri-rectal abscess.

FISTULA

A fistula can be identified by small circles of granulation tissue, which often exudate pus if compressed. There are four categories of fistulas based on their relationship to the sphincter muscles: intersphincteric, transsphincteric, suprasphincteric, and extrasphincteric (Fig. 17.2). Fistulas

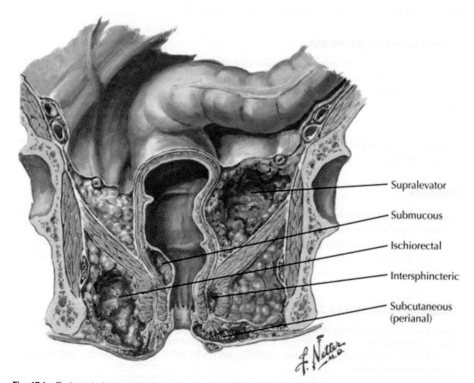

Supralevator

Submucous

Ischiorectal

Intersphincteric

Subcutaneous
(perianal)

Fig. 17.1 Perirectal abscess locations (perianal, ischiorectal, supralevator, intersphincteric). (From Bleier J IS, Moloo H: Perirectal abscess and fistula in ano. In *Netter's surgical anatomy and approaches*, 2014, Elsevier Saunders, Chapter 27, pp 327–338.)

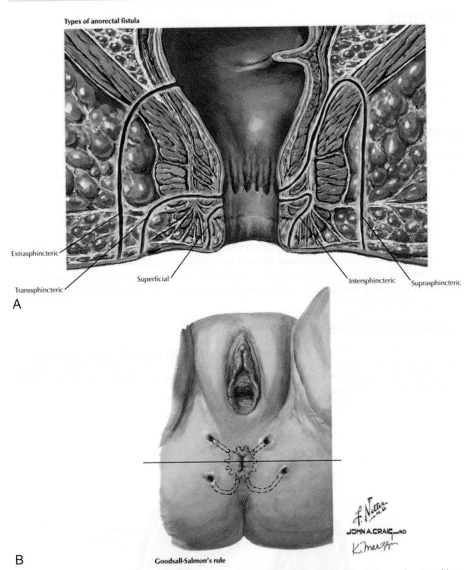

Fig. 17.2 Perirectal fistula locations (intersphincteric, transsphincteric, suprasphincteric, and extrasphincteric). (From Bleier J IS, Moloo H: Perirectal abscess and fistula in ano. In *Netter's surgical anatomy and approaches,* 2014, Elsevier Saunders, Chapter 27, pp 327–338.)

happen typically due to the failure of the crypt gland to heal. Other causes of fistulas include proctitis when associated with Crohn's disease, malignancy, and foreign body.

PROLAPSE

A prolapse will protrude or become more prominent upon straining. The direction of mucosal folds on the bulge will help distinguish between a full- and partial-thickness prolapse: a full-thickness prolapse contains concentric mucosal folds whereas a partial-thickness prolapse will have radial mucosal folds.

PROCTITIS

Patients with proctitis will have a fairly unremarkable physical examination. Based on the etiology, the patient may have abdominal pain or be unable to tolerate a rectal examination as a result of tenderness. There are several different etiologies to proctitis, including inflammatory bowel disease (IBD), infectious organisms (*Neisseria gonorrhea, Salmonella, Shigella*), and other noninfectious causes (radiation, ischemia, diversion).

HEMORRHOIDS

Hemorrhoids can be visualized as a bulge or protrusion in the anal canal. External hemorrhoids are often painful, whereas internal hemorrhoids are painless and more associated with itching and difficulty with anal hygiene. It is important to note the location, presence or absence of thrombosis, necrosis, gangrene, ulceration, or active bleeding of the hemorrhoid.

Hemorrhoids are classified by both axial and radial location. Hemorrhoidal cushions, which are a normal part of anal anatomy and contribute to physiologic continence mechanisms, are located in three anatomic locations: right anterior, right posterior, and left lateral (Fig. 17.3). External hemorrhoids are located distal to the dentate line and are covered by squamous cell epithelium. Internal hemorrhoids are located proximal to the dentate line and are covered in columnar/transitional epithelium (Fig. 17.4). Hemorrhoids can be internal, external, or mixed and can involve one, two, or three hemorrhoidal piles.

CLINICAL PEARL (STEPS 2/3)

A digital rectal examination and anoscopy/proctosigmoidoscopy are contraindicated if a fissure is identified with visual inspection and the patient is experiencing extreme pain. If there is no cause identified upon visual inspection and the patient cannot tolerate a rectal examination, an examination under anesthesia is indicated.

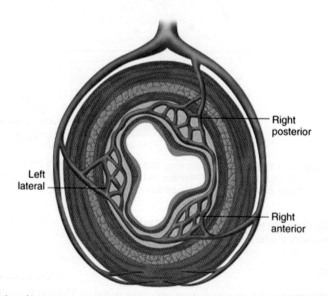

Fig. 17.3 Location of hemorrhoidal cushions (right anterior, right posterior, left lateral). Rossi, Daniel C., et al. "Hemorrhoids." *Colorectal Surgery.* Pages 95-116. January 1, 2013. Fig. 6.1 Anatomic location of hemorrhoidal vascular cushions (Redrawn from Cameron AM, editor: *Current surgical therapy*, ed 9, Philadelphia, 2007, Elsevier, p 262)

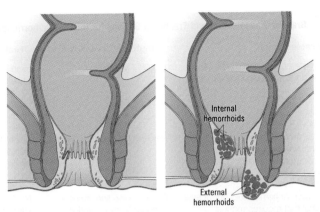

Fig. 17.4 External and internal hemorrhoids and location relative to dentate line. (From Hemorrhoids, *Clinical Gastroenterology and Hepatology* 16(3):A16–A16, 2018.)

Upon visual inspection, there is a swollen mass that is soft and cannot be reduced upon manual manipulation. There are no obvious tears, drainage, or fluctuance in the surrounding perianal region. Anoscopy reveals a mass that is extremely tender and originates proximal to the dentate line on the left side of the anal canal. The patient is told that the cause of his pain is likely due to a hemorrhoid.

How Are Hemorrhoids Classified and What Are the Treatment Options?

External hemorrhoids are classified by their location distal to the dentate line. A major complication of external hemorrhoids includes thrombosis. Thrombosis is classified by the length of time the hemorrhoid has been thrombosed at the time of presentation. Acute thrombosis is a thrombus that has occurred within 72 hours of presentation. A subacute thrombus is longer than 72 hours old and still exhibits inflammatory changes.

Internal hemorrhoids are proximal to the dentate line and are described by a grading system on a scale from I to IV (Table 17.2). Pain associated with internal hemorrhoids is indicative of strangulation that can lead to complications of necrosis and sepsis.

Treatment options for hemorrhoids range from nonoperative management to surgical resection. Patients with external thrombosed hemorrhoids that present within 72 hours are candidates for incision and enucleation of the thrombus. This can be accomplished under local anesthesia in the office or emergency department. An elliptical excision is made along the entire mass, extending through the skin and subcutaneous tissue and removal of the thrombus. The wound is left open without packing with instructions to care for the wound with analgesics and warm sitz baths several times a day and after bowel movements. Patients presenting with thrombosed hemorrhoids longer than 72 hours old are treated conservatively, as the thrombus will begin to be reabsorbed by this time, and the pain will resolve spontaneously. Occasionally the thrombus causes pressure on the adjacent skin, forming an area of necrosis and perforation within the hemorrhoidal cushion and may require intervention.

Nonoperative management is often the initial treatment of internal hemorrhoids and is indicated for: grades I, II, and potentially III; patients who are pregnant, coagulopathic, HIV positive; and those who have underlying IBD. Nonoperative management includes sitz baths, stool softeners, and dietary modifications, including a high-fiber diet (at least 25–35 g daily) with increased fluid intake in order to reduce constipation and straining. Topical treatments with glycerin suppositories

TABLE 17.2 ■ **Grading Classification and Treatment Options for Internal Hemorrhoids**

Grade	Characterization	Symptoms/Complications	Treatment options
I	Hemorrhoid bulges into anal canal but does not protrude past anus	Painless bleeding	High fiber diet Local pharmacotherapy Sclerotherapy Rubber band ligation Infrared coagulation
II	Protrusion of hemorrhoid out of anal canal that occurs with bowel movements or straining, reduces spontaneously	Painless bleeding, swelling	Sclerotherapy Rubber band ligation Infrared coagulation Excisional hemorrhoidectomy
III	Protrusion of hemorrhoid out of anal canal that requires manual reduction	Painless bleeding, swelling, possible strangulation	Rubber band ligation Infrared coagulation Excisional hemorrhoidectomy
IV	Irreducible protrusion or instantaneous reprolapse of hemorrhoid out of anal canal	Painless bleeding, swelling, high risk of strangulation with pain, necrosis, sepsis	Excisional hemorrhoidectomy

with or without topical steroids or local anesthetics can be used short term for patients that have failed conservative management. Procedural management of hemorrhoids is based on the grade (see Table 17.2) and patient factors as summarized in the box below.

Sclerotherapy

Sclerotherapy can be used for first-, second-, or third-degree hemorrhoids. This technique includes injecting a sclerosing agent (phenol in olive oil, sodium morrhuate, or quinine urea) into the submucosa of each respective hemorrhoidal tissue. Complications with this procedure are rare, but instances of infection and fibrosis have been reported to occur.

Rubber Band Ligation

Elastic ligation of hemorrhoidal tissue is a simple in-office procedure that can be performed on first-, second-, and third-degree hemorrhoids. The hemorrhoidal tissue is first visualized through an anoscope and grasped with forceps. The tissue is pulled through a double-sleeved cylinder, and two latex bands are placed on the hemorrhoidal bundle to strangulate the underlying tissue. This results in scarring and prevention of further bleeding or progression of hemorrhoidal disease. It is important to place the bands at least 1 to 2 cm higher than the dentate line to avoid extreme postprocedural pain. Usually only one or two hemorrhoidal cushions are ligated at a time. Another complication includes urinary retention, which occurs in approximately 1% of patients. Ligations can be performed in 2 to 4-week intervals until symptoms of bleeding or prolapse are resolved.

Infrared Coagulation

Infrared coagulation is an effective office treatment for first- and second-degree hemorrhoids. An instrument that uses infrared wavelengths is applied to each hemorrhoidal cushion to coagulate the underlying plexus. As opposed to rubber band ligation, all three quadrants can be treated at the same visit. Contraindications to this approach include large hemorrhoids and hemorrhoids with a high degree of prolapse (third or fourth degree).

Hemorrhoidectomy

Excisional hemorrhoidectomy includes a number of surgical procedures that can be performed for elective resection of symptomatic grade II, III, or IV hemorrhoids. Surgical techniques include an open (Milligan-Morgan), closed (Ferguson), and Whitehead's hemorrhoidectomy and are performed under local, regional, or general anesthesia. All procedures are aimed at ligating blood flow to the hemorrhoidal cushion and excising redundant tissue. The hemorrhoidal tissue is identified with the patient in the lithotomy position and with an anal speculum inserted into the anal canal. The hemorrhoidal tissue is excised using an elliptical incision, starting distal to the anal verge and extending proximally to the anal ring. During the dissection of the tissue, it is important to identify the fibers of the internal sphincter and to brush them away from the dissection in order to prevent injury to the muscle. Once the tissue is ligated, hemostasis is achieved, and the wound is either left open (open hemorrhoidectomy) or closed with a running absorbable suture (closed hemorrhoidectomy). Excision to all three hemorrhoid cushions can be performed in one operation.

Stapled hemorrhoidectomy is another surgical method that can be used to treat hemorrhoids. This technique can only be used on external hemorrhoids as opposed to open and closed methods. Compared with conventional techniques, the use of staple ligation has been shown to result in less postoperative pain in the initial 6 weeks after surgery. However, many disadvantages have been described, such as worse incontinence, tenesmus, and hemorrhoidal recurrences. Due to these outcomes, stapled hemorrhoidectomy has failed to gain popularity as a utilized technique.

What Are the Treatment Modalities for Other Causes of Perianal Pain?

FISSURE

Anal fissures are managed in three ways: symptomatic, medical, and surgical. Symptomatic management includes diet modification (high-fiber diet, increased fluid intake) and stool softeners to prevent constipation that is often associated with fissures. Constipation is common due to patients resisting the urge to defecate secondary to pain. Topical anesthetics may also be applied if the patient is having severe pain. Anal hygiene is extremely important—patients should be instructed to perform sitz baths daily and after defecation. Pharmacologic management includes topical nitrates and calcium channel blockers to vasodilate local blood vessels to promote healing. Botulinum toxin injections may also be used to reduce anal sphincter tone.

Although approximately one-half of anal fissures will heal with nonoperative management in 2 to 4 weeks, surgical treatment is indicated when conservative treatment fails. Surgical management includes a lateral internal sphincterotomy (LIS), anal dilation, or fissurectomy.

ABSCESS

An anorectal abscess requires surgical incision and drainage. Although antibiotics are often used in addition to surgical management, antibiotic administration alone is inadequate to treat an abscess. Surgical drainage should be performed as soon as an abscess is identified, as delayed intervention can result in chronic tissue destruction, fibrosis, and stricture formation that may impair anal continence. The use of CT or MRI to further characterize the location and extent of an abscess is often necessary for determination of further management.

A superficial or perianal abscess may be able to be drained at bedside. This is performed by making an incision over the area of fluctuance and performing adequate drainage of the abscess by manual compression. The abscess contents should be sent for culture, and the abscess cavity should be packed with gauze that can be removed after 24 hours. More complex abscesses include ischiorectal, intersphincteric, and supralevator abscesses and require operative drainage. Drain placement is indicated for complex or bilateral abscesses.

CLINICAL PEARL (STEPS 2/3)

A horseshoe abscess is an anorectal abscess that tracks from the deep postanal space into the ischiorectal fossae bilaterally (Fig. 17.5). Because these abscesses are deep, they are typically diagnosed on CT scan and require operative drainage with an incision into the deep postanal space and bilateral counter incisions to assure drainage of the ischiorectal fossae.

FISTULA

The treatment of a fistula depends on a number of factors including its location, the degree of involvement of the sphincter complex, the sex of the patient, as well as any association with Crohn' disease. Antibiotics should be given in the setting of overlying cellulitis or for patients with sepsis, diabetes, or other states of immune compromise. Surgical management is usually required for definitive treatment, and there are several surgical approaches.

Fistulotomy is the most definitive therapy with the highest success rate, but can only be performed for fistulas without sphincter involvement, or when only the distal third of the sphincter is involved in patients with an otherwise normal sphincter complex and with no evidence of Crohn's disease. A **draining seton,** a non-absorbable suture inserted directly into the fistula tract, allows the fistula to drain and possibly to close, and it may be used initially to allow the inflammation to settle prior to definitive surgical treatment.

When a fistula is thought to involve too much of the sphincter complex and it is felt that fistulotomy would lead to incontinence, there are other options which should be considered. Note, however, that each of the following, which can be used for such trans-sphincteric fistulae that cannot be treated by fistulotomy, is recognized to have a success rate inferior to that of fistulotomy:

- A **cutting seton** is a procedure whereas a tight suture is tied and sequentially tightened over time and it slowly cuts through the fistula.
- An **endoanal advancement flap** includes completely excising the granulation tissue associated with the fistula tract, suture ligating the internal opening at the sphincter, and covering the internal opening with an elevated mucosal flap.
- Fibrin glue - a **biological fistula plug** can be placed in the track and sutured in place, allowing for a creation of a scaffolding in which healing of the fistula can take place by granulation.
- A **LIFT procedure (Ligation of the Intersphincteric Fistula Tract)** is performed by dissecting the intersphincteric plane and suture-ligating the fistula track in this location.

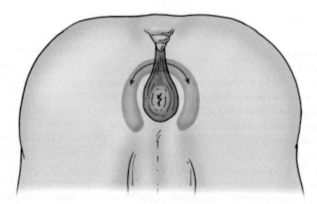

Fig. 17.5   A horseshoe abscess tracking from the deep postanal space in the midline to the ischiorectal fossae bilaterally *(arrows).*

PROLAPSE

Rectal prolapse can be manually reduced at bedside. Sphincter relaxation is required for a successful reduction as manual pressure is applied to the prolapsed tissue. The reduction may take several minutes and is complete when the rectal tissue is proximal to the anal sphincter. Sucrose is often applied to the prolapsed mucosa if edema is present, acting as an osmotic agent to reduce the extent of swelling. If gangrenous bowel is present before reduction, then surgery should be urgently performed.

There are a variety of surgical procedures performed for rectal prolapse. Transabdominal procedures include rectal mobilization and rectopexy (fixation of the rectum to the sacral promontory by mesh or nonabsorbable sutures). Sigmoid resection may also be indicated if the patient has redundancy in the colon with chronic constipation and subsequent prolapse. Perineal procedures have the advantage of sparing the pelvic nerves but have higher recurrence rates and potential bowel dysfunction from a decreased rectal reservoir. These procedures are performed on patients who are poor surgical candidates, had prior pelvic surgery or radiation, or have significant comorbid illnesses. A common perineal procedure is the Altemeier perineal rectosigmoidectomy, in which the redundant rectum is prolapsed through the anal canal and resected proximal to the dentate line. A handsewn anastomosis is performed, and a levatorplasty (suture approximation of the levator muscles) is often performed anterior to the anal canal to provide additional support.

PROCTITIS

The treatment for proctitis is generally nonsurgical. The treatment options vary based on the etiology of the proctitis. IBD proctitis warrants a colonoscopy to determine the extent of the inflammation. The first-line treatment is medical therapy; however, surgery may be indicated in patients who fail medical management. Infectious proctitis treatment is aimed at treating the underlying infectious cause. Treatment for radiation proctitis is based on its symptomology and grade. The presence of strictures, perforation, fistulas, or chronic bleeding despite endoscopic and medical treatments warrants surgical intervention.

For symptom management, a low-fiber, low-residue diet should be recommended in addition to antispasmodic agents and stool softeners to reduce abdominal complaints and protect the friable rectal mucosal from damage.

After informed consent is obtained, the patient is taken to the operating room the next day for an open hemorrhoidectomy. On examination under anesthesia, he is found to have a grade IV hemorrhoid in the left lateral position that is excised without complication. He tolerates the procedure well and is discharged to home the same day with instructions related to analgesia, a bowel regimen, and wound care with sitz baths. He is seen in the office 3 weeks postoperatively and is found to be healing well and having normal bowel movements without pain.

BEYOND THE PEARLS

- The differential diagnosis for perianal pain is broad and includes etiologies requiring both surgical and nonsurgical intervention.
- Hemorrhoids are categorized as internal or external based on their relationship to the dentate line.
- Chronicity, the degree of thrombosis or prolapse, and patient factors dictate the therapeutic options for symptomatic hemorrhoids.
- The size and location in relation to the internal and external sphincter dictate the treatment of perirectal/perianal abscesses and anal fistulae. Effective therapy while maintaining fecal continence is the primary goal of treatment.
- Rectal prolapse can have significant effects on patient quality of life. There are multiple operative approaches for treating recurrent rectal prolapse.

Suggested Readings

Bullard Dunn, K. M., & Rothenberger, D. A. (2015). Colon, rectum, and anus. In *Schwartz's Principles of Surgery* (10th ed.): McGraw Hill Education.

Jacobs, D. (2014). Hemorrhoids. *N Engl J Med*, *371*(10), 944–951. https://doi.org/10.1056/nejmcp1204188.

Lin, A. Y., & Fleshman, J. W. , Jr. (2013). Benign disorders of the anorectum (pelvic floor, fissures, hemorrhoids, and fistulas). In M. J. Zinner & S. W. Ashley (Eds.), *Maingot's abdominal operations* (12th ed.). New York: McGraw-Hill. http://accesssurgery.mhmedical.com/content.aspx?bookid=531&sectionid=41808823.

Surgical Oncology

CHAPTER 18

Breast Mass in a 32-Year-Old Female

Austin D. Williams ▪ Alycia So ▪ Julia Tchou

A 32-year-old female without significant past medical history presents to her primary care physician with a complaint of a lump in her left breast. She states she first detected the lump during a breast self-examination when showering about 3 weeks ago. She denies any other breast abnormalities, including pain and nipple discharge. She is concerned that she may have breast cancer because her grandmother was diagnosed with breast cancer several years ago.

What Is the Differential Diagnosis for a Palpable Breast Mass?

Many women presenting with a complaint of a palpable breast mass will be very concerned about a potential diagnosis of breast cancer. The differential diagnosis for a palpable breast mass is broad and includes both benign and malignant etiologies. As such, the history and physical examination are important for discerning the most likely diagnosis. Table 18.1 lists the most common benign breast diagnoses along with features in history and on physical examination that may help to distinguish them from other potential diagnoses. Of note, not all benign lesions present as palpable masses, and many are first identified as abnormalities on screening mammography. Please refer to Chapter 19 for a discussion of malignant breast disease and screening mammography.

CLINICAL PEARL (STEP 2/3)

Approximately 90% of palpable breast masses in women in their 20s to early 50s are ultimately benign. Although it is important to reassure patients with this fact, it is even more important to rule out breast cancer.

What Are the Important Aspects to Taking a Thorough History for Breast Disease?

The clinician is tasked with evaluating not only the history of the presenting problem but also the patient's personal history as it relates to risk factors for breast cancer, including family history as well.

Related to the breast mass, the clinician should elicit the history of presenting symptoms, including:

- how and when the mass was first noted and if there have been any changes in size or quality of the mass, especially related to the menstrual cycle;
- the precise location of the mass;
- changes in breast appearance, including asymmetry, skin changes, nipple inversion, or skin dimpling; and
- presence of nipple discharge, whether it is unilateral or bilateral, if it is spontaneous, its duration, and the character of the discharge.

TABLE 18.1 ■ Summary of Benign Breast Diseases and Their Presentation, Diagnosis, and Treatment

	History	Physical	Radiology	Pathology	Treatment
Traumatic					
Hematoma	Recent trauma	Tender, potentially ecchymotic	Variable		Conservative
Fat necrosis	Remote trauma	Potentially palpable mass	Often spiculated mass on mammogram	Fibrosis and degenerated fat	Conservative; repeat mammogram/US in 6 weeks to ensure resolution
Inflammatory					
Abscess	Progressive pain	Erythema, tenderness, warmth, fluctuant	Fluid-filled cavity on US	Purulent material; culture - most common bacteria are Staphylococci and Streptococci	Incision and drainage; antibiotics
Non-proliferative					
Cyst	Breast pain or palpable mass	Palpable abnormality; may wax and wane with menstrual cycle	Fluid-filled cavity on US; simple or complex	Serous or bloody fluid	Observation; aspiration if symptomatic (e.g. pain); fluid cytology if bloody, otherwise discard cyst fluid
Fibroadenoma	Palpable mass; reproductive age	Rubbery mobile mass	Well-circumscribed mass on mammogram or US	Benign fibroepithelial lesion	Observation or excision (if mass is enlarging over time)
Mammary duct ectasia	Nipple discharge	Subareolar mass	Calcifications on mammogram, dilarted ducts on ultrasound	Dilated major subareolar ducts	Conservative, smoking cessation

Proliferative without atypia

Lesion					Management
Radial scar (complex sclerosing lesion)	Abnormal mammogram	Usually non palpable	Spiculated lesion with translucent center on mammogram; targeted US may detect a mass	flame like fibrotic lesion; Sclerosing ductal hyperplasia	Excision
Intraductal papilloma	Nipple discharge	Serous or bloody unilateral nipple discharge	May not be visible or detected as intraductal mass on ultrasound	Fibrovascular core with epithelial branches within duct	Excision
Pseudoangiomatous stromal hyperplasia	Palpable mass or abnormal mammogram; reproductive age	Single cicumscribed mass or undetectable	Circumscribed mass on mammogram or US	Dense keloid-like stroma with slit-like clefts lined by myofibroblasts (simulating vascular spaces)	Observation or excision

Proliferative lesions with atypia

Lesion					Management
Atypical ductal hyperplasia	Abnormal mammogram	Usually non palpable	Cacifications on mammogram	Ducts completely or partially filled with cells with punched out spaces	Excision
Lobular neoplasia					
Atypical lobular hyperplasia					
Lobular carcinoma in situ				Distension of acini within lobules or terminal duct lobular units	

Table 18.1 groups benign breast diseases based on the risk they confer for a current or future breast cancer. Traumatic and inflammatory lesions confer almost zero breast cancer risk, and nonproliferative lesions have a very minimal risk. These lesions can typically be managed conservatively with observation (with the exception of draining a breast abscess and treating with antibiotics). Proliferative lesions are associated with a slightly increased risk for breast cancer, and those with atypia confer a two- to fourfold increased risk of breast cancer and may harbor a current, yet undiagnosed, breast cancer in up to 15% of patients when a larger tissue sample is obtained on surgical excision.

Related to the patient's breast cancer risk, it is important to elicit:

- menstrual history, including age at menarche and age at menopause if applicable;
- the age at first live birth of a child;
- the use of oral contraceptives or history of combination hormone replacement (estrogen and progesterone) therapy;
- a history of any breast biopsies and their results (especially if there was an *in situ* or invasive cancer diagnosis);
- the family history of breast and/or ovarian cancer (especially in first-degree relatives) and other malignancies such as prostate and pancreatic cancer, etc., or genetic syndromes;
- radiation exposure (Chernobyl nuclear accident, e.g.); and
- a history of chest wall radiation for the treatment of breast cancer or other disease such as Hodgkin's lymphoma.

What Are the Important Aspects of a Complete Breast Physical Examination?

Although many techniques are described for evaluating the breasts on physical examination, all have a goal of fully evaluating both breasts, the neck (cervical, supraclavicular, and infraclavicular fossae), the chest wall, and both axillae. Despite the low sensitivity (approximately 50%) of clinical breast and axilla examination, it is important to be thorough.

The examination should start with the concurrent **inspection** of both breasts in a seated (with arms elevated and then with the patient's hands on her hips) and then in supine position. A thorough inspection in all positions allows the clinician to evaluate for asymmetry and skin changes of the breasts and nipples. **Palpation** of nodal basins and breasts follows inspection. Axillae can be palpated when the patient is in a seated position with the examiner supporting the ipsilateral arm and palpating the axilla to assess for lymph nodes that are palpable, fixed, or tender. Cervical, infraclavicular, and supraclavicular nodes are also palpated bilaterally with the patient in a seated position. Finally, each breast is palpated in the seated position followed by thorough palpation of each breast in the supine position with the ipsilateral arm raised overhead. For a thorough examination, the clinician uses both hands to compress the breast tissue against the chest wall in order to detect abnormalities. It is imperative to examine the entire breast from the sternum laterally to the breast's axillary tail and from the clavicle inferiorly to the inframammary fold (Fig. 18.1).

CLINICAL PEARL (STEP 2/3)

Any abnormalities on physical examination should be well documented to include the nature of the abnormality, its size, and location. The location of breast abnormalities has three components: the laterality of the breast, the distance from the nipple, and the location within the breast. The location within the breast can be denoted either using quadrants (e.g., upper outer quadrant) or, more specifically, describing the location as if the breast were a clock from the examiner's viewpoint (e.g., the 3 o'clock position).

The patient undergoes a complete breast examination, which reveals a palpable mass of approximately 2 cm in the left breast at the 10 o'clock position 3 cm from the nipple. The mass is smooth, rubbery, and mobile. There are no other masses in either breast, and there are no abnormalities detected on lymph node examination. The physician refers the patient for a bilateral diagnostic mammogram and a targeted ultrasound during which a core biopsy of the lesion is performed (Fig. 18.2). The patient is referred to a breast surgeon. A review of the pathologic analysis of the lesion reveals a fibroadenoma. The patient asks about her treatment options.

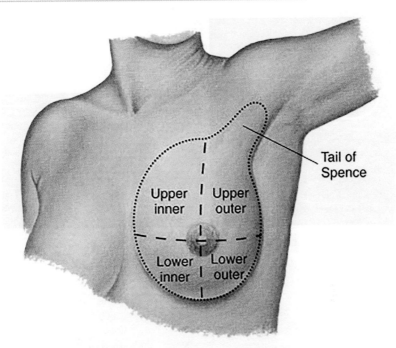

Fig. 18.1 Breast anatomy showing the axillary Tail of Spence and appropriate boundaries of breast examination *(red-dotted lines).* (From Ball JW, Dains JE, Flynn JA et al: Breasts and axillae. In *Seidel's guide to physical examination,* St. Louis, 2015, Mosby, pp 350–369.)

What Are the Steps in Working Up a Newly Detected Breast Lesion?

Most breast abnormalities detected on physical examination and/or radiographic imaging (mammogram, ultrasound, magnetic resonance imaging [MRI]) require additional diagnostic workup. The goal of the workup is to rule out the presence of breast cancer. Additional radiographic studies, such as additional mammographic views, may determine that the lesion is clearly benign, obviating the need for biopsy. Many lesions, however, will require biopsy under ultrasound or mammographic guidance. Core biopsy is preferred over fine-needle aspiration (FNA) for most breast lesions so the pathologist is able to evaluate the tissue architecture of the specimen more accurately. The location of a biopsy should be marked with a metallic clip so the area can be identified on subsequent radiographic studies and, if required, during surgical excision of the area.

Do All Benign Breast Lesions Require Surgery?

The decision to biopsy or excise breast lesions found on physical examination or screening radiology studies is predicated on the risk that the lesion harbors a current or future breast cancer. Despite their benign nature, lesions that are large or abnormally shaped on radiographic studies and those that demonstrate atypical cells on pathologic analysis are more likely to be upstaged to a malignant process upon surgical excision and should therefore be excised.

CLINICAL PEARL (STEPS 2/3)

The "upgrade rate" for benign lesions is the number of patients who, after being diagnosed with a benign breast disease on core needle biopsy, ultimately have breast cancer in the surgical excision specimen. For example, studies have demonstrated that patients with atypical ductal hyperplasia can have up to a 15% upgrade rate.

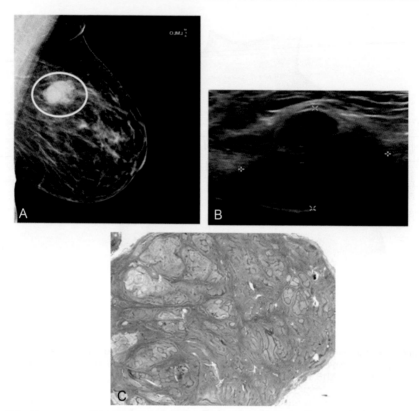

Fig. 18.2 Mammogram (A), ultrasound (B), and histologic (C) views of a fibroadenoma. (A, B, from Lee S, Mercado CL, Cangiarella JF, Chhor CM: Frequency and outcomes of biopsy-proven fibroadenomas recommended for surgical excision, *Clin Imaging* Jul–Aug;50:31–36. 2018. C, from Koerner FC: Fibroadenoma. In *Diagnostic problems in breast pathology,* Philadelphia, 2009, Saunders, pp 307–319.)

The surgeon reassures the patient that her fibroadenoma is benign and that she does not need surgery unless subsequent imaging studies show increasing size. The patient indicates that she would prefer to have the fibroadenoma removed, because she is concerned about developing breast cancer and wants to be vigilant about self-breast examination. Even though the fibroadenoma is benign, she does not want its presence to interfere with her ability to self-examine. She is taken to the operating room and undergoes excision of the mass. The patient does well postoperatively and is discharged the same day.

How Are Breast Lesions Identified in the Operating Room?

Unlike many other organs, the breast parenchyma is mainly comprised of adipose tissue and lacks specific anatomic landmarks. Palpable lesions are often easily and accurately identified in the operating room. Those that are not palpable, however, require preoperative identification involving the placement of localization wires or radio signal–emitting clips under ultrasound or mammographic guidance (Fig. 18.3). The surgeon then utilizes preoperative imaging to inform the location of the wire or clip to guide placement of the incision and excision of the tissue specimen. Commonly, a specimen radiograph is performed before the conclusion of the operation in order to verify that the wire, the metallic biopsy clip, and/or abnormality of interest are included in the specimen.

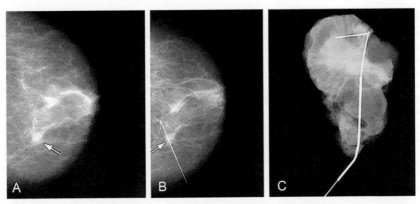

Fig. 18.3 Preoperative needle localization of a nonpalpable breast lesion. The lesion is seen on mammogram (A) (arrow), and a wire is placed in the lesion preoperatively (B). After excision, a specimen radiograph (C) demonstrates that the lesion of interest has been excised. (A, B, H, from Mahoney MC, Jackson VP: Presurgical needle localization. In Bassett LW, Mahoney MC, Apple SK, D'Orsi CJ, editors: *Breast imaging,* Philadelphia, 2011, Elsevier, pp 605–610. C, D, from Breast biopsy with or without needle localization. In Velasco JM, editor: *Essential surgical procedures,* Philadelphia, 2015, Elsevier, pp e821–e853.)

Partial Mastectomy

1. Appropriately identify the laterality and location of the targeted lesion.
2. Make an incision from which the lesion is readily accessible; incisions at the areolar margin or inframammary crease can be well hidden when healed.
3. Dissect sharply and/or using electrocautery to the location of the lesion and excise the specimen circumferentially.
4. If there is a concern for cancer, excise additional tissue at the anterior, posterior, superior, inferior, lateral, and medial margins (so-called "shave" margins).
5. Verify with a specimen radiograph that the target has been excised.
6. Irrigate the excision cavity and close the incision with subcuticular sutures.

The patient returns to the surgeon in 2 weeks. She has no complaints; her incision is healing well, and pathology confirms a benign fibroadenoma. She is counseled to resume routine breast cancer screening (see Chapter 19).

BEYOND THE PEARLS

- The vast majority of palpable breast masses in young female patients represent benign breast disease.
- Ruling out the presence of breast cancer and assessing breast cancer risk are the major responsibilities of a physician when diagnosing a benign breast disease.
- Complete history and physical examination are imperative to working up a breast mass, though most patients will undergo radiographic and pathologic workup also.
- The decision to excise a benign breast mass depends on the lesion's risk of harboring a current or future breast cancer.
- Surgical excision of a benign breast mass may also be performed based on patient preference.
- For benign breast diseases that confer no additional risk of breast cancer, subsequent normal breast cancer screening protocols are recommended.

Suggested Readings

Guray, M., & Sahin, A. A. (2006). Benign breast diseases: Classification, diagnosis, and management. *Oncologist, 11*, 435.

Menes, T. S., Rosenberg, R., Balch, S., et al. (2014). Upgrade of high-risk breast lesions detected on mammography in the Breast Cancer Surveillance Consortium. *Am J Surg, 207*, 24.

Morrow, M., Schnitt, S. J., & Norton, L. (2015). Current management of lesions associated with an increased risk of breast cancer. *Nat Rev Clin Oncol, 12*, 227.

Santen, R. J., & Mansel, R. (2005). Benign breast disorders. *N Engl J Med, 353*, 275.

Schnitt, S. J. (2003). Benign breast disease and breast cancer risk: Morphology and beyond. *Am J Surg Pathol, 27*, 836.

CHAPTER 19

Abnormal Screening Mammogram in a 48-Year-Old Female

Jonah D. Klein ■ Robin Ciocca

A 48-year-old female without significant past medical history presents to the breast surgeon's office after being informed by a radiologist of findings of an abnormal screening mammogram. She was told she had new areas of suspicious calcifications noted over a 1-cm area in the upper outer quadrant of her right breast (Fig. 19.1). She does not have any breast complaints, denying breast masses, nipple discharge, and breast pain.

What Are the Recommendations for Breast Cancer Screening?

A screening mammogram differs from a diagnostic mammogram in that its objective is early preclinical identification of suspicious lesions in an otherwise asymptomatic patient. For low risk women, current US Preventative Services Task Force recommendations are to start screening between 40 and 50 years of age and screen biennially to 74 years of age. Screening is not recommended in women of average risk younger than 40, given a low breast cancer rate and high prevalence of dense breast tissue leading to false positives and unnecessary testing. Women with dense breast tissue are at increased risk for developing breast cancer compared with those with fatty breast tissue, yet other screening tools such as ultrasound have not been universally accepted. Although recommendations vary, women at increased risk, such as those with strong family history or those with known genetic mutations, should initiate screening between the ages of 25 and 40 with annual mammography or MRI. It is not recommended to screen women older than age 75; however, if they are in good health, women may choose to continue mammographic screening and are encouraged to discuss this with their primary care physician or breast surgeon.

CLINICAL PEARL (STEPS 2/3)

Recommendations for screening mammography have been variable, but consensus is that mammograms should be performed at least every two years starting at age 40 to 50 through age 69 to 74. MRI can be used in patients with genetic susceptibility to breast cancer. Breast self-examination as screening has not consistently demonstrated effectiveness in detection.

What Mammographic Findings Are Concerning for Breast Cancer?

The goal of screening mammography is to detect and characterize abnormalities of concern for breast cancer and inform further diagnostic studies and/or tissue biopsy. The American College of Radiology Breast Imaging Reporting and Data System (BI-RADS) is a radiographic classification system that categorizes mammographic findings and recommends next steps (Table 19.1). Generally, BI-RADS category 3 is an indication for short-term follow-up, and BI-RADS

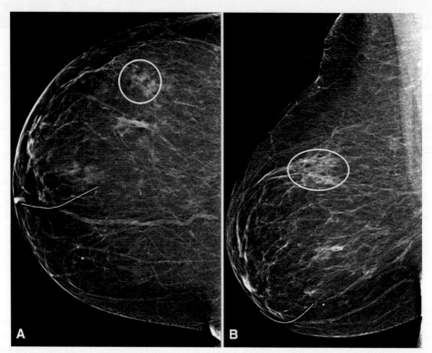

Fig. 19.1 (A) Right breast mammogram in craniocaudal (CC) and (B) mediolateral oblique (MLO). Areas of suspicious calcification are circled. (From Atkins KA, Kang C: Practical breast pathology: a diagnostic approach, Philadelphia, 2013, Elsevier, pp 25–54.)

categories 4 and 5 are an indication for tissue biopsy due to a greater than 2% and up to 95% risk of malignancy. Mammographic findings that are concerning include masses, calcifications, distortions, and asymmetries. Masses that are lobulated, spiculated, or stellate are most concerning. Calcifications that are small, heterogeneous, clustering, and/or linear branching are also particularly suggestive of malignancy (see Fig. 19.1).

TABLE 19.1 ■ BI-RADS Assessment Categories: Mammography

BI-RADS Category	Assessment	Comments/Recommendation
Category 1	Negative	Nothing suspicious; continue routine screening
Category 2	Benign	e.g., Benign calcifications, cysts; continue routing screening
Category 3	Probably benign	e.g., Focal asymmetry, noncalcified mass; 6-month follow-up mammogram
Category 4	Suspicious	Some malignant features, divided 4A,B,C; core needle biopsy
Category 5	Highly suggestive	> 95% likelihood malignant; core needle biopsy
Category 6	Biopsy proven	Imaging performed before definitive therapy
Category 0	Nondiagnostic	Spot compression, magnification, ultrasound

What Is Necessary in the Clinical Evaluation of a Newly Diagnosed Breast Mass?
Generally, a patient presenting with concerning findings on a screening mammogram will be asymptomatic, yet the evaluation still necessitates a focused history and physical examination. Relevant history should include personal history of palpable breast masses, nipple discharge, prior cancers and respective treatments, breast biopsies and pathologies, upper body radiation exposure, age at menarche, gravidity, parity, menopausal status, and any use of hormone replacement therapy. Family history of breast cancer, age of diagnosis and if it was unilateral or bilateral are also important. Breast examination findings concerning for malignancy include asymmetry, skin or nipple retractions, edema of the skin (peau d'orange), architectural distortion, and any palpable mass. The axilla should also be evaluated for palpable, fixed masses.

If a clinically detected mass or radiographic abnormality is identified in the breast, the next step in workup is core needle biopsy (CNB) with or without image-guidance. For abnormalities found on screening imaging, ultrasound is often needed for guidance of CNB. If calcifications are present on mammography, yet no mass is identified on ultrasound, a stereotactic biopsy is beneficial. Fine needle aspiration (FNA) can be used for axillary lesions of concern; CNB, however, is far superior for tissue sampling of the breast in order to evaluate tissue architecture and distinguish between invasive and *in situ* lesions, which the cytology obtained by FNA cannot do. A radiographically dense clip is usually deployed after biopsy to enable accuracy of future excision.

What Is the Differential Diagnosis for Abnormalities on Screening Mammogram?
Benign. Please see Chapter 18 for a detailed discussion of benign breast disease. In brief, the entities to be considered include lesions that are not associated with the development of breast cancer (such as fibroadenoma) and lesions that, although not *precursors* of malignancy, are *markers* for increased risk of future malignancy (such as lobular neoplasia and radial scar).

DUCTAL CARCINOMA *IN SITU*

Ductal carcinoma *in situ* (DCIS) is an intraductal neoplastic lesion that generally presents as asymptomatic mammographic calcifications. DCIS is characterized by cellular proliferation and atypia confined to the ductal-lobular system with propensity for progression to invasive cancer. It can be classified as low grade (often estrogen receptor positive) or high grade (often estrogen receptor negative). Treatment generally involves surgical excision to negative margins, radiation therapy, and hormone chemoprophylaxis. Clinical predictors of recurrence or development of invasive cancer include comedo pattern (necrotic), positive margins, and high nuclear grade.

INVASIVE CARCINOMA

Invasive breast cancer involves proliferation of the terminal duct lobular unit. There are several histologic subtypes with varying prognoses and malignant characteristics, the most common being ductal carcinoma followed by lobular carcinoma. The category of ductal carcinoma includes tubular, medullary, mucinous, and papillary subtypes. Unlike ductal carcinoma, lobular carcinoma does not form calcifications and is more often bilateral and multicentric. Additional prognostication of breast cancer involves subdivision into grade as determined by tubule formation, mitotic figures, and nuclear pleomorphisms. Metaplastic features and signet ring cells confer a worse prognosis. Surgical treatment as discussed later in this chapter generally involves mastectomy versus breast conservation therapy, plus sentinel lymph node biopsy with or without axillary dissection. Inflammatory breast cancer is a very aggressive form of invasive breast cancer, conferring a poorer prognosis. It is marked by dermal lymphatic invasion with a peau d'orange or cellulitic appearance and is generally treated with neoadjuvant chemotherapy followed by mastectomy.

OTHER MALIGNANT CONDITIONS

- Paget's disease—a clinical entity presenting as crusting, eczematous, ulcerative skin lesions on the nipple, histologic epidermal infiltration by Paget cells. It is indicative of an underlying DCIS or invasive ductal carcinoma.
- Phyllodes tumor—a fibroepithelial breast tumor with varying aggressiveness that presents as a mass or mammographic abnormality. Histologic hallmarks are leaf-like papillary projections.
- Male breast cancer—represents up to 1% of all breast cancers and is associated with other conditions including Klinefelter's syndrome and prior radiation therapy.

What Are the Inherited and Genetic Risks for the Development of Breast Cancer?

Mutations in BRCA1 on chromosome 17 and BRCA2 on chromosome 13 are the most discussed genetic mutations increasing the risk of patients for the development of breast cancer as well as ovarian cancer. The estimated lifetime risk of breast cancer in female patients harboring a BRCA mutation ranges from 40% to 60%. BRCA2 mutations are also associated with a higher risk of male breast cancer. Patients with a family history of breast cancer and/or a personal or family history, where the diagnosis has been at a young age, should be considered for genetic testing. Women of Ashkenazi Jewish descent have a higher likelihood of carrying BRCA mutations. Other genes implicated in the development of breast cancer include TP53, ATM, PTEN and PALB2.

The patient does not have any personal or family history of breast cancer and is not of Ashkenazi Jewish descent. After focused history and physical examination and review of the patient's mammographic studies, the patient undergoes an ultrasound-guided core needle biopsy under local anesthesia in the office. The pathology returns as ductal carcinoma in situ with foci of invasive ductal carcinoma. Her cancer is estrogen receptor, progesterone receptor, and HER2 positive. The patient states she had a friend with breast cancer that had spread to her lymph nodes and she asks about her surgical options for treatment.

BASIC SCIENCE PEARL (STEP 1)

Breast Anatomy

The breast parenchyma is composed of fibrofatty glandular tissue with the proportion of fatty tissue increasing with age. Blood supply to the breast comes via the internal mammary perforators, thoracoacromial artery, lateral thoracic artery, and terminal branches of the third through eighth intercostal perforators (Fig. 19.2). Sensory innervation is derived from branches of T3–T5 intercostal nerves and supraclavicular nerves from the cervical plexus. The breast overlies the pectoralis muscles between the second and sixth rib, with the inferior border being the rectus abdominus, and is anchored by Cooper suspensory ligaments.

Axillary Anatomy

The axilla is a triangular space bordered by the chest wall medially, latissimus dorsi posteriorly, the pectoralis major muscle anteriorly, and the axillary vein superiorly (see Fig. 19.2). There are three levels of axillary nodes. Level I nodes are inferior and lateral to the pectoralis minor muscle. Level II nodes are beneath the pectoralis minor muscle and adjacent and inferior to the axillary vein. Level III nodes are medial to the pectoralis minor muscle and adjacent to the subclavian vein (Fig. 19.3). Rotter's nodes is the name given to the nodes between the pectoralis major and minor muscles. Level I has the highest volume of nodes, followed by level II then III.

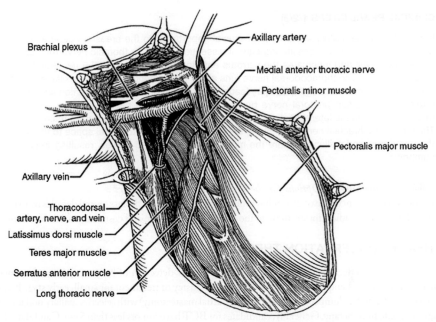

Fig. 19.2 Breast and axillary anatomy. (Redrawn from Chapter 44 *Essential surgical procedures,* Elsevier: Philadelphia, 2015, 6, e790–e820.)

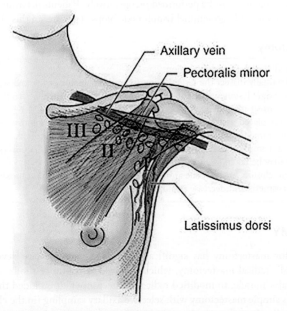

Fig. 19.3 Axillary lymph nodes in levels I–III. (From Prati R, Chang HR, Chung MA: Therapeutic value of axillary node dissection and selective management of the axilla in small breast cancers. In Bland KI, Copeland EM III, Klimberg VS, Gradishar WJ, editors: *The breast: comprehensive management of benign and malignant diseases,* ed 5, Philadelphia, 2018, Elsevier, pp 590–603.)

CLINICAL PEARL (STEPS 1/2/3)

Knowledge of the axillary anatomy is of crucial importance to the breast surgeon as it contains critical structures necessitating careful dissection. The long thoracic nerve runs parallel to the chest wall and innervates the serratus anterior muscle; injury to the nerve leads to a winged scapula. The thoracodorsal nerve runs along the posterior wall of the axilla and innervates the latissimus dorsi muscle; injury leads to weakness of shoulder adduction and internal rotation. The median pectoral nerve bundle supplies both the pectoralis major and minor muscles, whereas the lateral pectoral nerve bundle supplies only the pectoralis major muscle. The intercostal brachial nerves run along the second and third intercostal space to the skin of the upper arm and axilla; these are the most commonly injured nerves, resulting in sensory numbness.

What Are the Surgical Options for the Treatment of Breast Cancer?

The surgical treatment of breast cancer has evolved substantially over the last several decades from invasive and disfiguring radical mastectomy to more minimally invasive and cosmetic partial mastectomy.

BREAST CONSERVATION THERAPY

Better radiographic techniques have resulted in the earlier detection of breast cancer, and as such, breast conservation therapy (BCT) has become the mainstay of treatment for small, early stage breast cancers. BCT involves lumpectomy (also termed partial mastectomy) with selective axillary nodal sampling and radiation therapy. Generally, candidates for BCT have tumors less than 5 cm. Candidates for BCT may have lesions that are not palpable and have been identified on imaging studies. If the lesion is palpable, no preoperative localization is necessary; otherwise mammographic or ultrasound-guided wire localization techniques must be performed preoperatively. Patients determined to have invasive cancers will also need to undergo sentinel lymph node biopsy (see later in this chapter).

Partial Mastectomy

1. Make a radial or periareolar incision.
2. Circumferentially dissect the target lesion (whether palpable or marked with a guide wire).
3. Excise the target lesion and orient the specimen with marking stiches so the pathologist can assess the correct margins.
4. If a clip was placed at the time of the preoperative core needle biopsy, perform specimen radiograph immediately after excision to assess successful clip retrieval.
5. To ensure complete excision, additional specimens at each margin (so-called "shave" margins) may be taken.
6. Before skin closure, breast tissue around the excision cavity may be approximated in order to improve cosmesis and decrease postoperative seroma formation.

MASTECTOMY

The procedure for mastectomy has significantly evolved over the past several decades from William Halstead's radical mastectomy, which involved resection of the breast, axillary tissue, and pectoralis major muscle, to modified radical mastectomy that excluded the pectoralis major muscle, to today's simple mastectomy with selective axillary sampling (in the clinically node negative patient). Indications for simple mastectomy as opposed to breast conservation therapy include multicentric disease, extensive microcalcifications, inability to obtain negative margins, inability to receive radiation therapy (i.e., pregnancy), prior breast irradiation, inflammatory breast cancer, or chest wall involvement.

Simple Mastectomy

1. Make an elliptical transverse incision around the nipple areolar complex.
2. Raise skin flaps either sharply or with electrocautery
3. Dissect off breast parenchyma to the clavicle superiorly, rectus sheath insertion inferiorly, latissimus dorsi laterally, pectoralis major fascia posteriorly, and sternal border medially.
4. Remove breast parenchyma, place a drain at the mastectomy site and close skin.

Alternatives to simple mastectomy include skin-sparing mastectomy for immediate breast reconstruction or nipple sparing mastectomy for improved cosmesis (with ongoing debated oncologic results).

SENTINEL LYMPH NODE BIOPSY

Sentinel lymph node biopsy (SLNB) has replaced axillary lymph node dissection (ALND) for staging in clinically node-negative patients. Axillary status remains the most important prognostic factor for survival in breast cancer. Studies have demonstrated that there is no survival difference between patients who have undergone axillary lymph node dissection versus SLNB alone, if the nodes were tumor free. It has been further shown that patients with T1 or T2 tumors and up to two positive nodes in their SLNB have no additional survival benefit by completion Axillary Lymph Node Dissection (ALND).

Sentinel Lymph Node Biopsy

1. Inject blue dye and/or radioactive technetium sulfur colloid around the tumor or deep to the areola.
2. Make a curvilinear incision in the axilla and dissect through subcutaneous tissue and through the axillary fascia.
3. Identify sentinel nodes visually (with blue dye) or via gamma detection probe (with technetium sulfur colloid) and excise them.
4. Excise any suspicious palpable lymph nodes.
5. Excised nodes can be analyzed under frozen section to determine need for further dissection.
6. Irrigate the cavity and close the incision.

AXILLARY LYMPH NODE DISSECTION

With SLNB, the prevalence of ALND is decreasing. The current indications for ALND are T4 tumors, clinically positive axillary nodes, biopsy-proven nodal metastasis, more than two positive SLNs, inflammatory breast cancer, prior inadequate axillary dissection, failed SLN biopsy, axillary local recurrence, and inability to perform SLNB. Generally, ALND is defined as excision of levels I and II nodes and sometimes level III. Lymphedema is the complication of most concern after ALND and, though it may occur after SLNB, it is rare.

Axillary Lymph Node Dissection

1. Make a radial incision in the axilla or extend an existing mastectomy incision laterally.
2. Dissecting skin flaps should be performed to anatomic boundaries of the axillary vein superiorly, serratus inferiorly, latissimus dorsi laterally, and pectorals major superomedially.
3. After incising the clavopectoral fascia, identify the axillary vein lateral to the pectoralis major, and mobilize the axillary contents inferolaterally exposing the axillary vein and medial pectoral bundle.
4. Retract the pectoralis muscles medially and dissect the axillary contents continue inferiorly and off the chest wall with identification and preservation of the long thoracic nerve and thoracodorsal nerve.
5. Place a drain in the axilla and close the incision.

CONTRALATERAL PROPHYLACTIC MASTECTOMY

Patients with invasive breast cancer or DCIS are increasingly opting for contralateral prophylactic mastectomy (CPM). CPM decreases the risk of contralateral cancer but has not been proven to increase survival. CPM may be indicated for patients with BRCA mutation or strong family history of breast cancer, though current recommendations are to discuss alternate options for risk reduction with patients, such as endocrine therapy.

BREAST RECONSTRUCTION AFTER MASTECTOMY

After mastectomy, immediate or delayed reconstruction may be considered. Options include no reconstruction, prosthetic reconstruction with tissue expanders and/or implants and autologous tissue reconstruction. Factors driving the decision of whether and how to reconstruct include patient preference, body habitus, plans for management of the contralateral breast, and comorbid conditions such as diabetes, tobacco use, and obesity. Prosthetic reconstruction can be performed in one stage with implant insertion at the time of mastectomy or in two stages with tissue expander placement, followed by gradual expansion, and implant exchange when the breast has expanded to the desired size. Autologous tissue reconstruction is performed at the time of mastectomy and involves a musculocutaneous flap that is either *pedicled* (connected to its original vascular supply) or *free* (requiring vascular anastomosis). Examples include the *pedicled* Transverse Rectus Abdominus Myocutaneous (TRAM) flap, based off the superior and inferior epigastric arteries, and the *free* Deep Inferior Epigastric Perforator (DIEP) flap, based off of the inferior epigastric artery and vein.

CLINICAL PEARL (STEPS 2/3)

Breast conservation therapy has become the standard for most women with invasive cancers. Contraindications include multicentric disease, persistent positive margins, pregnancy or other conditions prohibiting breast irradiation, prior chest irradiation, and large tumors with unfavorable cosmetic outcome.

The patient opts for breast conservation therapy and undergoes an ultrasound-guided wire localized partial mastectomy with sentinel lymph node biopsy. Intraoperative frozen section of the sentinel nodes is negative for carcinoma. Final pathologic analysis demonstrates a 1.2-cm invasive ductal carcinoma with negative margins and negative nodes—pathologic stage T1N0. She returns to the office for surgical follow-up and has an appointment scheduled to meet with the radiation oncologist so that radiation treatment can begin when surgical healing is complete.

How Is Breast Cancer Staged?

Until recently breast cancer was staged according to an anatomic tumor, node and metastasis (TNM) staging system (Table 19.2). The American Joint Committee on Cancer (AJCC) staging guide (8th edition) added biological factors as adjuncts to the staging of breast cancer in order to provide more precise and personalized prognostic information. These biological factors include tumor grade, hormone receptor and epidermal growth factor receptor 2 (HER2) positivity, and multigene tumor signature profiles. Multiple tools are available to assist in calculation of a patient's comprehensive prognostic stage.

Anatomic criteria continue to play into the overall prognostic stage and are used alone for patients in whom no biomarker data are available. The TNM definitions for breast cancer are found in Table 19.2.

TABLE 19.2 ■ **TNM Breast Cancer Staging**

Tumor	
0	No tumor identified
in situ (is)	Carcinoma in situ
1	≤ 2 cm
2	> 2 cm and ≤ 5 cm
3	> 5cm
4	Extension into chest wall or skin

Nodes	
0	No regional nodal metastasis
1	1–3 positive ipsilateral axillary lymph nodes
2	4–9 positive ipsilateral axillary nodes or positive ipsilateral internal mammary nodes
3	≥ 10 positive ipsilateral axillary nodes or positive infraclavicular nodes

Stage	Tumor	Node	Metastasis
0	in situ	0	0
I	0 or 1	0	0
II	0 or 1	1	0
	2 or 3	0	0
III	3 or 4	1	0
	Any	2 or 3	0
IV	Any	Any	1

What Are the Current Standards for Radiation Therapy, Chemotherapy, and Hormonal Therapy for Breast Cancer?

- **Radiation therapy** is indicated for nearly all patients undergoing breast conservation therapy. It involves daily treatment for approximately 6 weeks and generally targets the ipsilateral breast and level I and II lymph nodes. There are times when radiation is required even after a patient has undergone mastectomy. Postmastectomy radiation is indicated for findings of four or more positive axillary lymph nodes, tumors greater than 5 cm, tumors with involvement of the skin or chest wall, positive surgical margins, or inflammatory breast cancer. Note that radiation of a breast which has been reconstructed can adversely affect form and function due to fibrosis and contraction of the irradiated tissue.

- **Chemotherapy** is standard for patients with triple-negative breast cancer, tumor size larger than 0.5 cm, or pathologically involved lymph nodes. If micro invasive disease is present or the tumor is 1 to 3 mm in size, the use of adjuvant chemotherapy has to be weighed against its risks. At present, most chemotherapy regimens involve a combination of cyclophosphamide, an anthracycline, and a taxane. Neoadjuvant therapy can be used to downstage disease to make patients with large tumors or a high tumor-to-breast ratio candidates for breast conservation therapy. There are also genetic profile tests that can be used to predict response to endocrine and adjuvant chemotherapy.

ENDOCRINE AND TARGETED THERAPY

Endocrine therapy is indicated for patients with hormone receptor positive tumors, which account for about 75% of all invasive cancers. Many studies indicate improved overall survival with use of endocrine therapeutic agents such as selective estrogen receptor modulators (SERMs, e.g., tamoxifen) and aromatase inhibitors (AIs, e.g., anastrozole, letrozole). Endocrine therapy is generally used for postmenopausal women and high-risk premenopausal women. In general, for hormone receptor positive disease, postmenopausal women are treated with AIs and premenopausal women are treated with SERMs. Recent evidence has shown additional benefit from treating premenopausal women with ovarian suppression and an AI.

Approximately 15% of invasive cancers are epidermal growth factor receptor 2 (HER2) positive. For these patients (identified by immunohistochemical analysis), treatment with adjuvant trastuzumab and/or pertuzumab, a monoclonal antibody to HER2, has improved survival.

The patient elects to undergo radiation therapy and is treated with hormone therapy in addition to HER2 monoclonal antibody therapy. On surgical follow-up, her incisions are well healed, and she is happy with the cosmetic outcome of her partial mastectomy.

BEYOND THE PEARLS

- Screening for breast cancer in average risk women should begin at age 40 to 50 and continue through age 74.
- Concerning mammographic findings include spiculations, calcifications, distortions, and asymmetries; further biopsy, imaging, or surgery will be based on BI-RADS criteria.
- Regarding axillary anatomy, care is taken for preservation of the long thoracic, thoracodorsal, median and lateral pectoral bundles and intercostobrachial nerves.
- Breast conservation therapy with or without SLNB is used for most DCIS and invasive cancers less than 5 cm.
- Postmastectomy radiation therapy is used for patients with four or more involved axillary lymph nodes, tumor greater than 5 cm, tumors with skin or chest wall involvement, positive margins, or inflammatory breast cancer.
- Adjuvant chemotherapy and endocrine therapy utilized for patients depend on the specific pathologic endocrine receptor and HER2 profile.

Suggested Readings

Bromham, N., Schmidt-Hansen, M., Astin, M., Hasler, E., & Reed, M. W. (2017). *Axillary treatment for operable primary breast cancer, Cochrane Database Syst Rev 1:CD004561.*

Chan, B. K., Wiseberg-Firtell, J. A., Jois, R. H., Jensen, K., & Audisio, R. A. (2015). Localization techniques for guided surgical excision of non-palpable breast lesions. *Cochrane Database Syst Rev.* CD009206.

Darby, S., McGale, P., Correa, C., Taylor, C., Arriagada, R., Clarke, M., et al. (2011). Effect of radiotherapy after breast-conserving surgery on 10-year recurrence and 15-year breast cancer death: meta-analysis of individual patient data for 10,801 women in 17 randomised trials. *Lancet, 378*(9804), 1707–1716.

Giuliano, A. E., Ballman, K. V., McCall, L., Beitsch, P. D., Brennan, M. B., Kelemen, P. R., et al. (2017). Effect of axillary dissection vs no axillary dissection on 10-year overall survival among women with invasive breast cancer and sentinel node metastasis: the ACOSOG Z0011 (Alliance) randomized clinical trial. *JAMA, 10,* 918–926.

von Minckwitz, G., Procter, M., de Azambuja, E., Zardavas, D., Benyunes, M., Viale, G., et al. (2017). Adjuvant pertuzumab and trastuzumab in early HER2-positive breast cancer. *N Engl J Med, 377,* 122–131.

Krag, D. N., Anderson, S. J., Julian, T. B., Brown, A. M., Harlow, S. P., Costantino, J. P., et al. (2010). Sentinel-lymph-node resection compared with conventional axillary-lymph-node dissection in clinically node-negative patients with breast cancer: overall survival findings from the NSABP B-32 randomised phase 3 trial. *Lancet Oncol,* (10), 927–933.

Lakhani, S. R., Ellis, I. O., Schnitt, S. J., Tan, P. H., & van de Vijver, M. J. (Eds.), (2012). *WHO classification of tumours of the breast.* (ed 4). Lyon, France: International Agency for Research on Cancer.

Plitas, H. S. (2014). Axillary dissection. In J. R. Harris, M. E. Lippman, M. Morrow, & C. K. Osborne (Eds.), *Diseases of the breast.* (ed 5, pp. 570–578). Philadelphia: Wolters Kluwer Health.

Sickles, E. A., D'Orsi, C. J., Bassett, L. W., et al. (2013). ACR BI-RADS mammography. In *ACR BI-RADS atlas, breast imaging reporting and data system.* Reston, VA: American College of Radiology.

Siu, A. L. (2016). Screening for breast cancer: U.S. Preventive Services Task Force recommendation statement. *Ann Intern Med, 164*(4), 279–296.

Warner, E., Plewes, D. B., Hill, K. A., Causer, P. A., Zubovits, J. T., Jong, R. A., et al. (2004). Surveillance of BRCA1 and BRCA2 mutation carriers with magnetic resonance imaging, ultrasound, mammography, and clinical breast examination. *JAMA, 292*(11), 1317–1325.

Wolff, A. C., Hicks, D. G., Dowsett, M., McShane, L. M., Allison, K. H., Allred, D. C., et al. (2013). Recommendations for human epidermal growth factor receptor 2 testing in breast cancer: American Society of Clinical Oncology/College of American Pathologists clinical practice guideline update. *J Clin Oncol, 31,* 3997–4013.

CHAPTER 20

Pigmented Skin Lesion in a 58-Year-Old Female

Madalyn Neuwirth ■ Giorgos C. Karakousis

A 58-year-old Caucasian female presents to her physician with a pigmented skin lesion on her right shoulder. She has multiple pigmented nevi of the skin including this lesion; however, she has noticed recent enlargement of this particular lesion with associated itching and intermittent bleeding. Her past medical history is significant only for hypertension, and she denies any family and personal history of cancer. She does state that she has had significant sun exposure as she works as a gardener but that she tries to always wear a hat and sunscreen.

What Is the Differential Diagnosis for a Pigmented Skin Lesion?

There are a number of pathologies that can present as a pigmented skin lesion. The first step is to distinguish between benign and cancerous etiologies. This task is generally approached by assessing the lesion for concerning features, as well as by recognizing typical appearances of common pigmented neoplasms.

BENIGN LESIONS

Common benign lesions are shown in Fig. 20.1.

Seborrheic keratosis is a common noncancerous skin growth that classically has a "stuck-on" appearance. These lesions appear round, are usually elevated, and have a waxy or scaly surface. The color of these lesions ranges from tan to dark brown.

Actinic keratosis or "solar keratosis" is a precancerous skin lesion caused by chronic sun damage. These lesions appear on sun-exposed areas of skin, can be flat or elevated, typically have a rough surface, and can present with a variety of colors, including red, pink, tan, and brown.

Benign melanocytic nevus is a common acquired nevus that appears within the first 6 months to 1 year of life on sun-exposed areas of skin. These lesions reach maximum size in young adulthood and often disappear with advanced age. They are typically small with even pigmentation and smooth borders.

Dysplastic nevi are atypical benign nevi that tend to be larger and more irregular than the common mole, with variations in color, border, and surface texture. These lesions usually occur in sun-exposed areas. Because a small percentage of dysplastic nevi may develop into melanoma, more concern is given to these lesions based on the severity of the dysplasia. The risk of melanoma in dysplastic nevi increases in patients with the number of lesions. Dysplastic nevus syndrome, or familial atypical multiple mole (FAMM) syndrome, is a hereditary cutaneous condition in which patients have more than 100 melanocytic nevi, nevi in atypical locations, and two or more clinically atypical nevi.

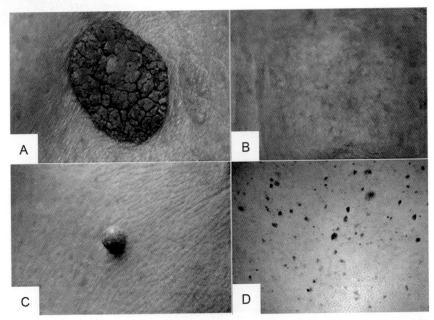

Fig. 20.1   Benign pigmented skin lesions. (A) Seborrheic keratosis. (B) Actinic keratosis. (C) Melanocytic nevi. (D) Dysplastic nevi. (A, from Brinster NK, Liu V, Diwan AH, et al: Seborrheic keratosis. In *Dermatopathology: high-yield pathology,* Philadelphia, 2011, Elsevier. B, from Soyer PH, Rigel DS, McMeniman E: Actinic keratosis, basal cell carcinoma, and squamous cell carcinoma. In Bolognia JL, Schaffer JV, Cerroni L, editors: *Dermatology,* ed 4, Philadelphia, 2018, Elsevier. C, from Luzur B, Bastian BC, Calonje E: Melanocytic nevi. In Calonje E, Brenn T, Lazar A, McKee PH, editors: *McKee's pathology of the skin,* Philadelphia, 2012, Elsevier. D, from Clark LE: Dysplastic nevi, *Surgical Pathology Clinics* 2(3):447–456, 2009.)

CANCEROUS LESIONS

Common cancerous lesions are shown in Fig. 20.2.

Basal cell carcinoma (BCC) is the most common form of skin cancer and arises from basal cells in the basal layer of the epidermis. BCCs typically present as red or pink patches, which can have a shiny or waxy appearance, and occur in skin areas with high cumulative sun exposure.

Squamous cell carcinoma (SCC) is the second most common cause of skin cancer and arises from the superficial squamous cells of the epidermis. SCC is closely related to sun exposure, occurring in areas that have prolonged or chronic exposure to UV light. These lesions can present as pink or brown rough scaly patches on the skin, which may ulcerate or bleed.

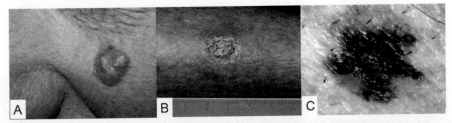

Fig. 20.2   Cancerous skin lesions. (A) Basal cell carcinoma. (B) Squamous cell carcinoma. (C) Malignant melanoma. (A, B, from Bolognia JL, Schaffer JV, Duncan KO, Ko CJ: Actinic keratosis, basal cell carcinoma, and squamous cell carcinomas. In *Dermatology essentials,* Philadelphia, 2014, Elsevier. C, from)

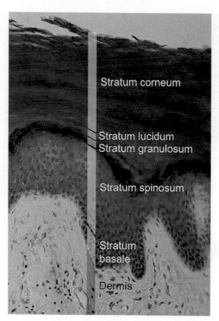

Fig. 20.3 Histologic view of the epidermal strata and the superficial dermis. (From Gantwerker EA, Hom DB: Skin: histology and physiology of wound healing, *Facial Plastic Surg Clin North Am* 19(3):441–453, 2011.)

Malignant melanoma (sometimes referred to as just melanoma) is less common than other skin cancers (accounting for about 1%); however, its incidence increasing, and it is currently the leading cause of mortality due to skin cancer. These tumors arise from the melanocytes, melanin-producing cells in the epidermis. Similar to other skin cancers, melanoma is closely related to sun exposure; other risk factors specific for melanoma include the presence of numerous melanocytic nevi, fair skin, and family history. These lesions are typically black or brown and appear irregular compared with typical benign moles.

There are several other types of rare skin cancers, such as *Merkel cell carcinoma* and *adnexal or sweat gland carcinomas,* that are typically diagnosed after excision and are difficult to diagnose on physical examination alone.

BASIC SCIENCE PEARL (STEP 1)

The skin is composed of multiple cell types, most of which can transform into benign and cancerous lesions (Fig. 20.3). Overall the skin is composed of the epidermis and dermis. The epidermis is a keratinized stratified squamous epithelium and is arranged in strata ordered deep to superficial: basale (most mitotically active), spinosum, granulosum, lucidum, and corneum (completely filled with keratin). The epidermis also contains melanocytes (pigment cells), and Langerhans cells (immune cells). The dermis consists of connective tissue, capillaries, nerve endings, and glands.

What Are the Key Aspects of a Physical Examination in a Patient With a Pigmented Skin Lesion?
Although examination of the lesion of primary concern is paramount, a full physical examination of the patient's skin is also imperative in order to identify any other suspicious lesions and document the presence of benign lesions that may confer subsequent risk of malignancy. Documentation of lesions with photographs is helpful for evaluating any changes in the lesion on subsequent visits.

The lesion and surrounding skin should be inspected for concerning features of a cancerous lesion. This should include the "ABCDE" evaluation for melanoma: **A**symmetry, **B**orders (irregular), **C**olor (uneven distribution), **D**iameter (larger than 6 mm), and **E**volution (change in appearance over time).

Any pigmented lesion should be evaluated for cutaneous/subcutaneous nodules or satellite lesions (less than 2 cm proximity to lesion) or in-transit disease (greater than 2 cm from lesion). These are thought to represent dermal lymphatic metastases. The regional lymph node basins should also be palpated for masses and/or lymphadenopathy. Multiple basins may need to be examined for evidence of regional spread of disease depending on the location of the primary lesion in question (e.g., bilateral axillae for central trunk lesion or low cervical for upper trunk lesions).

What Is the Preferred Method of Diagnosis for Pigmented Skin Lesions?

Physical examination is often all that is required for the diagnosis of benign skin lesions. Patients with skin lesions that are clearly benign can be reassured and instructed in proper skin self-examination and follow up for complete skin examination. Biopsy or excision can be undertaken at the patient's request and/or clinician's judgment, and pathologic evaluation will yield a definitive diagnosis.

Patients with a suspicious lesion should undergo skin biopsy. Punch biopsy or excisional biopsy is superior to the shave biopsy technique because the full thickness of the lesion, which is a major component of staging and surgical management for melanoma, must be assessed with a full thickness biopsy of skin. Shave specimens often have tumor extending to the deep margins of the biopsy, and therefore depth of invasion can be difficult to determine. Punch biopsy may also be useful in evaluating subcutaneous nodules arising in a patient with a history of melanoma. For lymphadenopathy with a history of melanoma or without a primary lesion identified, fine needle aspiration is recommended for initial pathologic assessment of the lymph node.

On physical examination the lesion on her right shoulder is noted to be 8 mm in diameter, with dark brown pigmentation and asymmetric borders; it is slightly raised without gross evidence of ulceration. There is no axillary lymphadenopathy, and a full skin examination does not reveal any other suspicious lesions. A punch biopsy of the lesion is performed. Pathology shows a 0.9 mm malignant melanoma, superficial spreading type with 1 mitosis per high-powered field, and no ulceration.

What Are the Most Common Types of Cutaneous Melanoma?

Most melanomas can be classified into four subtypes: superficial spreading, nodular, lentigo maligna, and acral lentiginous. *Superficial spreading* is the most common subtype, accounting for 70% to 75% of cases, and seen most often in younger patients. It presents as a flat or slightly raised pigmented lesion with a prolonged horizontal growth phase and typically invades deeper layers of the epidermis in later stages. Conversely, *nodular type* melanoma develops a vertical growth phase early on and is usually thicker in appearance with invasion of deeper layers at the time of diagnosis. These tend to be more aggressive lesions overall and are seen more frequently in older patients. *Lentigo maligna* is also commonly seen in the elderly and has a flat appearance similar to the superficial spreading type and arises in chronically exposed areas of skin. *Acral lentiginous* melanoma is a pigmented lesion found in atypical locations, such as under the nail beds, on soles of feet, or palms of hands. These tumors are rare and, because of their abnormal locations, are often diagnosed in later stages, having invaded into the deeper layers of the skin by the time of detection. These occur more commonly in African American and Asian populations.

CLINICAL PEARL (STEPS 2/3)

Amelanotic and desmoplastic melanoma are two less common but potentially aggressive cutaneous melanoma subtypes. Although upward of 95% of melanomas are pigmented lesions, amelanotic melanomas can develop from melanocytic cells but often mimic the appearance of other benign lesions or squamous or basal cell cancers. Desmoplastic melanoma (DM) is a spindle cell variant, which is often amelanotic, and demonstrates variability in presentation and histologic characteristics. Desmoplastic melanomas are often thicker at time of diagnosis but interestingly appear to have a lower predilection for lymphatic metastasis.

What Are the Current Guidelines for Surgical Approach to Malignant Melanoma of the Skin?
The main role of surgery for the primary melanoma lesion is local control. This is accomplished by achieving gross and macroscopic margins in resection of the primary tumor by means of wide local excision. An elliptical incision (to facilitate primary closure without tension) is made that includes the lesion and margins of unaffected skin. Based on randomized trials of recurrence after excision, the requirements for radial gross margins depend on the Breslow thickness for invasive lesions (Table 20.1). Radial margins of 5 mm may be sufficient for the management of melanoma *in situ.*

For high-risk, clinically localized, melanoma lesions, sentinel lymph node biopsy (SNB) may be recommended to assess whether there has been regional dissemination of disease, offering important prognostic and staging information, as well as opportunity for regional control of disease. For intermediate thickness lesions (1.01–4.0 mm), SNB is routinely recommended because the rate of lymph node involvement in this group ranges from approximately 15% to 20%. For thin melanomas (1.0 mm or less), the SNB positivity rate is relatively low (approximately 5%); consequently, sentinel node biopsy is generally only recommended selectively for those lesions with more concerning features, such as thickness 0.76 mm or greater, with mitotic rate greater than 1 per high-power field, or presence of ulceration. If a sentinel lymph node biopsy is positive for metastatic melanoma, patients traditionally undergo completion lymphadenectomy to determine extent of lymphatic involvement, as well as for locoregional control of disease. Recent studies suggesting no survival benefit in patients who undergo lymphadenectomy may cause a shift toward decreasing the rates of patients undergoing this additional surgery. Indeed, with the results of two recent large randomized trials (DECOG and MSLT2), practice patterns are now favoring observation with ultrasound in select patients with a positive sentinel node.

The patient undergoes wide local excision and inguinal sentinel lymph node biopsy using blue dye and a radiotracer. Final pathology shows no residual melanoma, negative margins, and one of three lymph nodes positive (3 mm metastatic focus in the node) for metastatic melanoma. Discussion with the patient results in decision to proceed with completion inguinal lymph node dissection.

TABLE 20.1 ■ Recommended Surgical Excision Margins for Cutaneous Melanoma

Primary Tumor Thickness	Excisional Margin
Melanoma *in situ*	5 mm
< 1.0 mm	1 cm
1.0–2.0 cm	1–2 cm
> 2.0 cm	2 cm

What Is the Relevant Anatomy for a Superficial (Inguinofemoral) Lymphadenectomy?
The primary draining lymphatics of the lower extremity are the inguinal basins, which can be separated into deep and superficial by anatomic location. The superficial nodal basin is bounded primarily by femoral triangle, which includes superiorly the inguinal ligament (although occasionally some nodes may extend more superiorly anterior to the external oblique muscle), medially the adductor longus muscle, and laterally the sartorius muscle. The most cephalad node in the dissection is also known as Cloquet's node. The inguinal nodes are situated deep to the Camper's fascia and superficial to the fascia lata of the thigh and drain into the external iliac lymph nodes. The deep inguinal lymph nodes in the femoral triangle are located posterior to the fascia lata primarily along the femoral vein. The deep or pelvic nodal basin includes the external iliac nodes and the obturator nodes and, when dissected out in conjunction with the superficial nodal basin, is referred to as a radical groin dissection. Typically, a superficial (inguinofemoral) lymphadenectomy is performed in the setting of a positive inguinal sentinel lymph node.

Superficial Inguinal Lymphadenectomy

1. Make an incision inferior to the inguinal ligament or medial to anterior superior iliac spine toward the apex of the femoral triangle.
2. Raise flaps medially and laterally to the adductor longus and sartorius muscles respectively, exposing the contents of the femoral triangle (Fig. 20.4).
3. Identify and excise the femoral lymph node package (medial to both femoral vessels).
4. A sartorius transposition flap may be performed by dividing the muscle at its origin at the anterior superior iliac spine and rotating the muscle medially to cover the exposed femoral vessels.

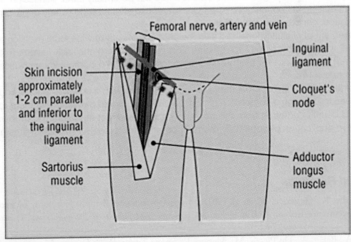

Fig. 20.4 Boundaries of the femoral triangle, and operative approach to superficial lymphadenectomy. (Redrawn from Sharma P, Zargar-Shoshtari K, Spiess PE: Current surgical management of penile cancer, *Curr Probl Cancer.* 2015;39(3):147–157, 2015.)

CLINICAL PEARL (STEPS 2/3)

Cloquet's node (or Rosenmuller's node), named after the French surgeon Jules Cloquet, is the deepest most proximal draining superficial inguinal node whose status may offer predictive value for the status of nodes in the deep pelvic (external iliac/obturator) nodal basin. This node is typically located within the femoral canal and therefore may be important to harvest during superficial inguinal dissections for staging to help in decision making for deep nodal dissection. Other common indications for deep (pelvic) nodal dissection include clinically apparent superficial nodal disease, or microscopic metastases in three or more superficial nodes. Secondary lymphoscintigraphy drainage to the deep nodal basin that has not been sampled in the setting of a positive superficial inguinal sentinel node is another indication for consideration of a deep nodal dissection at time of completion lymphadenectomy.

What Are the Potential Complications of an Inguinal Lymph Node Dissection?

The most common complications associated with superficial inguinal lymphadenectomy include seroma (25%), wound infection (20%), wound dehiscence (15%), skin necrosis (10%), hematoma (5%), and, perhaps most clinically significant, lymphedema (20%–40%). Less common complications include acute postoperative bleeding, deep venous thrombosis, and nerve injury. More recently, experience with minimally invasive inguinal lymphadenectomy has been described by some centers as a technique to further reduce the morbidities associated with this procedure. Of note, superficial and deep inguinal lymphadenectomies are performed at increasingly less frequent rates in the setting of more effective adjuvant therapies.

The patient has no complications related to the lymph node dissection, and there is no tumor seen in any of the excised nodes. She is asked to continue skin self-examinations and to continue preventative measures.

BEYOND THE PEARLS

- Primary cutaneous malignant melanoma is a rare but potentially lethal skin lesion, which has been increasing in frequency in recent years, and can affect a wide variety of patients across age groups, gender, and ethnicities.
- Management of clinically localized skin melanoma consists of wide local excision as well as sentinel lymph node biopsy for staging and prognosis in higher-risk lesions (melanomas >1.0 mm or those <1 mm with concerning features ($\geq$0.76 particularly with ulceration or mitotic rate $\geq$1/mm^2).
- Although the standard approach for melanoma patients with a positive sentinel node biopsy has been to undergo a completion lymphadenectomy, recent data suggest there may be no survival benefit conferred from this approach; this may effect a paradigm shift toward more selective application of potentially morbid operation for patients with SLN metastasis.

Suggested Readings

Baur, J., Mathe, K., Gesierich, A., et al. (2018). Impact of extended lymphadenectomy on morbidity and regional recurrence-free survival in melanoma patients. *The Journal of Dermatological Treatment, 29*(5), 515–521.

Cesmebasi, A., Baker, A., Du Plessis, M., Matusz, P., Shane Tubbs, R., & Loukas, M. (2015). The surgical anatomy of the inguinal lymphatics. *The American Surgeon, 81*(4), 365–369.

Faries, M. B., Thompson, J. F., Cochran, A. J., et al. (2017). Completion dissection or observation for sentinel-node metastasis in melanoma. *The New England Journal of Medicine, 376*(23), 2211–2222.

Gershenwald, J. E., Scolyer, R. A., Hess, K. R., et al. (2017). Melanoma staging: Evidence-based changes in the American Joint Committee on Cancer eighth edition cancer staging manual. *CA: A Cancer Journal for Clinicians, 67*(6), 472–492.

Jakub, J. W., Terando, A. M., Sarnaik, A., et al. (2017). Safety and feasibility of minimally invasive inguinal lymph node dissection in patients with melanoma (SAFE-MILND): Report of a prospective multi-institutional trial. *Annals of Surgery, 265*(1), 192–196.

Madu, M. F., Franke, V., Bruin, M. M., et al. (2017). Immediate completion lymph node dissection in stage IIIA melanoma does not provide significant additional staging information beyond EORTC SN tumour burden criteria. *European Journal of Cancer, 87*, 212–215.

Thomson, D. R., Rughani, M. G., Kuo, R., & Cassell, O. C. S. (2017). Sentinel node biopsy status is strongly predictive of survival in cutaneous melanoma: Extended follow-up of Oxford patients from 1998 to 2014. *Journal of Plastic, Reconstructive & Aesthetic Surgery: JPRAS, 70*(10), 1397–1403.

Verstijnen, J., Damude, S., Hoekstra, H. J., et al. (2017). Practice variation in sentinel lymph node biopsy for melanoma patients in different geographical regions in the Netherlands. *Surgical Oncology, 26*(4), 431–437.

CHAPTER 21

Dysphagia in a 62-Year-Old Male

Courtney L. Devin ■ Michael J. Pucci

A 62-year-old man presents to the gastroenterology clinic after a referral from his primary care physician with a 3-month history of progressive dysphagia and a 10-pound weight loss. He reports heartburn for many years that has been treated with over-the-counter antacids and a proton pump inhibitor. He also has a history of hypertension that is medically managed. He denies abdominal pain, hematemesis, or melena. His social history is significant for a 25 pack/year smoking history, though he quit over 10 years ago, and infrequent alcohol use. His physical examination is unremarkable, showing no evidence of lymphadenopathy.

What Is the Differential Diagnosis for Dysphagia?

The differential diagnosis for dysphagia includes benign and malignant causes. Benign causes of dysphagia in an adult can be divided into esophageal obstruction and esophageal motility disorders. Benign causes of esophageal obstruction include peptic strictures, Schatzki ring, benign neoplasms, and foreign body. Esophageal motility disorders include achalasia, diffuse esophageal spasm, hypercontractile esophagus, ineffective esophageal motility, and scleroderma. Benign causes of dysphagia are detailed in Case 9. Importantly, a primary concern with new-onset dysphagia in an adult who is experiencing weight loss is esophageal carcinoma.

BASIC SCIENCE PEARL (STEP 1)

The distal esophagus is lined with squamous epithelium. Chronic reflux disease may result in a histologic change of the esophageal mucosa to a columnar Barrett's metaplasia (Fig. 21.1), and further exposure to reflux can result in dysplasia and ultimately the development of adenocarcinoma. Barrett's esophagus has a 30- to 40-fold increased risk of progressing to adenocarcinoma.

CLINICAL PEARL (STEP 2/3)

Squamous cell carcinoma, which is the most common type worldwide, can arise anywhere along the length of the esophagus, as it arises from native squamous epithelium and not from metaplastic esophageal mucosa. Risk factors for squamous carcinoma include smoking, alcohol use, consumption of hot beverages, and poor nutrition.

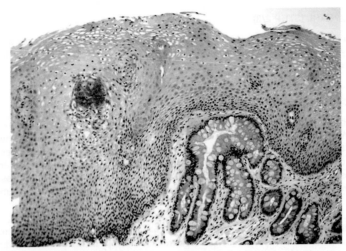

Fig. 21.1 Squamous epithelium of the esophagus overlying developing metaplasia in the crypts *(bottom right)* consistent with early Barrett's metaplasia. (From Lisovsky M, Srivastava A: Barrett esophagus: evolving concepts in diagnosis and neoplastic progression, *Surg Pathol Clin* Sep;6(3):475–496, 2013. doi: 10.1016/j. path.2013.05.002. Epub 2013 Aug 6.)

What Are the Primary Physical Examination Techniques and Workup to Evaluate a Suspected Diagnosis of Esophageal Cancer?

A careful physical examination should be performed. Oftentimes, early-stage tumors may have no physical examination abnormalities or secondary signs related to the obstruction such as dehydration or signs of recent weight loss. More advanced disease states may show evidence of cachexia, cervical and supraclavicular lymph nodes, including an enlarged left supraclavicular (Virchow's) lymph node, and nodular hepatomegaly from hepatic metastases.

Laboratory studies may show nonspecific findings such as anemia due to chronic gastrointestinal (GI) bleeding, hypoalbuminemia from impaired nutrition, and elevated liver enzymes from hepatic metastases. New-onset dysphagia should be evaluated with a barium swallow initially. This esophagram may show an irregular mucosal narrowing or ulceration. The classic "apple core" filling defect may be seen if there is a symmetric, circumferential narrowing. More often, though, an asymmetric, infiltrative bulge is seen in the area of the esophagus affected by the tumor. (Note that a barium swallow may show no evidence of a discrete tumor and may be suggestive of a motility disorder.) In this case an endoscopy should be performed, and multiple biopsies should be performed on any lesion or abnormality noted. The endoscopist should note the location of the tumor relative to the incisors and esophagogastric junction, the length of the tumor, and the degree of obstruction caused by the tumor.

Once the diagnosis of esophageal carcinoma has been established, staging of the disease is needed to determine treatment options and prognosis. A computed tomography (CT) of the chest and abdomen helps define the extent of the tumor and identify any obvious metastatic disease to mediastinal or upper abdominal lymph nodes or distant organs. A positron emission tomography (PET) scan supplements a CT scan and can help determine whether the tumor is localized or has distant metastatic disease. If there is no evidence of metastatic disease, an esophageal endoscopic ultrasonography (EUS) should be performed to define the depth of the intramural tumor invasion as well as the involvement of paraesophageal and upper abdominal lymph nodes.

CLINICAL PEARL (STEP 2/3)

Dysphagia in an adult must always be fully evaluated with endoscopy. Additional workup with manometry, barium esophagram, gastric-emptying study, and pH evaluation can be added based on clinical scenario and symptoms.

CLINICAL PEARL (STEP 2/3)

The incidence of esophageal carcinoma in the United States is approximately 17,000 new cases per year. Worldwide, squamous cell carcinoma is the most common histologic type whereas in the United States, adenocarcinoma has a higher incidence. The incidence in adenocarcinoma has increased dramatically in recent years and has risen faster than any other cancer in the United States. This is likely caused by the increased prevalence of obesity and chronic gastroesophageal reflux in Americans. There has been an associated decline in squamous cell carcinoma.

The patient undergoes a barium swallow (Fig. 21.2) that demonstrates a circumferential narrowing in the distal third of the esophagus. Esophagogastroduodenoscopy is then performed, which identifies a mass in the distal esophagus that is biopsied. On pathologic evaluation, the biopsy is

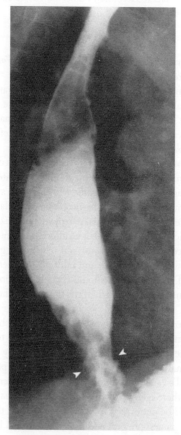

Fig. 21.2 Barium swallow demonstrating circumferential narrowing in the distal third of the esophagus *(arrows)*. (From Meyerhardt JA, Kulke MH, Turner JR: Cancer of the gastrointestinal tract and neuroendocrine tumors. In *Atlas of Diagnostic Oncology*, Philadelphia, 2010, Elsevier, pp 169–232.)

consistent with esophageal adenocarcinoma. Imaging using CT and PET scans and endoscopic ultrasound does not identify any sites of local invasion beyond the esophageal wall, no evidence of distant metastasis, and no abnormally enlarged lymph nodes. The patient is referred to an esophageal surgeon to discuss options for resection.

How Is Esophageal Cancer Staged and How Does Staging Affect Treatment Nodalities?

Staging of esophageal cancer is based on a standard tumor, lymph node, and metastasis (TNM) system in which evaluation of the depth of tumor invasion into the esophageal wall or beyond, the presence of affected regional lymph nodes, and distant metastases (Fig. 21.3) are considered. Additionally, the degree of cellular differentiation, known as grade, also affects the overall stage of the cancer.

The cancer stage directly influences the initial treatment options in patients with esophageal cancer. Although the algorithm is ever changing, with more patients receiving neoadjuvant chemoradiation therapy, there is still a role for upfront surgical resection. In patients with early-stage IA disease or who may not tolerate neoadjuvant treatment, an esophagectomy is recommended. For those patients who are 75 years and younger with stage IB through III tumors, neoadjuvant chemoradiation therapy is recommended with definitive surgical resection after completion of therapy. Patients with stage IV disease are not candidates for esophagectomy. There is generally no role for resection for palliation in esophageal cancer; however, either surgical enteral access or endoscopic esophageal stenting may help with nutrition requirements.

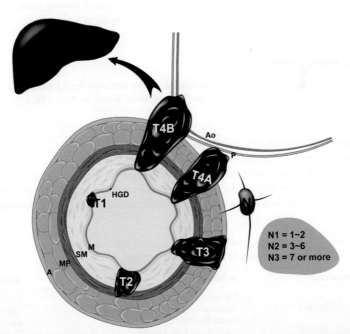

Fig. 21.3 Staging of esophageal adenocarcinoma. The tumor stage is determined by the depth of invasion of the esophageal wall and local extension. (HGD, high grade dysplasia; M, mucosa; SM, submucosa; MP, muscularis propria; A, adventitia; P, pleura; Ao, aorta). (From Shin KE, Lee KS, Choi JY, et al: Esophageal malignancy and staging, *Semin Roentgenol* 48(4):344–353, 2013.)

BASIC SCIENCE PEARL (STEP 1/2/3)

The lymphatic drainage from the proximal third of the esophagus drains into the deep cervical lymph nodes and ultimately into the thoracic duct. The lymphatics from the middle third of the esophagus drain into the superior and posterior mediastinal nodes. From the distal third of the esophagus the lymphatics follow the left gastric artery to the gastric and celiac lymph nodes. The extensive interconnections among the three regions of lymph drainage and the bidirectional lymph flow are responsible for the spread of malignancy from the lower esophagus to the upper esophagus.

What Are the Surgical Approaches Used for Resecting Esophageal Cancers?

There are several approaches to esophageal resection. The specific approach must be individualized to the patient, to the location of disease, and to the surgeon's experience and preference. The different approaches to esophagectomy include: transhiatal esophagectomy; combined abdominal and right transthoracic esophagectomy with intrathoracic anastomosis (Ivor Lewis); resection via combined abdominal, right transthoracic, and left neck incision with cervical anastomosis (McKeown); and large left thoracoabdominal resection (Table 21.1). All of these can be performed via any combination of laparoscopic and thoracoscopic minimally invasive techniques based on the surgeon's experience and preference. Regardless of the approach, the goal of surgical resection is to remove the carcinoma and reestablish gastrointestinal continuity. The latter goal is typically accomplished by utilizing a portion of the stomach pulled into the chest and anastomosed to the proximal esophageal resection margin. If the stomach is not able to reach, colon can be used as a conduit. Additionally, an en bloc lymphadenectomy should be included with the esophageal specimen with the goal to include all surrounding lymphatic tissue from the carina to the celiac axis.

Esophagectomy is also frequently accompanied by a pyloroplasty or pyloromyotomy due to inadvertent vagotomy that can result in gastric outlet obstruction. A feeding jejunostomy tube is placed for postoperative enteral nutrition if not already performed as a preoperative measure.

CLINICAL PEARL (STEP 2/3)

It is imperative to preserve the right gastroepiploic artery and vein during esophagectomy and gastric conduit creation as this will likely be the only blood supply to the conduit.

What Are the Contraindications to Surgical Resection?

Contraindications to surgical resection of esophageal carcinoma include: biopsy-proven stage IV (distant metastatic) disease; intraoperative stage IV (distant metastatic) disease either found on EGD, diagnostic laparoscopy, or during open surgical resection; tracheobronchial invasion by the tumor proven at bronchoscopy; and evidence of aortic invasion. In addition, given the potential

TABLE 21.1 ■ Naming and Types of Esophageal Resections

Surgical Approach	Incisions	Anastomosis
Ivor Lewis	Abdomen, right thoracotomy	Thoracic
Three-hole (McKeown)	Abdomen, right thoracotomy, left neck	Cervical
Transhiatal	Abdomen, left neck	Cervical
Left thoracoabdominal	Large thoracoabdominal	Thoracic

morbidity and adverse effect on quality of life associated with recovery from an esophagectomy, the procedure may be contraindicated in a patient who shows poor surgical fitness with regard to age, frailty, nutritional status, and comorbidities. The goal of treatment in patients who are considered poor surgical candidates secondary to functional status or who have distant metastatic disease at the time of diagnosis is palliation of current symptoms and prevention of potential complications. Palliative treatment is individualized to the patient's symptoms, extent of disease process, and goals of care. Options include supportive care for symptom control, palliative chemotherapy or radiation, esophageal stent placement for dysphagia, and enteral nutrition.

What Are the Potential Complications of Esophagectomy?

As with any large gastrointestinal operation, there are many complications possible and they must be carefully assessed for in order to salvage patients. Aspiration from conduit delay/dysfunction and pneumonia commonly occur, and thus postoperative pain control and aggressive pulmonary toilet with postoperative pain control are essential. Atrial fibrillation may commonly occur on postoperative days 2 through 5, requiring rate control to avoid decreasing perfusion to the gastric conduit. Anastomotic leak is one of the most feared complications and will typically manifest itself as new-onset fever, tachycardia, and leukocytosis, and may first manifest as septic shock. It is generally managed with antibiotics and appropriate drainage. Chyle leaks, occurring by injury or ineffective ligation of the thoracic duct or its branches, are identified by milky drain output, typically when feeding starts. Drain outputs of less than 500 mL per day can be managed with total parenteral nutrition and NPO status. Chyle leaks with greater than 1 L per day typically require surgical exploration of the thoracic cavity to ligate the thoracic duct. Additional complications include myocardial infarction, gastric emptying problems, and laryngeal nerve dysfunction secondary to injury.

CLINICAL PEARL (STEP 2/3)

Most esophageal cancer recurrences occur within 12 to 18 months, and more than 90% by 3 years. Surveillance should include clinical follow-up every 3 to 4 months for the first 2 years, every 6 months up to 5 years, and then annually. CT is the preferred imaging for detecting recurrence after an esophagectomy.

The surgeon discusses with the patient and his wife that due to the low stage of his cancer, he is a candidate for immediate surgical resection. After informed consent is obtained, the patient is taken to the operating room and undergoes an Ivor Lewis esophagectomy and feeding jejunostomy placement. There are no intraoperative complications, and he is extubated in the operating room. The patient does well postoperatively and tolerates jejunostomy feeds at goal. A barium swallow on postoperative day 5 demonstrates no anastomotic leak and good gastric emptying. The patient is started on liquids, his diet is advanced and he is discharged to home on postoperative day 7. He is set up with follow-up with the surgeon and oncology team to discuss final pathology and a plan for adjuvant therapy and surveillance.

BEYOND THE PEARLS

- Dysphagia may be due to benign and malignant conditions, and a full workup is essential to determine the etiology of a patient's dysphagia.
- Barium swallow and esophagogastroduodenoscopy are mainstay modalities in the workup of patients with dysphagia.

- Squamous esophageal cancer is most common worldwide, but adenocarcinoma is most common in the Western world.

- Neoadjuvant chemoradiotherapy is standard of care for most resectable and potentially resectable esophageal cancers, with the exception of early-stage disease and those patients with a contraindication to chemoradiation therapy.
- There are many different approaches to an esophagectomy, and the appropriate approach should be tailored to the patient presentation and the surgeon's experience.
- Anastomotic leak is one of the most feared complications after esophagectomy.

Suggested Readings

Cunningham, D., Allum, W. H., Stenning, S. P., et al. (2006). Perioperative chemotherapy versus surgery alone for resectable gastroesophageal cancer. *N Engl J Med, 355*, 11–20.

Jones, D. R. (2013). Minimally invasive Ivor Lewis esophagectomy. *Oper Tech Thorac Cardiovasc Surg, 18*, 254–263.

Luketich, J. D., Pennathur, A., Awais, O., et al. (2012). Outcomes after minimally invasive esophagectomy: Review of over 1000 patients. *Ann Surg, 256*, 95–103.

Reed, C. E. (2009). Technique of open Ivor Lewis esophagectomy. *Oper Tech Thorac Cardiovasc Surg, 14*, 160–175.

van Hagen, P., Hulshof, M. C., van Lanschot, J. J., Steyerberg, E. W., van Berge Henegouwen, M. I., Wijnhoven, B. P., et al. (2012). Preoperative chemoradiotherapy for esophageal or junctional cancer. *N Engl J Med, 366*(22), 2074–2084.

CHAPTER 22

Thyroid Nodule in a 48-Year-Old Female

Ujwal Yanala ▪ Abbey Fingeret

A 48-year-old female with a past medical history of well-controlled diabetes and hypertension presents to the surgery clinic after a thyroid nodule was incidentally found on a recent CT scan obtained during a motor vehicle accident workup. She states that she had not previously noticed the nodule and that she cannot feel it when she palpates her neck. She denies any symptoms of cold or heat intolerance, unintended weight loss or gain. She also denies any radiation exposure and family and personal history of cancer.

What Are the Important Anatomic and Physiologic Considerations of the Thyroid Gland?

Anatomy The thyroid gland is found in the neck. It is shaped like a shield and garners its name from the Greek word for shield, *thyros*. The thyroid gland lies in the neck anterior to the trachea and posterior to the platysma muscle and is comprised of two lobes connected by the thyroid isthmus at approximately the second tracheal ring. The thyroid is supplied by two main arteries: the superior thyroid artery is the first branch of the external carotid artery, and the inferior thyroid artery is a branch of the thyrocervical trunk that arises from the subclavian artery. Venous drainage occurs through the superior, middle, and inferior thyroid veins (Fig. 22.1). The thyroid gland is covered anteriorly by the skin, subcutaneous fat, and platysma muscle and anterolaterally by the sternocleidomastoid, sternohyoid, and sternothyroid muscles.

The thyroid gland is closely associated with the parathyroid glands (see Chapter 23). The thyroid gland is also closely associated with two branches of the vagus nerve: the external branch of the superior laryngeal nerve (EBSLN) and the recurrent laryngeal nerve (RLN). The EBSLN courses from the vagus in the carotid sheath medially near the upper pole of the thyroid gland where it enters and innervates the cricothyroid muscle that controls voice pitch and projection. The RLNs supply all of the intrinsic muscles of the larynx, with the exception of the cricothyroid muscle, including the posterior cricoarytenoid muscles, the only muscles that can open the vocal cords. They also provide sensation of the larynx inferior to the vocal cords. The left RLN recurs around the arch of the aorta whereas the right recurs around the subclavian artery.

PHYSIOLOGY

The primary function of the thyroid gland is to produce thyroid hormone, which regulates the basal metabolic rate. The thyroid gland has two distinct groups of hormone-producing cells. Follicular cells produce, store, and release thyroxine (T4) and triiodothyronine (T3). Additionally, the parafollicular C cells of the thyroid secrete calcitonin, a hormone that has a minor role in maintaining calcium homeostasis.

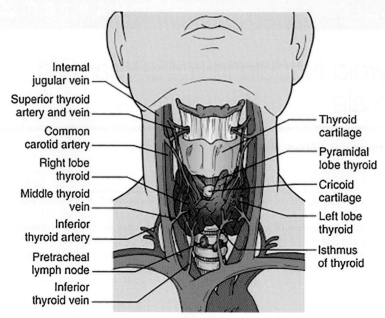

Internal jugular vein
Superior thyroid artery and vein
Common carotid artery
Right lobe thyroid
Middle thyroid vein
Inferior thyroid artery
Pretracheal lymph node
Inferior thyroid vein

Thyroid cartilage
Pyramidal lobe thyroid
Cricoid cartilage
Left lobe thyroid
Isthmus of thyroid

Fig. 22.1   Thyroid vascular anatomy. (Ahmadi S, Fish S: Thyroid gland. Ch 32. In Soni NJ, Arntfield R, Kory R (eds): *Point-of-Care Ultrasound*. Philadelphia: Elsevier, 2015, p. 254.)

Follicular cells actively uptake iodide from the circulation using a sodium-iodine transporter, which is the rate-limiting step in thyroid hormone synthesis. The tyrosine residues of thyroglobulin are iodinated forming monoiodotyrosine (MIT) and diiodotyrosine (DIT), which then couple to form the iodothyronines T3 (MIT + DIT) and T4 (DIT + DIT). This iodinated thyroglobulin is the storage form of the thyroid hormones that are kept in the follicle (Fig. 22.2) and can be hydrolyzed to the active forms T3 and T4, which are then released into the circulation. The majority of the circulating hormone is T4 (roughly 80%), but T3, which is generated by the peripheral conversion of T4 to T3, is the most active form of thyroid hormone. Every nucleated cell in the body has receptors for thyroid hormone, and thus its effects are ubiquitous.

Follicular cell function is regulated by thyroid-stimulating hormone (TSH, or thyrotropin), which is secreted by the anterior pituitary and stimulates the thyroid to release T3 and T4. TSH also stimulates the cell to increase the means of producing thyroid hormones, which includes increasing both thyroglobulin synthesis and iodide transport efficiency. TSH production, in turn, is controlled by thyrotropin-releasing hormone (TRH), which is secreted by the hypothalamus into the hypothalamic-pituitary portal venous system and increases TSH release. There is a negative feedback system whereby excessive concentrations of T3 and T4 decrease the secretion of TSH and TRH.

The other hormone-producing cells in the thyroid, the parafollicular C cells, are stimulated by high serum calcium levels to secrete the hormone calcitonin, which inhibits osteoclast activity, thus decreasing the calcium level. Calcitonin secretion is not primarily responsible for regulating serum calcium levels. Its function probably is to protect the skeleton from excessive scavenging during times of high calcium demand such as growth, pregnancy, or lactation. The absence of calcitonin production after total thyroidectomy does not have a physiologic effect.

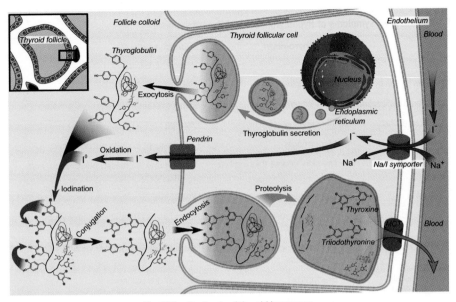

Fig. 22.2   Synthesis of thyroid hormones.

In embryology, the thyroid gland begins as a tissue ridge on the floor of the pharynx at the base of what will become the tongue. This endodermal thickening grows caudally as the thyroglossal duct into the neck, passing ventral to the embryonic hyoid bone and thyroid cartilage. The duct disappears by the 50th day of gestation but may persist anywhere along its migratory pathway as the pyramidal lobe of the thyroid, which is found in up to 50% of adults, or as a thyroglossal duct cyst.

What Are the Important Components Within the History and Physical Examination for Evaluation of a Thyroid Nodule?

The evaluation of a patient with a thyroid nodule begins with a complete history and physical examination focusing on symptoms of hyper- or hypothyroidism, historical risk factors, local or compressive symptoms, and lymphadenopathy. Risk factors for thyroid carcinoma include a history of ionizing radiation to the head and neck, exposure to radiation from nuclear fallout, familial thyroid carcinoma, or syndromes associated with thyroid carcinoma including Cowden's disease, familial adenomatous polyposis (FAP), Carney complex, Werner syndrome, or multiple endocrine neoplasia (MEN) 2. Compressive symptoms may include dysphagia, globus sensation, throat clearing or coughing, dyspnea, or neck pressure especially when supine or arms extended. Local symptoms may include voice change with breathless hoarseness or lymphadenopathy. Often patients are asymptomatic. A complete history should also include relevant age- and sex-related malignancy screening. Assessment for euthyroid status should include evaluation for musculoskeletal, gastrointestinal, temperature tolerance, menstrual, integumentary, neurologic, and cardiovascular complaints (Table 22.1).

TABLE 22.1 ■ Symptoms of Hypothyroidism and Hyperthyroidism

	Hypothyroidism	Hyperthyroidism
General	Fatigue	Tremors, irritability
Weight	Weight gain	Weight loss
Temperature tolerance	Cold intolerance	Heat intolerance
Gastrointestinal	Constipation	Diarrhea
Menstruation	Menorrhagia	Less frequent periods with less flow
Integumentary	Dry skin, coarse thinning hair	Thinning skin, increased perspiration, and brittle hair
Weight	Weight gain	Weight loss
Neurologic	Depression, difficulty concentrating	Nervousness, irritability, restlessness, insomnia
Musculoskeletal	Muscle cramps, muscle weakness	Muscular weakness and tremor
Cardiovascular	Bradycardia	Tachycardia, palpitations

Physical examination should start with visual inspection and proceed to careful palpation. The thyroid gland should be examined at rest and with swallowing. Palpable nodules should be characterized by their texture, mobility, and borders. A full cervical lymph node examination should be performed. If the patient exhibits signs of symptoms of voice change, perform a vocal fold examination with mirror or flexible fiberoptic laryngoscopy to assess vocal fold mobility.

What Is the Differential Diagnosis of a Thyroid Nodule?
A thyroid nodule is a discrete lesion within the thyroid gland that is radiographically distinct from the surrounding thyroid parenchyma. Some palpable lesions may not correspond to a radiographically distinct region of the thyroid gland by ultrasonography and do not meet the definition of thyroid nodule. Other nodules may be nonpalpable and detected incidentally on imaging.

A thyroid nodule can be broadly classified in two ways: benign or malignant, and "hot" or "cold." Table 22.2 describes the most common diagnoses grouped as benign or malignant; benign lesions are more common than malignant lesions. Classifying lesions as hot or cold refers to whether the lesion is functioning or not and is so named for the ability to detect radioactive iodine uptake within the lesion. Malignancies are more likely to be cold lesions and do not typically cause hyperthyroidism.

What Is the Workup of a Thyroid Nodule?
The evaluation of a thyroid nodule begins with a serum TSH assay to determine thyroid function and ultrasonography of the thyroid gland and cervical lymph nodes. If the TSH is suppressed or elevated, follow up testing with free T3 and free T4 levels should be obtained. If the TSH is suppressed, the workup should proceed with radioactive iodine uptake scanning to determine whether the nodule is hyperfunctioning. Thyroid ultrasound is useful to characterize the thyroid parenchyma and gland size as well as thyroid nodules, including the number, size, echogenicity, vascularity, and features of thyroid nodules, including composition (cystic, solid or mixed structure, wide or tall shape, margins) and presence of microcalcifications. Ultrasound can identify suspicious

TABLE 22.2 ■ Thyroid Pathologies That May Present as a Solitary Nodule and Important Associated History or Symptoms

Benign

Adenoma	Follicular more common than papillary; may have potential for microinvasion
Hyperplastic nodule	Highly cellular; may be congenital
Thyroid cyst	Fluid-filled with epithelial lining; may harbor a malignancy
Thyroiditis	Goiter formation as a result of inflammation

Malignant

Papillary	Most common; metastasizes to lymph nodes
Follicular	Hematogenous metastasis
Medullary	Arises from C cells; associated with MEN 2A and MEN 2B
Anaplastic	Rare; undifferentiated and aggressive
Metastatic	Rare

TABLE 22.3 ■ The Bethesda System for Reporting Thyroid Cytopathology and Recommended Clinical Management

Diagnostic Category	Rate of Malignancy	Usual Management
I: Nondiagnostic or unsatisfactory	5%–10%	Repeat FNA
II: Benign	0%–3%	Clinical follow up
III: Atypia of undetermined significance (AUS) or follicular lesion of undetermined significance (FLUS)	10%–30%	Repeat FNA, molecular testing, or surgical lobectomy
IV: Follicular neoplasm (FN), suspicious for follicular neoplasm (SFN) or Hürthle cell neoplasm (HCN)	25%–40%	
V: Suspicious for malignancy	50%–75%	Surgical lobectomy or total thyroidectomy
VI: Malignant	97%–99%	

lymphadenopathy in the central or lateral neck regions. Fine-needle aspiration biopsy (FNA) is performed based on the sonographic features of the thyroid nodule and the corresponding risk of malignancy. Table 22.3 outlines the Bethesda reporting guidelines for thyroid FNA results and the associated risk of malignancy. It is important to note that FNA is not able to distinguish between benign and malignant follicular neoplasms when the results reveal high follicular cellularity, so surgical management may be necessary.

Because the incidence of malignancy in toxic nodules is low and biopsy of toxic nodules can precipitate thyrotoxicosis, toxic nodules should be treated with surgical excision—either thyroid lobectomy or total thyroidectomy, depending on the multiplicity and location of toxic nodule(s).

The patient undergoes laboratory analyses that reveal a normal TSH. She also has a thyroid ultrasound performed, which reveals a hypoechoic nodule in the right lobe of her thyroid (Fig. 22.3). A fine-needle aspiration is performed of the lesion and is sent for pathologic analysis, which is consistent with a follicular neoplasm. She discusses these results with her surgeon, and after they review the risks and benefits of surgery, the patient consents to undergo a right thyroid lobectomy with the possibility of converting to a total thyroidectomy.

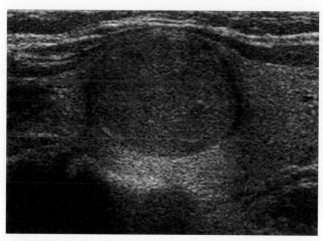

Fig. 22.3 Thyroid ultrasound demonstrating a hypoechoic nodule. (From Desser TS, Kamaya A: Ultrasound of thyroid nodules, *Neuroimaging Clin North Am* 18(3):463–478, 2008.)

CLINICAL PEARL (STEPS 2/3)

It is important to remember that follicular cancers of the thyroid spread to distant sites hematogenously, whereas papillary cancers spread to lymph nodes.

What Are the Management Options for Patients With Thyroid Nodules?

Management of a patient with a thyroid nodule depends on both factors related to the nodule (e.g., pathology on biopsy as outlined in Table 22.3, presence of compressive symptoms) and patient (e.g., operative risk, thyroid cancer risk factors). Benign and asymptomatic lesions in low-risk patients should be observed. Surgical options for treating benign symptomatic nodules or those that are malignant on FNA biopsy include thyroid lobectomy, total thyroidectomy, and total thyroidectomy with lymph node dissection. The extent of surgery is dictated by multiplicity and location of nodules, current thyroid function, operative risk, and patient preference. Patients with nodules with repeated nondiagnostic FNAs or suspicious molecular testing results may also undergo operative management.

The goal of surgical treatment of malignant lesions is to remove the primary tumor and clinically significant lymph node metastases. Although some thyroid cancers can be treated with lobectomy, those larger than 4 cm, cancers with high-risk features, bilateral thyroid nodules, hypothyroid patients, or those with clinically significant lymph node metastases benefit from total thyroidectomy. Adjuvant therapy with radioactive iodine is indicated for high-risk tumors, with the possibility of the addition of radiation and/or chemotherapy.

How Is Thyroid Cancer Staged?

Thyroid cancer staging is unique because it is dependent on whether the cancer is well differentiated or anaplastic and it includes age at diagnosis in the staging algorithm. For example, all patients under the age of 55 years without distant metastases have stage 1 disease and those with distant metastases have stage 2 disease, regardless of tumor or nodal stage. For patients older than 55, the staging for well-differentiated thyroid cancer follows a more traditional tumor, node, metastasis (TNM) staging algorithm. This staging is based on the excellent overall prognosis and survival for well-differentiated thyroid cancer.

What Are the Potential Complications of Thyroid Surgery?

The extent of surgery and the experience of the surgeon both play important roles in determining the risk of surgical complications. Due to the operative location in the neck, complications from thyroid surgery must be taken seriously in order to avoid respiratory compromise. The most concerning complication of thyroid surgery is recurrent laryngeal nerve injury that when unilateral causes hoarseness and when bilateral causes airway obstruction requiring tracheostomy. Bleeding in the operative site can cause hematoma, which, if rapidly expanding, can lead to compression on surrounding structures including the trachea. Hematomas must be taken seriously and often require reoperation. Hypoparathyroidism causing hypocalcemia is also possible, so patients must be assessed for tetany and paresthesias in the post-operative period.

The patient undergoes right thyroid lobectomy without any complications. No suspicious lymph nodes are palpated intraoperatively. She has no alterations in her serum calcium and experiences no hoarseness of her voice and only minimal neck swelling. She is discharged home the first postoperative day and presents one week later to review her pathology. Her surgeon discusses that the lesion was consistent with a benign follicular adenoma and that she requires no further treatment. Additionally, her TSH remains normal at this visit, and she requires no thyroid hormone supplementation.

Suggested Readings

Cibas, E. S., & Ali, S. Z. (2017). The 2017 Bethesda system for reporting thyroid cytopathology. *Thyroid, 27* (11), 1341–1346.

Haugen, B. R., Alexander, E. K., Bible, K. C., et al. (2015). American Thyroid Association management guidelines for adult patients with thyroid nodules and differentiated thyroid cancer: The American Thyroid Association guidelines task force on thyroid nodules and differentiated thyroid cancer. *Thyroid, 26*(1), 1–133.

Remonti, L. R., Kramer, C. K., Leitao, C. B., & Pinto, L. C. (2015). Thyroid ultrasound features and risk of carcinoma: A systematic review and meta-analysis of observational studies. *Thyroid, 25*(5), 538–550.

Yip, L., & Sosa, J. A. (2016). Molecular-directed treatment of differentiated thyroid cancer: Advances in diagnosis and treatment. *JAMA Surg, 151*(7), 663–670.

CHAPTER 23

Hypercalcemia in a 56-Year-Old Female

Michael Kochis ▪ Roy Phitayakorn

A 56-year-old female with a history of kidney stones presents to her primary care physician for an annual physical examination. She has no complaints, and there have been no changes in her health in the previous year, including having a normal mammogram and normal colonoscopy. There are no issues identified on physical examination, but she is found to have an elevated total serum calcium to 11.3 mg/dL on laboratory analysis.

What Are the Main Mediators of Calcium Homeostasis?

Over 98% of the body's total calcium is stored in bones. Of the approximately 1% of calcium that circulates in the body, half is bound to proteins (albumin) or ions (phosphate), whereas the other half is unbound in its ionized form. Only this "free" ionized calcium exerts physiologic effects. The free serum calcium level is usually tightly controlled between 8 and 10 mg/dL. It is primarily regulated by parathyroid hormone (PTH) and vitamin D.

The parathyroids are four pea-sized glands located posteriorly on the thyroid gland's lateral lobes (Fig. 23.1). Parathyroid chief cells produce PTH, which acts on the bones, kidneys, and intestines to increase calcium levels in the body (Fig. 23.2). In addition to those mechanisms, PTH also increases phosphate release from bones and absorption from the gastrointestinal tract. Because calcium and phosphate form a complex in the serum, PTH's effect on those tissues does not affect free calcium concentrations. It is PTH's unique effect of decreasing phosphate reabsorption in the kidneys that allows free serum calcium levels to rise.

Finally, thyroid parafollicular cells (or simply "C cells") produce a hormone called calcitonin that functions to decrease calcium levels. It does not play a significant role in routine calcium homeostasis.

How Is Parathyroid Hormone Secretion Regulated?

PTH secretion is normally regulated on a minute-to-minute scale via negative feedback from the parathyroid cells' calcium sensing receptor (CaSR). Low levels of free calcium in the blood result in reduced CaSR stimulation and increased PTH secretion. In the longer term, PTH secretion can be increased via mRNA upregulation and even parathyroid cellular hyperplasia.

Gain-of-function mutations result in constitutive activation of CaSR and reduced PTH secretion, even in low calcium states. On the other hand, inactivating CaSR mutations may lead to PTH secretion even in the presence of high free serum calcium. Such mutations are a cause of the condition familial hypocalciuric hypercalcemia.

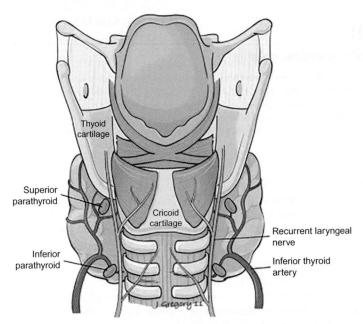

Fig. 23.1 Posterior schematic of the neck revealing the normal location of the parathyroid glands, as well as the recurrent laryngeal nerve and inferior thyroid artery in close proximity. (Redrawn from Policeni BA, Smoker WRK, Reede DL: Anatomy and embryology of the thyroid and parathyroid glands, *Semin Ultrasound CT MRI* 33;104–114, 2012.)

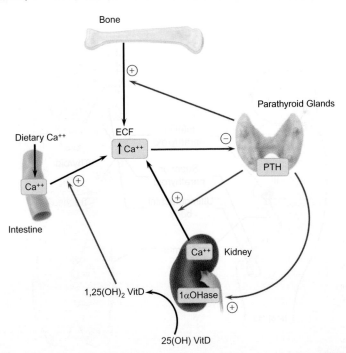

Fig. 23.2 PTH's effect on extracellular fluid (ECF) calcium is mediated through the bones, kidneys, and intestines. In bones, PTH increases osteoclastic activity, which releases calcium. In the kidneys, PTH increases the reabsorption of calcium in the distal tubule. A second function of PTH in the kidney is to increase transcription of 1-alpha hydroxylase. This enzyme converts a vitamin D precursor, 25-OH-vitamin D, into its active form, 1,25-OH_2-vitamin D (also called calcitriol). Calcitriol increases calcium absorption in the gut. High levels of calcium in the blood decrease PTH secretion. (Adapted from Thakker R. (2016). The parathyroid glands, hypercalcemia and hypocalcemia. In *Goldman-Cecil medicine,* 25th ed., pp. 1649–1661. Philadelphia, PA: Saunders.)

BASIC SCIENCE PEARL (STEP 1)

The parathyroid glands are formed from the embryologic endoderm, which also gives rise to the gastrointestinal tract and lungs. Specifically, the parathyroid glands develop out of the third and fourth branchial (also called pharyngeal) pouches. Interestingly, the glands that arise from the cranial third pouch eventually migrate to become the inferior glands, whereas the glands that arise from the caudal fourth pouch migrate to become the superior glands (Fig. 23.3).

This embryologic migration has two main clinical implications. First, failure of migration results in ectopic parathyroid glands and may be a cause of sustained hyperparathyroidism after parathyroidectomy. Second, failure to develop the third and fourth branchial pouches, which occurs in DiGeorge syndrome, results in absence of the parathyroid glands and hypocalcemia.

What Is the Differential Diagnosis for Hypercalcemia?

Hypercalcemia due to increased PTH activity (lack of negative feedback) represents primary hyperparathyroidism. Eighty percent of cases of primary hyperparathyroidism are due to a single parathyroid adenoma, whereas multiglandular hyperplasia accounts for most of the remainder. Carcinoma is rare, accounting for less than 1% of cases.

The second most common cause of hypercalcemia is malignancy. For one, myeloma or metastatic disease can infiltrate bones and increase osteoclastic activity via cytokine secretion. Secondly, tumors, such as squamous cell lung carcinoma or renal cell carcinoma, may secrete a protein called

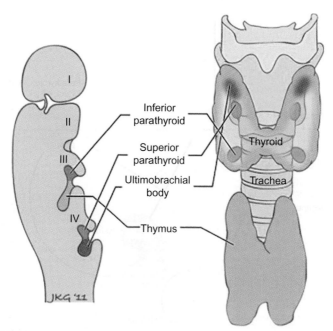

Fig. 23.3 The third branchial pouch gives rise to the inferior parathyroid glands and the thymus, and the fourth pouch gives rise to the superior glands and ultimobranchial body, which becomes part of the thyroid gland. (Redrawn from Policeni BA, Smoker WRK, Reede DL: Anatomy and embryology of the thyroid and parathyroid glands, *Semin Ultrasound CT MRI* 33:104–114, 2012, Fig. 13.)

parathyroid hormone-related peptide (PTHrP), which has structural and functional similarity to PTH.

Hypercalcemia can also be due to states of elevated vitamin D. This can be due to overconsumption of dietary supplements or as a manifestation of granulomatous diseases like sarcoidosis. An additional cause of hypercalcemia is immobilization, but the mechanism is poorly understood.

CLINICAL PEARL (STEPS 1/2/3)

An easy mnemonic for the causes of hypercalcemia is "chimpanzees":
<u>C</u>alcium supplementation (excess can lead to milk-alkali syndrome)
<u>H</u>yperparathyroidism
<u>I</u>atrogenic: hydrochlorothiazide, lithium, or immobility after surgery
<u>M</u>ultiple myeloma or metastases
<u>P</u>aget's disease of bone
<u>A</u>drenal insufficiency
<u>N</u>eoplasm (remember PTHrP)
<u>Z</u>ollinger-Ellison Syndrome
<u>E</u>xcessive vitamin D
<u>E</u>xcessive vitamin A
<u>S</u>arcoidosis

What Are the Clinical Manifestations of Hypercalcemia?

Mild hypercalcemia may be asymptomatic. More severe hypercalcemia has myriad manifestations encapsulated in the mnemonic, "Stones, bones, groans, thrones, and psychiatric overtones."

- Stones: nephrolithiasis, which arise when hypercalciuria results in the precipitation of calcium stones
- Bones: pain secondary to increased osteoclastic activity. A related condition is osteitis fibrosis cystica, in which cystic spaces in the bone fill with brown fibrous tissue
- Groans: abdominal pain and constipation. High calcium levels stabilize cell membranes, thereby decreasing neuromuscular excitability and slowing peristalsis
- Thrones: polyuria, possibly related to nephrogenic diabetes insipidus.
- Psychiatric overtones: ranging from impaired concentration to lethargy to coma, these are also due to impaired neuronal excitability

What Underlying Genetic Conditions Should Be Considered in a Patient With Primary Hyperparathyroidism?

In a minority of cases, hyperparathyroidism is associated with the familial cancer syndromes multiple endocrine neoplasia (MEN) types 1 and 2A. These are autosomal-dominant conditions with high penetrance characterized by tumors in multiple endocrine glands.

MEN1 results from inactivating mutations in the menin tumor suppressor gene on chromosome 11. It is associated with tumors of the three "Ps": parathyroids, pancreas, and pituitary. In fact, over 95% of MEN1 patients have hyperparathyroidism, and asymptomatic hypercalcemia often appears early, in the second or third decade of life. The pancreatic tumors are often functional (hormone-secreting), such as gastrinomas or insulinomas.

MEN2A is caused by inactivating mutations in the *RET* proto-oncogene (a receptor tyrosine kinase) on chromosome 10. Its manifestations include medullary thyroid cancer, pheochromocytomas (catecholamine-secreting adrenal tumors), and parathyroid hyperplasia/adenomas. Hyperparathyroidism is less common in MEN2A, occurring in only about 10% to

20% of cases. Although MEN2B is a familial cancer syndrome also caused by *RET* mutations, MEN2B is not associated with hyperparathyroidism.

The patient is referred to an endocrine surgeon, who performs a complete hypercalcemia-directed history and physical examination. The patient has had two previous episodes of nephrolithiasis and notes occasional forgetfulness that has been worse over the last several months during the summer. She has no family history of hypercalcemia or endocrine neoplasms. Additional laboratory analyses are sent that reveal a serum parathyroid hormone (PTH) level of 147 pg/mL (normal 10–65 pg/mL) and a 25-hydroxy-vitamin D level of 60 ng/mL (normal 20–100 ng/mL). The surgeon orders a 24-hour urine calcium and creatinine, which demonstrates a complete 24-hour collection with elevated urine calcium levels, consistent with a diagnosis of primary hyperparathyroidism. She asks whether she needs to undergo any treatment for her hypercalcemia.

What Is the Treatment for Primary Hyperparathyroidism?

If patients are symptomatic or have calcium levels higher than 14 mg/dL, they should be immediately treated with IV fluids with loop diuretics, calcitonin, and bisphosphonates. In general, primary hyperparathyroidism is treated with parathyroidectomy and can occur via a traditional bilateral neck exploration or more targeted "minimally invasive" approaches. Preoperative imaging can be used to localize abnormal parathyroid glands; options include ultrasound and technetium-99m sestamibi with single photon emission computed tomography (SPECT). Some centers also have access to four-dimensional computed tomography (4D-CT) scans, which are traditional CT scans with the added dimension of constrast attenuation over time. This technology has increased sensitivity for both single and multigland disease, but a disadvantage is the increased radiation and cost over ultrasound or sestamibi imaging.

Using the preoperative imaging findings to direct the intial approach, the surgeon will remove the suspected abnormal gland(s) and then verify that there are no additional abnormalities using intraoperative PTH testing, which takes advantage of PTH's very short half-life—under 5 minutes. Venous blood is drawn from either the patient's arm or leg, and a drop in the patient's PTH to less than half of preoperative levels and into the normal range is strongly predictive of complete cure, in which case the surgery can end. If the PTH does not drop, the surgeon will typically explore the other side of the neck.

If the patient is underoing a total parathyroidectomy or it is found that all four glands are hyperplastic, pieces of a gland are autotransplanted into the forearm in order to provide easy access for ongoing surveillance and to avoid subsequent neck surgeries. The glands develop a blood supply and begin functioning in approximately 4 to 6 weeks.

What Are Potential Concerns After Parathyroidectomy?

Parathyroidectomy cures over 95% of primary hyperparathyroidism. However, persistent hypercalcemia can arise from an overlooked parathyroid adenoma (perhaps in an ectopic location) or an incomplete resection of hyperplastic parathyroid tissue. These errors most often occur with multiglandular disease. Repeat parathyroidectomy is indicated, and although these operations may be associated with higher complication rates, they are often successful when performed by experts.

On the other hand, if too much parathyroid tissue is removed (most relevant with suspected multiglandular disease), patients can suffer from permanent postoperative hypocalcemia, which requires treatment with high dosages of oral calcium and vitamin D several times a day. Patients must be counseled about the signs and symptoms of hypocalcemia, such as tetany and perioral numbness and tingling.

Immediately preoperatively it is also important to assess the patient for any hoarseness, stridor, or respiratory distress, as the recurrent laryngeal nerves are at risk for injury. Unilateral injury may not manifest for days to weeks postoperatively, but the affects of bilateral injury present immediately.

The surgeon orders a 4D-CT, which demonstrates a 0.9-cm low-attenuation lesion in the upper right quadrant of the thyroid gland with intense arterial-phase enhancement and delayed washout. The patient undergoes open removal of the suspect gland, and intraoperative PTH levels drop from 120 pg/mL to 20 pg/mL. Postoperatively, the patient feels well and has no voice hoarseness; her pain is controlled, and she is discharged home that afternoon.

The patient presents to her follow-up appointment 2 weeks after the surgery with no complaints and a well-healing incision. Pathological evaluation of the removed gland revealed a benign parathyroid adenoma. Her calcium measurement at this time is 8.1 mg/dL.

BEYOND THE PEARLS

- Only unbound ionized serum calcium exerts a physiologic effect.
- PTH increases serum calcium via increased osteoclastic activity in bones, increased calcium reabsorption and decreased phosphate reabsorption in the kidneys, and increased vitamin D activation, which increases calcium absorption in the gut.
- The parathyroid glands arise from the endodermal third and fourth pharyngeal pouches, which fail to develop in DiGeorge syndrome.
- Hyperparathyroidism is associated with the familial cancer syndromes MEN1 and MEN2A but not MEN2B.
- Severely hypercalcemic patients should be immediately treated with IV fluids and diuresis.
- Parathyroidectomy cures over 95% of cases of primary hyperparathyroidism.

Suggested Readings

Carroll, M. F., & Schade, D. S. (2003). A practical approach to hypercalcemia. *Am Fam Physician*, *67*, 1959–1966.

Craven, B. L., Passman, C., & Assimos, D. G. (2008). Hypercalcemic states associated with nephrolithiasis. *Rev Urol*, *10*, 218–226.

Dowthwaite, S. A., Young, J. E., Pasternak, J. D., & Yoo, J. (2013). Surgical management of primary hyperparathyroidism. *J Clin Densitom*, *16*, 48–53.

Kukar, M., Platz, T. A., Schaffner, T. J., Elmarzouky, R., Groman, A., Kumar, S., … Cance, W. G. (2015). The Use of Modified Four-Dimensional Computed Tomography in Patients with Primary Hyperparathyroidism: An Argument for the Abandonment of Routine Sestamibi Single-Positron Emission Computed Tomography (SPECT). *Ann Surg Oncol*, *22*, 139–145.

Liew, V., Gough, I. R., Nolan, G., & Fryar, B. (2004). Re-operation for hyperparathyroidism. *ANZ J Surg*, *74*, 732–740.

Policeni, B. A., Smoker, W. R. K., & Reede, D. L. (2012). Anatomy and embryology of the thyroid and parathyroid glands. *Semin Ultrasound CT MRI*, *33*, 104–114.

Ryan, S., Courtney, D., Moriariu, J., & Timon, C. (2017). Surgical management of primary hyperparathyroidism. *Eur Arch Oto-Rhino-Laryngology*, *274*, 4225–4232.

Thakker, R. (2016). The parathyroid glands, hypercalcemia and hypocalcemia. In *Goldman-Cecil medicine* (25th ed., pp. 1649–1661). Philadelphia, PA: Saunders.

CHAPTER 24

Lateral Neck Mass in a 67-Year-Old Male

D. George Ormond ■ Royd Fukumoto

A 67-year-old male with no significant past medical history presents to the surgery clinic after referral from his primary care provider for malaise and multiple neck masses. The masses are nonpainful and have slowly grown over the past 6 months. The patient denies any neurologic symptoms or recent upper respiratory illness but has experienced a general feeling of fatigue over the last 2 months.

What Is the Differential Diagnosis for a Neck Mass and What Elements of the Patient's History Are Important for Narrowing the Differential?

The differential diagnosis of a neck mass is wide and includes congenital, inflammatory, and malignant lesions (Table 24.1). A thorough and detailed history can be useful in determining the suspicion of malignancy; however, all new neck masses in adults should be considered malignant until proven otherwise. The lesion's growth characteristics are of importance because those with rapid growth raise higher concerns for malignancy. Associated general symptoms of malignancy, such as unexplained weight loss, generalized malaise/weakness, or fever, may also be present. Determination of risk factors for cancer, including radiation exposure, smoking, alcohol use, and sun exposure, is critical. The concern for metastatic disease to the neck is also significant, and prior malignancies (even if reported as treated or in remission) are important. Cancers of the skin, head and neck, throat, breast, gastrointestinal tract, and lung are common primary sites. Inflammatory symptoms such as pain, fevers, recent trauma, dental issues, and so forth indicate malignancy is much less likely. Location, in addition to age of the patient, can also aid in differentiation between congenital and neoplastic or inflammatory masses.

What Are the Primary Physical Examination Techniques to Evaluate a Neck Mass?

Evaluating a neck mass on physical examination can be difficult due to the hidden nature of a large component of the structures of interest. Special instruments and techniques are required to examine difficult-to-visualize anatomic areas such as a fiberoptic endoscope and a nasopharyngoscope.

Even without these specialized tools, a good physical examination can help narrow the diagnosis. Begin the physical examination with a general inspection of the face for any general asymmetry, swellings, or discolorations. Continue observing the scalp, ears, and finally the neck, which should also be observed during a swallow. After inspection, the head and neck should be palpated using a systematic top-down approach. The scalp is felt for any lesions, swellings, or other abnormalities. Moving caudally, the salivary glands, including the parotid, sublingual, and submandibular, should all be palpated. Within the neck are the cervical lymph nodes and the thyroid. The lymph nodes themselves should be examined in a routine fashion with a common progression being submental,

TABLE 24.1 ■ **Differential Diagnosis of Neck Mass**

Congenital	Branchial cleft cyst
	Thyroglossal duct cyst
	Vascular malformation (hemangioma)
	Lymphangiomas
	Teratoma
	Dermoid cyst
	Thymic cyst
Inflammatory	Bacterial/viral lymphadenopathy (Epstein-Barr, toxoplasmosis, tularemia, brucellosis, tuberculosis)
	Noninfective lymphadenopathy (Castleman, Rosai-Dorfman, Kawasaki)
	HIV-related infections (all the previously listed)
Benign neoplasm	Salivary gland tumor
	Thyroid nodule/goiter
	Soft tissue tumor (lipoma/sebaceous cyst)
	Neurogenic tumor (neurofibroma, neurilemoma)
	Carotid body tumor
	Laryngeal tumor (chondroma)
Malignant	**Primary**
	• Salivary gland tumor
	• Thyroid cancer
	• Upper gastrointestinal tract cancer
	• Soft tissue sarcoma
	• Skin cancer (melanoma, squamous cell carcinoma, basal cell carcinoma)
	• Lymphoma
	Metastatic
	From any of the previously listed lesions
	From breast, lung, or unknown primary

submandibular, jugulodigastric, preauricular, anterior cervical, posterior occipital, posterior cervical, to finally the supraclavicular lymph nodes (Fig. 24.1). The thyroid is best examined from behind with light palpation and should also be palpated during a swallow. The gland should rise under the examiner's fingers just lateral to both sides of the trachea.

Upon completion of palpation, the motor and sensory function of the cranial nerves should be assessed. Cranial nerve 5, the trigeminal nerve, is responsible for the muscles of mastication, tested by palpating either the masseter or the temporalis muscle, as well as the sensation over the ophthalmic, maxillary, and mandibular regions of the face. Cranial nerve 5 is also responsible for sensation over the entire face. Cranial nerve 7, the facial nerve, is responsible for the intrinsic muscles of the face, which are tested by having the patient close their eyes against resistance, puff out their cheeks, and smile. Cranial nerve 8, the auditory nerve, is tested with the Rinne and Weber tests. Cranial nerve 11, the spinal accessory nerve, is examined by having the patient attempt to turn their heads laterally with the examiner providing resistance against the chin and a shoulder shrug against resistance.

CLINICAL PEARL

Facial palsy is a startling physical examination finding. Care must be taken on physical examination to elucidate the locations of the lesion due to the remarkable innervation of cranial nerve 7. Due to the bilateral innervation of both of the facial motor nuclei, any upper motor lesions (i.e., cerebral infarction) result in paralysis of the contralateral lower face. By contrast, any lesion in a lower motor neuron (i.e., trauma, Bell's palsy) generates a full ipsilateral facial paralysis.

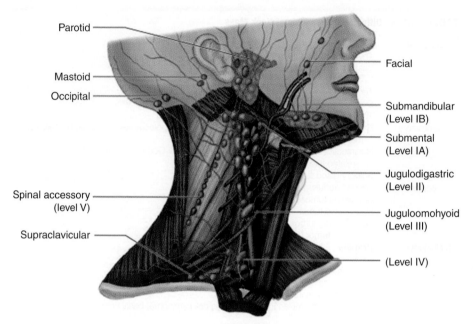

Fig. 24.1 Lymph nodes of the neck. (From Som PH, Brandwein-Gensler MS: Lymph nodes of the neck. In Som PH, Curtin HD, editors: *Head and neck imaging*, ed 5, Philadelphia, Elsevier, pp 2287–2383.)

Once the external examination is complete, the oropharynx should be examined, including all surfaces of the tongue, tonsils, and hard and soft palates. Also, within the mouth, Wharton ducts (orifice of the submandibular gland) and the Stensen ducts (orifice of the parotid gland) should be visualized. The uvula should be visualized midline (cranial nerve 9), and the patient should be asked to stick out their tongue to assess any deviation (cranial nerve 12). It is important to remember to examine the vasculature by palpation and auscultation of the carotid arteries. Both the ears and nares should be examined with an otoscope. The corneal reflex (testing cranial nerves 5 and 7) and the gag reflex (testing cranial nerves 9 and 10) complete the head and neck examination.

What Is the Relevant Anatomy in the Neck?

The central neck consists of the hyoid bone, thyroid isthmus, thyroid and cricoid cartilages, and the trachea. The lateral neck is divided into anterior and posterior triangles (Fig. 24.2) by the sternoclei-domastoid muscle (SCM). The borders of the anterior triangle are the angle of the jaw, the midline, and the SCM. This is then divided by the digastric muscle into the submental and submandibular triangles. Masses within the anterior triangle are commonly lymph nodes, either inflammatory or metastatic. The posterior triangle is bordered by the SCM medially, the trapezius posteriorly, and the clavicle anteriorly. Masses in the posterior triangle are highly suspicious for malignancy.

CLINICAL PEARL

It is important to remember that all muscles of the larynx are innervated by the recurrent laryngeal branch of the vagus nerve **except** the cricothyroid muscle that is innervated by the external laryngeal branch of the superior laryngeal nerve. Clinically, this is important, as injury to the recurrent laryngeal branch results in paralysis of the vocal cord at midline, possibly causing airway obstruction, compared with superior laryngeal nerve injury, resulting in voice changes but no danger to the patient.

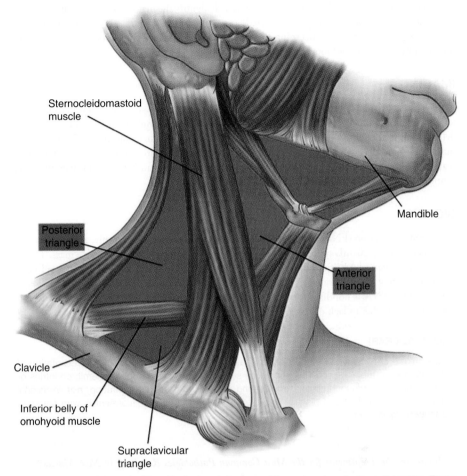

Sternocleidomastoid
muscle

Mandible

Posterior
triangle

Anterior
triangle

Clavicle

Inferior belly of
omohyoid muscle

Supraclavicular
triangle

Fig. 24.2   Triangles of the neck. (From Deslauriers J: Anatomy of the neck and cervicothoracic junction, *Thorac Surg Clin* 17(4):529–547, 2007.)

On further questioning, the patient reports a 30-pack/year smoking history and a drinking history of 1 to 2 beers per week. Physical examination reveals three masses, all less than 1 cm, in the left posterior triangle of the neck. The masses are nontender, rubbery, and slightly mobile. There are no neurologic deficits.

What Additional Diagnostic Testing Should Be Considered in the Evaluation of a Neck Mass?
History and physical examination can be suggestive of diagnosis and can determine the next course of diagnostic testing. Soft, multiple, or tender nodes portend to inflammatory causes in contrast to fixed, firm, solitary, or nontender lymph nodes that are more likely to represent a malignant process. Multiple regions tend to indicate a more systemic disease (i.e., lymphoma, infectious mononucleosis).

Systematic examination of the skin and oral cavity will identify the majority of potentially malignant skin lesions. If infectious etiology is suspected, a trial of antibiotics and observation is appropriate. Most masses in adults are concerning enough to warrant further evaluation with a computed tomography (CT) scan or biopsy.

IMAGING

Ultrasound is a valuable noninvasive technique in differentiating cystic from solid masses, specifically thyroid, parathyroid, or vascular lesions. CT scan is commonly employed and is useful in delineating the anatomic location, consistency, vascularity, and tissue involvement of head and neck masses. Because the neck contains many vital structures, a CT scan can provide important information about whether the mass is affecting other structures and can help inform operative intervention if indicated.

BIOPSY

Fine-needle aspiration (FNA) is the initial diagnostic test of choice. Commonly, a small-gauge (25 or 27) needle and a 20-mL syringe are used to collect tissue and fluid samples from a mass. The test is highly sensitive and specific with very low complication rates. Several studies have shown FNA to be approximately 90% accurate in establishing a definitive diagnosis. An excisional biopsy may be required if the FNA is nondiagnostic. Also, if lymphoma suspected, FNA is unable to determine the specific type due to lack of tissue architecture, so an excisional biopsy is required.

CLINICAL PEARL

Tuberculosis cervical lymphadenitis, also known as scrofula, is a rare primary presentation of Mycobacterium tuberculosis. This should be suspected in patients from endemic countries or those who are immunocompromised. Testing involves fine needle aspiration, *not* excisional biopsy, as this may spread disease and lead to fistula formation. Treatment is with standard antituberculosis drugs.

What Are the Treatments for the Most Common Pathologies Resulting in Neck Masses?

LYMPHONA

Hodgkin's and non-Hodgkin's lymphoma commonly present with cervical lymphadenopathy; however, they tend to be nontender, rubbery, and more mobile than lymph nodes containing metastatic disease. Affected lymph nodes can grow rapidly. Diagnosis is usually suggested by FNA and then confirmed through open excisional biopsy. The eventual treatment involves chemotherapy, radiotherapy, or both.

CLINICAL PEARL

Diffuse large B-cell lymphoma (DLBCL) is one of the most aggressive forms of lymphoma and accounts for approximately 35% of non-Hodgkin lymphomas. Clinical presentation varies and can range from being asymptomatic to having symptoms related to compression of adjacent organs, such as the spinal cord. Patients classically have the typical "B" symptoms: unexplained weight loss, night sweats, fevers. This disease requires excisional tissue biopsy for proper diagnosis, as well as routine laboratory examinations (including lactate dehydrogenase, human immunodeficiency virus (HIV), and hepatitis B and C serologies), chest radiograph, and CT of the chest, abdomen, and pelvis. Treatment of DLBCL is with chemotherapy, commonly involving cyclophosphamide, doxorubicin, vincristine, prednisone (CHOP), and the recently added rituximab (R-CHOP).

PRIMARY SKIN CANCERS

Primary skin cancers may present as neck masses and require biopsy and staging, including whether they have metastasized to local lymph nodes. They may be treated with chemotherapy, radiation, or both. See Chapter 20 for a full discussion of primary skin cancers.

SALIVARY GLAND TUMORS

Any slow-growing mass in the preauricular area, in the angle of the jaw, or superior neck arouses concern for salivary gland neoplasm. Benign lesions are usually asymptomatic, with the most common being a pleomorphic adenoma (mixed histology). Warthin's tumor is a monomorphic papillary cystic adenoma that is a common benign parotid tumor found in elderly males.

Malignant salivary tumors commonly cause neurologic entrapment symptoms such as numbness, paresthesia, or motor dysfunction. CT or magnetic resonance imaging (MRI) can be obtained, but the final diagnosis is dependent on biopsy, most commonly open excision, which also serves as treatment for the mass. Mucoepidermoid carcinoma and adenoid cystic carcinoma are the most common histologic varieties.

Removal of the tumor with negative surgical margins is the cornerstone of treatment, with malignant lesions being additionally treated with radiotherapy. If clinically or radiographically evident neck metastasis is present, the patient should undergo a radical or modified radical neck dissection.

METASTIC CARCINOMA

If the lymph node is nontender, firm, or immobile, metastatic cancer should be suspected. The most common source of primary cancer is the upper aerodigestive tract with alcohol use and/or smoking being the highest risk factors. A thorough examination to locate the primary lesion should be undertaken, and diagnosis can be confirmed with an FNA. Imaging should be considered to further delineate the primary site of disease as well as detect other metastatic lesions. Treatment depends on the type of metastatic disease present and focuses on addressing the primary lesion. The extent of disease and the response to treatment will dictate the management of the metastasis.

BENIGN LYMPHADENOPATHY

Cervical lymph node enlargement is a common sign of head and neck infectious disease. A thorough history and physical examination should elucidate most infectious etiologies. Often the patient presents with fevers, chills, or malaise, single or multiple tender cervical lymph nodes, and a nidus for infection. The diagnosis is established, and appropriate medical therapy can be initiated. Chronic infections, such as tuberculosis or AIDS, may also cause cervical lymphadenopathy. Biopsy is occasionally needed if lymph node enlargement is chronic.

The patient undergoes a fine-needle aspiration of one of the lesions in the office, and cytology is suggestive of lymphoma. Excisional biopsy for lymph node architecture is performed, and the patient is diagnosed with diffuse large B-cell lymphoma (DLBCL). The patient is discussed at the multidisciplinary oncology meeting and decides with his physicians to undergo chemotherapy and radiotherapy.

BEYOND THE PEARLS

- Neck masses presenting in adults are most commonly malignant but have a wide differential.
- If infectious etiology suspected, an assessment should focus on the likely causative organism, and, if bacterial, a trial of antibiotics is appropriate.
- Fine-needle aspiration provides sufficient tissue for diagnosis in most cases, but excisional biopsy may be necessary to assess tissue architecture and establish the diagnosis of some pathologies.
- Surgery for salivary gland tumors should have negative surgical margins to minimize risk of recurrence.

Suggested Readings

Alvi, A., & Johnson, J. T. (1995). The neck mass: A challenging differential diagnosis. Postgrad Med. 97(5), 87–90, 93–84, 97.

Andry, G., Hamoir, M., Locati, L. D., Licitra, L., & Langendijk, J. A. (2012). Management of salivary gland tumors. *Expert Rev Anticancer Ther*, *12*(9), 1161–1168.

Bell, R. B., Dierks, E. J., Homer, L., & Potter, B. E. (2005). Management and outcome of patients with malignant salivary gland tumors. *J Oral Maxillofac Surg*, *63*(7), 917–928.

Dunleavy, K., & Wilson, W. (2013). Diagnosis and treatment of diffuse large B-cell lymphoma and Burkitt lymphoma. In *Hematology: basic principles and practice* (pp. 1236–1241). Philadelphia: Saunders Elsevier.

Ruhl, C. (2004). Evaluation of the neck mass. *Med Health R I*, *87*(10), 307.

Roseman, B. J. (2008). *Clark OH: 3 NECK MASS.*

Tiemstra, J. D. (2007). Khatkhate N: Bell's palsy: diagnosis and management. *Am Fam Physician*, *76*(7), 997–1002.

CHAPTER 25

Thigh Mass in a 35-Year-Old Male

Madeline B. Torres ■ Colette Pameijer

A healthy 35-year-old male presents to the physician's office complaining of a painless left anterior thigh mass. The mass has been present for 3 months and has slowly grown in size. The patient denies a history of radiation or injury to the area. The patient denies smoking and IV drug use and reports occasional alcohol consumption. His family history is significant only for hypertension in both of his parents.

What Are Key Portions of the History to Elicit From a Patient Presenting With a New Mass?
A complete and detailed history must be obtained from a patient presenting with a new mass, as it may provide key information in characterizing the mass as either benign or malignant. Important information to obtain during the visit includes the rate at which the mass has been growing, presence of overlying skin changes, pain at the site of the mass, any trauma or injury to the area, and any deficits in sensation or movement to the limb when it is present in an extremity. Changes in the character of the mass, such as its mobility and texture, are also essential. It is additionally important to elicit personal history of radiation therapy and personal or family history of cancer or syndromes such as Li-Fraumeni syndrome, familial adenomatous polyposis (FAP), Gardner's syndrome, neurofibromatosis, and hereditary retinoblastoma.

What Is the Differential Diagnosis for Extremity Masses?
There are many causes for masses in the extremity, and it is important to obtain a complete history and physical examination before narrowing the differential diagnosis. Any of the soft tissue lineages in the limb are capable of forming benign soft tissue tumors (Table 25.1), including the more common lipomas, fibromas, and neurofibromas. Malignant degeneration of the mesenchymal tissues of the limb form sarcomas, of which there are many. A hematoma is likely to result from a traumatic injury of the extremity, especially in a patient who is anticoagulated.

BASIC SCIENCE PEARL (STEP 1)

The embryologic lineage of the tissues within the limb are the ectoderm (skin) and mesoderm (muscle, cartilage, bone, and blood vessels), also known as mesenchymal tissues. Malignancies of the skin are discussed in Chapter 20. Malignant degeneration of the mesenchyme leads to the development of sarcomas.

On examination, there is a 10 cm × 20 cm ovoid mass in the left anterior thigh. The lesion is firm and fixed to the surrounding tissue. There are no skin changes and no obvious signs of trauma. There is no tenderness on palpation of the mass, and the patient has full range of motion in his left hip and knee with no obvious neurovascular deficits. There are no palpable lymph nodes in the leg or groin.

TABLE 25.1 ■ Differential Diagnosis of Extremity Masses

Benign Soft Tissue Tumor	Malignant Soft Tissue Tumor (Sarcoma)
Lipoma	Liposarcoma
Fibroma	Fibrosarcoma
Rhabdomyoma	Rhabdomyosarcoma
Leiomyoma	Leiomyosarcoma
Lymphangioma	Lymphangiosarcoma
Neurofibroma	Neurofibrosarcoma
Benign mesothelioma	Malignant mesothelioma
Benign fibrous histiocytoma	Malignant fibrous histiocytoma
Hemangioma	Angiosarcoma
Hemangiopericytoma	Chondrosarcoma
Chondroma	Synovial sarcoma
Synovioma	
Benign Hard Tissue Tumor	**Malignant Hard Tissue Tumor**
Osteoma	Osteosarcoma
Other	**Other**
Hematoma	Ewing sarcoma
	Alveolar soft part tumor
	Epithelioid sarcoma

What Are Key Findings on Physical Examination for Extremity Masses?
When examining soft tissue masses, one should pay attention to the size of the mass (masses > 5 cm are concerning), its location in relation to other structures such as joints and vessels, the appearance of the overlying skin including any ulceration, and the overall characteristics of the mass (firm, rubbery, soft, fixed, or mobile). Additionally, a neurovascular examination and assessment of range of motion can help elucidate involvement of other structures. Finally, a complete examination for palpable lymph nodes should be undertaken to assess for potential metastases.

CLINICAL PEARL (STEPS 2/3)

The most common site of sarcoma metastasis is the lung. Only about 3% of sarcomas metastasize to regional lymph nodes. The sarcoma subtypes that more commonly metastasize to the lymph nodes are synovial, epithelioid, rhabdoid, and clear cell. Sentinel node biopsy can be considered in these cases, although the role and benefit of early detection of nodal disease remain unclear.

What Are the Diagnostic Steps in Evaluating an Extremity Mass?
Imaging studies are crucial in the evaluation of soft tissue masses in order to characterize the size, extent, and nature of the mass. The imaging study of choice for an extremity mass is magnetic resonance imaging (MRI), as it delineates muscle compartments, vasculature, and the tumor's location in relation to other structures. If MRI is not readily available, too costly, and/or contraindicated (e.g., the patient has a metal join replacement or other metallic implant), a computed tomography (CT) scan with IV contrast should be obtained. On MRI, sarcomas appear heterogeneous and enhance on T2-weighted images, whereas benign tumors appear similar to the surrounding tissues and tend not to cross anatomic barriers such as fascial compartments.

The next step in the workup is a biopsy of the tumor. A core needle biopsy is preferred, but if a core needle biopsy cannot be performed, an experienced surgeon can perform an incisional biopsy. When performing incisional biopsy, it is important to make the incision along the longitudinal axis of the extremity in a location that can be reexcised at the time of formal resection of the mass (see later in this chapter).

The patient undergoes a magnetic resonance imaging (MRI) of the left thigh (Fig. 25.1). The mass measures 6 cm, is confined to the quadriceps femoris, and is irregular and heterogeneous in character. The physician reviews the images with the patient and describes these features as concerning for sarcoma. After discussion of next steps, the patient proceeds to biopsy of the mass.

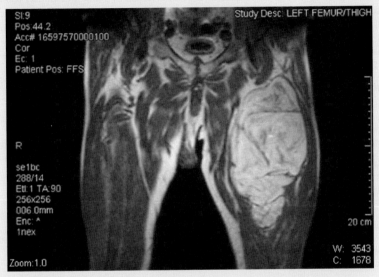

Fig. 25.1 MRI demonstrates a large lipomatous mass in the anterior left thigh.

CLINICAL PEARL

Sarcomas are painless, rapidly growing masses. Oftentimes a history of trauma is reported, although the trauma merely brings attention to the area. Trauma does not cause sarcoma.

CLINICAL PEARL

Nodal metastasis is rare with sarcoma, except for synovial, epithelioid, rhabdoid, and clear cell subtypes. Sentinel node biopsy can be considered in these cases, although the role and benefit of early detection of nodal disease remain unclear.

The patient returns 1 week later to review the results of the core needle biopsy. Pathologic analysis of the tissue sample reveals a low-grade liposarcoma, without evidence of necrosis. The patient undergoes a CT scan of his chest.

What Is the Staging System for Sarcomas?

The essence of sarcoma staging involves tumor size, location, grade, and metastasis. Histologic evaluation of the tumor should note the type of sarcoma (Table 25.2), histologic grade, and presence or absence of necrosis. In addition to biopsy to assess tumor characteristics, a chest radiograph (CXR) and/or a CT scan of the chest should be obtained to assess the presence of metastatic disease.

The tumor, node, and metastasis (TNM) staging system of the American Joint Committee on Cancer (AJCC) is used for sarcomas. Importantly, the staging of sarcomas also takes into consideration the grade of the tumor (Table 25.3).

What Is the Treatment for Sarcoma?

The treatment plan for patients with sarcoma is best developed by a multidisciplinary team of specialists composed of a surgeon, medical oncologist, and radiation oncologist and may include social workers, physical and occupational therapists, and even palliative care. A majority of sarcomas are

TABLE 25.2 ■ Histologic Classification of Sarcoma Based on Tissue of Origin

Connective Tissue of Origin	Sarcoma Subtype
Fat	Liposarcoma
Smooth muscle	Leiomyosarcoma
Unknown	Synovial sarcoma
Fibrohistiocytic	Undifferentiated pleomorphic sarcoma, formerly malignant fibrous histiocytoma
Skeletal muscle	Rhabdomyosarcoma
Fibrous tissue	Fibrosarcoma
Bone	Osteosarcoma
Cartilage	Chondrosarcoma
Blood vessels	Angiosarcoma
Lymphatic	Lymphangiosarcoma
Nerve	Malignant peripheral nerve sheath tumor (MPNST)
Uncertain	Ewing sarcoma
	Alveolar soft part tumor
	Epithelioid sarcoma

TABLE 25.3 ■ Primary Tumor (T), Lymph Node (N), Metastasis (M), and Histologic Grade (G) Classification

Tumor (T)	Tx: Primary tumor cannot be assessed
	T0: No evidence of primary tumor
	T1: Tumor 5 cm or less in greatest dimension
	T2: Tumor more than 5 cm in greatest dimension
Nodes (N)	Nx: Regional lymph nodes cannot be assessed
	N0: No regional lymph node metastasis
	N1: Regional lymph node metastasis
Metastasis (M)	M0: No distant metastasis
	M1: Distant Metastasis
Histologic grade[a]	Gx: Grade cannot be assessed
	G1: Grade 1
	G2: Grade 2
	G3: Grade 3

[a]The grade is assigned using a scoring system after assessing the tumor for differentiation, mitotic count and necrosis

treated with surgical resection, with or without radiation therapy. The sequence of modalities will depend on resectability of the tumor, tumor grade, and functional outcome, with no proven survival benefit to neoadjuvant therapy.

Patients with low-grade, resectable tumors (stage IA, IB) can be managed with surgery alone, provided a negative margin is obtained. If the margins are positive, reexcision and/or radiation therapy is recommended.

Patients with intermediate and higher-grade tumors that are resectable may benefit from neoadjuvant therapy, which results in a higher rate of margin negative resection but a higher rate of wound complications. These patients may also require adjuvant radiation therapy and/or chemotherapy depending on tumor histology and surgical margins.

Patients who present with unresectable tumors or tumors that are resectable with significant functional deficit should be managed with chemotherapy, radiation therapy, or a combination of the two. The treatment plan after primary therapy will depend on the patient's response to treatment. Surgery may be an option for these patients if resection with acceptable margins is possible. Lastly, it is recommended that patients with metastatic disease be managed based on the location of metastasis—for example, surgery, radiation, or ablation procedures for single-organ disease and chemotherapy for disseminated disease.

Recurrent disease is treated based on location of recurrence (local vs distant) and previous response to initial therapies with surgical resection preferred when possible.

What Are the Principles of Surgical Resection of Sarcomas

Surgical management includes wide local excision aimed toward a margin negative resection. The surgical incision should be made along the longitudinal axis of the extremity, and any biopsy scar should be excised (Fig. 25.2A). Margins should be at least 1 cm with inclusion of fascial planes if possible, as they provide an adequate barrier for tumor extension (see Fig. 25.2B). Neurovascular bundles should be preserved, unless they are grossly involved with the tumor (see Fig. 25.2C and D). Metallic clips should be placed in the surgical bed to help define the margins of the resection and help guide subsequent radiation therapy. As mentioned earlier, lymph node metastases rarely occur in soft tissue sarcoma; thus routine sentinel lymph node dissection is not performed. Radical lymphadenectomy is performed when regional lymph nodes are clinically positive on initial diagnosis or upon regional lymph node recurrence. The role of sentinel lymph node biopsy in the treatment of soft tissue sarcoma is unclear and currently not recommended.

Patients with large defects may require reconstructive flaps and/or skin grafts to repair defects and improve function.

CLINICAL PEARL

Limb-preserving, wide, local excision plus adjuvant radiation therapy became standard after a randomized trial in the 1970s by Rosenberg and his team at the National Cancer Institute, showing that limb-sparing resection plus adjuvant radiation therapy was comparable to amputation, with no difference in disease-free or overall survival rates.

The patient undergoes radical resection of his left anterior thigh mass without lymph node assessment. The mass is excised with good margins, and the incision is able to be closed primarily without the use of a flap or graft. He is discharged home the next day with physical and occupational therapy services and is scheduled to see medical radiation and surgical oncology in a multidisciplinary follow-up appointment in 1 week.

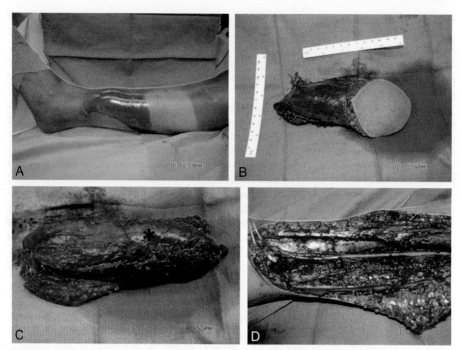

Fig. 25.2 (A) Preoperative planning for resection of left leg mass. (B) Anterior aspect of resected specimen, including skin excision to insure appropriate margin. (C) Posterior specimen, showing ample muscle margin, but also close margin of tumor capsule (*) where the tumor abutted the tibia. (D) Surgical bed after resection demonstrating intact neurovascular structures.

What Follow-up Is Required After Sarcoma Treatment?

After completing the appropriate treatment, patients enter a surveillance plan, undergoing local imaging (CT scan or MRI) of the primary site and chest imaging. Current follow-up recommendations include history and physical examination every 3 to 6 months for the first 2 to 3 years, then annually. Additionally, continued evaluation for physical and occupational therapy needs is encouraged to ensure maximal functional recovery.

> The patient returns 2 weeks after surgery for a follow-up appointment and to review final pathology. On examination, the surgical wound is healing well, and he has no neurovascular deficits. Pathologic evaluation of the resection specimen revealed negative margins. The patient is relieved to not need reexcision or radiation at this time and is scheduled for a follow-up in 3 months with imaging of his left lower extremity.

Suggested Readings

Andreou, D., et al. (2013). Sentinel node biopsy in soft tissue sarcoma subtypes with a high propensity for regional lymphatic spread: Results of a large prospective trial. *Ann Oncol, 24*(5), 1400–1405. https://doi.org/10.1093/annonc/mds650.

Chao, A. H., Mayerson, J. L., Chandawarkar, R., & Scharschmidt, T. J. (2015). Surgical management of soft tissue sarcomas: Extremity sarcomas. *J Surg Oncol, 111*(5), 540–545. https://doi.org/10.1002/jso.23810.

Maduekwe, U. N., Hornicek, F. J., Springfield, D. S., et al. (2009). Role of sentinel lymph node biopsy in the staging of synovial, epithelioid, and clear cell sarcomas. *Ann Surg Oncol, 16*, 1356–1363. https://doi.org/10.1245/s10434-009-0393-9.

Mulholland, M. W. (Ed.). (2006). *Greenfield's surgery: scientific principles and practice*. (5th ed.). Philadelphia: Lippincott Williams & Wilkins.

National Comprehensive Cancer Network (2017). *NCCN clinical practice guidelines in oncology: sarcoma (Version 2.2017)*. https://www.nccn.org/professionals/physician_gls/pdf/sarcoma.pdf. Accessed September 27, 2017.

Rosenberg, S. A., Tepper, J., Glatstein, E., et al. (1982). The treatment of soft-tissue sarcomas of the extremities: Prospective randomized evaluations of (1) limb-sparing surgery plus radiation therapy compared with amputation and (2) the role of adjuvant chemotherapy. *Ann Surg, 196*(3), 305–315.

CHAPTER 26

Jaundice in a 63-Year-Old Female

Ned Carp ■ Kei Nagatomo

A 63-year-old female presents to emergency department with a complaint of vague mid-abdominal pain, jaundice, and recent unintentional weight loss of 15 pounds over 4 months. She reports severe pruritus and noticed tea-colored urine and clay-colored stools. Her social history reveals that she is a social drinker and a former 20 pack/year smoker. Her past medical history includes a recent diagnosis of type 2 diabetes. On physical examination, the patient's vital signs are within normal range, but she is noted to have scleral icterus. Her abdomen is soft and nontender, though there is what appears to be a mass palpable in her right upper quadrant.

What Is the Differential Diagnosis for Jaundice?

The differential diagnosis for jaundice is broad. Causes can be categorized as prehepatic, hepatic, and posthepatic or those that are obstructive or nonobstructive. Prehepatic and many hepatic causes are considered nonobstructive because the biliary system is not affected. These include increased hemolysis, bacterial and viral infection, drugs, alcohol, steatohepatitis, disorders of bilirubin metabolism (such as Gilbert's disease), and vascular causes. Obstructing causes of jaundice are most frequently posthepatic and include both benign and malignant causes of biliary obstruction. The differential includes benign diseases such as cholecystitis and choledocholithiasis (see Chapter 6), hepatitis, pancreatitis, and benign strictures from the biliary tree, and malignancies of the pancreas and the biliary tree. It is important to elicit factors such as the chronicity or acuity of the jaundice, its association with other symptoms such as abdominal pain, and changes in bowel habits in order to help in differentiating these causes from one another.

What Are the History and Physical Examination Techniques in Evaluating Patients With Jaundice?

Although physical examination is important, a detailed medical history is paramount. Assessing the onset of jaundice, whether it has occurred before (metabolic causes), and eliciting its association with right upper quadrant abdominal pain are key. If the patient is experiencing pain, asking its duration and character, and whether it is constant (cholecystitis or choledocholithiasis) or colicky (biliary colic) can help differentiate causes of jaundice from one another. Itching is common in patients with sever jaundice, as bilirubin is deposited in the skin. A history of known biliary disease and previous endoscopic retrograde cholangiopancreatography (ERCP) are also important. Other symptoms such as itching are common in patients with severe jaundice as bilirubin is deposited in the skin. Additionally, a personal or family history of gallbladder, biliary tree, and pancreatic pathology, including malignancy, is important.

Physical examination in a patient with jaundice includes assessing the extent of jaundice (sclerae, skin, under the tongue) and a thorough abdominal examination to assess for tenderness and palpable masses. Jaundice may be clinically apparent when bilirubin levels rise higher than 2.0 mg/dL (normal serum bilirubin: 0.5–1.3 mg/dL). Patients often report "tea-colored" urine. This is because the excess amount of bilirubin in the body is converted to urobilinogen in the terminal ileum. Ten to 20% of urobilinogen is reabsorbed via the entero-portal circulation and undergoes either reexcretion into the bile or excretion into the kidney, producing dark urine.

CLINICAL PEARL (STEPS 2/3)

Unlike choledocholithiasis, simple biliary colic and cholecystitis do not typically present with abnormal liver function tests or jaundice. However, "Mirizzi syndrome" can occur when a gall-stone within a gallstone causes mechanical compression at the cystic duct–common bile duct junction and ultimately results in obstructive pathology, elevating the bilirubin and other liver function tests.

CLINICAL PEARL (STEPS 2/3)

The presence of a nontender, palpable gallbladder or RUQ mass along with mild painless jaundice is called Courvoisier's sign. In this situation, the pathology is more likely malignant from a biliary or pancreatic etiology rather than from a benign etiology of gallstones.

What Diagnostic Modalities Are Used in the Workup of Patients With Jaundice?

In addition to history and physical examination, laboratory tests (complete blood count, metabolic panel, and liver function tests) are important in the initial workup of patients with jaundice (Fig. 26.1). Specifically, determining the proportion of direct (conjugated) and indirect (unconjugated) bilirubin allows for the initial branch point for the workup, as increases in indirect bilirubin

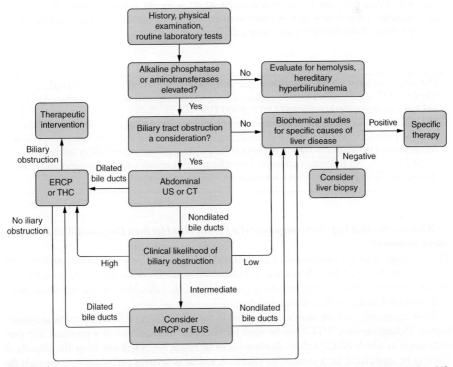

Fig. 26.1 Algorithm for the assessment of jaundice that includes laboratory analyses and imaging studies. (US, ultrasound; CT, computed tomography; MRCP, magnetic resonance cholangiopancreatogram; EUS, endoscopic ultrasound; ERCP, endoscopic retrograde cholangiopancreaticogram; THC, transhepatic cholangiogram. (Redrawn from Lidofsky SD: Jaundice. In Feldman M, Friedman LS, Brandt LJ, editors: *Sleisenger and Fordtran's gastrointestinal and liver disease*, Philadelphia, 2016, Elsevier, pp 336–348.)

are typically due to hemolysis. For patients with a direct hyperbilirubinemia, assessment of whether the etiology is hepatocellular or extrahepatic guides the necessity for imaging studies or serologic studies for hepatitis. A right upper quadrant ultrasound is the initial imaging study of choice to assess the extrahepatic biliary tree and gallbladder. An ultrasound can detect distension and edema of the gallbladder (cholecystitis) as well as dilation of the bile duct (possible extrahepatic obstruction, as in choledocholithiasis). Ultrasound may also reveal hepatic lesions such as cysts, primary tumors, and metastases. Magnetic resonance cholangiopancreatogram (MRCP) is a noninvasive method for visualizing the biliary tree to assess for stones in the bile ducts. ERCP is both diagnostic and therapeutic, as sphincterotomy and stone retrieval are able to be performed. ERCP, however, is an invasive test with risks including post-ERCP pancreatitis. When malignancy is suspected, a computed tomography (CT) scan of the abdomen and pelvis is indicated which enables visualization of masses in the pancreas. A CT scan will delineate vascular involvement, which is a key component to determining resectability of the pancreatic tumor or extrahepatic/intrahepatic bile duct tumors. Laboratory analyses should also include CA19-9 if a malignancy is suspected. CA19-9 is elevated in obstructive jaundice from malignant causes; however, a chronically dilated pancreatic or bile duct from benign causes might cause a falsely elevated CA19-9. CA19-9 is a good marker for tumor surveillance but cannot be used for diagnostic purposes.

CLINICAL PEARL (STEPS 2/3)

The common bile duct (CBD) diameter increases with age, so when assessing for dilation, it is important to take the patient's age into account. At 60 years old, a normal CBD is 6 mm. The CBD increases 1 mm in size for every additional decade of life. Additionally, patients who have had a previous cholecystectomy can have a CBD size up to 10 mm.

The patient undergoes laboratory analyses that reveal: a white blood cell count of 7000/µL; a total bilirubin of 13 mg/dL with a direct bilirubin of 8 mg/dL; an aspartate aminotransferase (AST) of 345 U/L; alanine aminotransferase (ALT) of 400 U/L; and an alkaline phosphatase of 320 U/L. The physician described to the patient that there is concern for a malignancy affecting her biliary tree. She orders a CA19-9, which is elevated, and a CT scan of the abdomen and pelvis, which demonstrates a heterogenous mass in the head of the pancreas with associated biliary and pancreatic ductal dilatation. An endoscopic ultrasound is performed that reveals a 4 cm pancreatic head mass, and fine-needle aspirate of the mass is consistent with adenocarcinoma.

What Are the Next Steps in Management of a Patient Who Has Been Diagnosed With Pancreatic Adenocarcinoma?

The two major steps in management of patients with a diagnosis of pancreatic adenocarcinoma are to relieve symptomatic biliary obstruction and to assess resectability of the pancreatic mass. Patients with symptomatic biliary obstruction (cholangitis, pruritus, etc.) should be treated either with proximal or distal drainage of their obstructed duct.

Most commonly a biliary stent can be placed in the CBD during ERCP. Percutaneous transhepatic cholangiography (PTC) can be used for temporal management of a proximal bile duct obstruction in which ERCP fails to decompress or technical issues will not allow the ampulla of Vater to be cannulated for a stent to be placed. A needle is inserted percutaneously through the liver to access bile ducts. In this way, biliary access is established to the proximal portion of biliary tree, and a drainage catheter can be placed for further biliary decompression. This can be very important to establish a biliary roadmap for intrahepatic bile duct tumors or proximal cholangiocarcinoma being considered for resection.

Criteria for whether a pancreatic mass is resectable are based on imaging findings of metastatic disease and invasion or encasement of surrounding structures. A CT scan of the abdomen and pelvis with pancreatic protocol is aimed at assessing the primary tumor, and a CT scan of the chest is performed to assess for metastatic disease. Although a CT scan can demonstrate abdominal carcinomatosis, 15% to 20% are missed by this modality. Staging laparoscopy can be performed to confirm that there are no disseminated intraabdominal metastases.

Related to resection of the primary tumor, the superior mesenteric artery and celiac artery are the arterial structures that must not be involved with tumor for pancreatic head and body/tail masses, respectively. The superior mesenteric and portal veins are the venous structures assessed. Tumor abutment does not prohibit resection. Some patients may, in fact, be considered "borderline resectable" even with invasion of these venous structures, provided their anatomy lends itself to resection and reconstruction. Patients with metastatic disease and significant involvement of surrounding vessels are deemed nonresectable.

Nonsurgical therapy should also be discussed, especially in patients who are not outright surgically resectable. Preoperative chemotherapy and/or radiotherapy are controversial, and management varies by institution and patient presentation. Chemotherapy is, however, recommended for adjuvant therapy in resected pancreatic carcinoma.

BASIC SCIENCE PEARL (STEPS 1/2/3)

Vascular anatomy is important not only for determining resectability of pancreatic cancer but also in operative planning. In 55% to 60% of patients, the celiac trunk gives rise to the common hepatic artery, from which the proper hepatic artery arises and branches into the right and left hepatic arteries (Fig. 26.2). One of the most common variants (10%–15%) is a replaced right hepatic artery, where the right hepatic artery arises from the superior mesenteric artery and traverses posterior to the pancreatic head (where it is at risk for injury) and emerges lateral to the cystic duct.

CLINICAL PEARL (STEPS 2/3)

The risk factors for pancreatic cancer include advanced age, smoking, history of pancreatitis, and family history. There are some weak associations with obesity, diabetes, and African American or Ashkenazi Jewish ancestry.

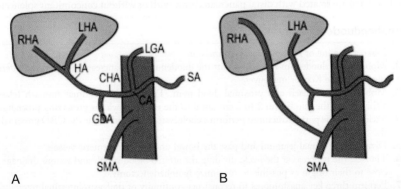

Fig. 26.2 Hepatic artery anatomy with normal variant (A) and replaced right hepatic artery (B). (CA, celiac artery; SMA, superior mesenteric artery; LGA, left gastric artery; CHA, common hepatic artery; GDA, gastroduodenal artery; HA, hepatic artery; LHA, left hepatic artery; RHA, right hepatic artery; SA, splenic artery.) (Redrawn from Kessel D, Robertson I: Achieving angiographic diagnosis. In *Interventional radiology: a survival guide*, London, 2017, Elsevier, pp 266–297.)

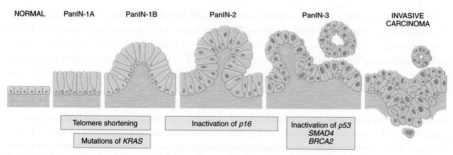

Fig. 26.3 Progression of normal pancreatic tissue to intraepithelial neoplasia (PanIN) and invasive carcinoma with associated genetic alterations and mutations. (Redrawn from Maitra A: Pancreas. In Kumar V, Abbas AK, Aster JC, editors: *Robbins basic pathology*, Philadelphia, 2018, Elsevier, pp 679–689.)

CLINICAL PEARL (STEPS 2/3)

Pancreatic cancer is believed to evolve in stepwise progression (Fig. 26.3). Pancreatic intraepithelial neoplasia (PanIN) progresses as a precursor, then transforms into adenocarcinoma with the accumulation of mutations. K-ras is a very common activation mutation found in pancreatic cancer, though there may be others (CDKN2A, BRCA2, TP53, p14, and SMAD4).

The patient is discussed at the pancreatic cancer tumor board. A review of her abdominal CT scan and endoscopic ultrasound shows that her 4 cm pancreatic head mass has no vascular involvement, and there is no obvious lymph node enlargement to suggest nodal metastasis. A CT of the chest reveals no findings concerning for metastatic disease. She is deemed resectable and is set up for surgery the next week.

What Are the Types of Surgery for Pancreatic Cancer?

The types of surgery for pancreatic cancer are predominantly based on the location of the tumor. For cancer in the pancreatic head or uncinate process, pancreaticoduodenectomy (also known as the Whipple procedure) may be performed for tumors deemed to be resectable. Tumors in the pancreatic body and tail are treated with distal pancreatectomy with or without concomitant splenectomy.

Pancreaticoduodenectomy (Fig. 26.4)

1. Make a midline or bilateral subcostal incision.
2. Mobilize the duodenum medially to lift the duodenum and pancreatic head off the inferior vena cava (the Kocher maneuver).
3. Mobilize the stomach and proximal duodenum. Transect the proximal stomach (classic Whipple) or the duodenum 2 to 3 cm distal to the pylorus (pylorus preserving procedure).
4. Skeletonize the portal structures: perform a cholecystectomy and divide the CBD proximal to the cystic duct.
5. Divide the proximal jejunum and pass the bowel under the mesenteric vessels.
6. Transect the pancreas at the neck, dividing the arterial blood supply and venous drainage as close to their origin as possible to maximize lymphadenectomy.
7. Perform three key anastomoses to reconstruct continuity of the gastrointestinal tract:
   - Pancreaticojejunostomy (PJ) anastomosis
   - Hepaticojejunostomy (HJ) anastomosis
   - Gastrojejunal (GJ) or duodenojejunal (DJ) anastomosis. The former is used in a pylorus preserving procedure.
8. Place Jackson-Pratt (JP) drains at the PJ and HJ anastomoses.
9. Place an optional feeding jejunostomy distal to the anastomoses.

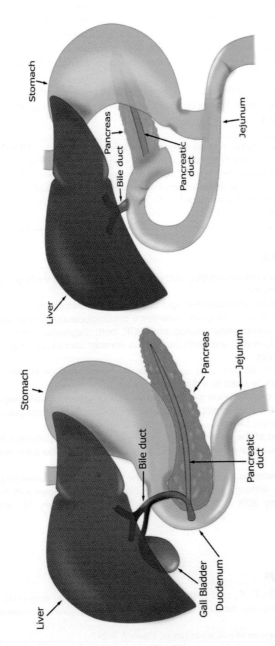

Fig. 26.4 Normal gastrointestinal anatomy (*left*) and reconstructed anatomy after pylorus-preserving pancreaticoduodenectomy (*right*). Note that a solitary loop of jejunum has anastomoses to the bile duct, pancreatic duct, and duodenum in order to reestablish continuity of the gastrointestinal tract.

What Are the Potential Complications After Pancreaticoduodenectomy?

Pancreaticoduodenectomy is a procedure that carries a substantial morbidity. Potential complications include pancreatic leak/fistula, delayed gastric emptying, marginal ulcers, pancreatic enzyme insufficiency, and insulin-dependent diabetes. Many of these complications can be detected in the immediate postoperative period, whereas others present in a delayed fashion and are recognized when the patient is unable to tolerate an oral diet. It is important to have these complications in mind and the ways in which they present as patients are assessed daily and advanced from nothing per os (NPO) to a diet.

Although not a morbidity of the operation itself, it must be mentioned that the risk of recurrence of pancreatic cancer after surgical resection is still relatively high, so adjuvant therapy and surveillance must be undertaken.

The patient undergoes a pylorus-preserving pancreaticoduodenectomy for her T3N0M0 pancreatic head adenocarcinoma, and the final pathology shows a negative margin. She is progressed from nothing by mouth to a regular diet over the next 5 days as she regained bowel function. Her pain was controlled, and her surgical drains removed on postoperative day 6, and she is discharged to home without complication. She continued to do well postoperatively, tolerated adjuvant chemotherapy well, and surveillance CA19-9 remains low.

BEYOND THE PEARLS

- Painless jaundice is classically associated with a tumor obstructing the biliary tree causing a direct hyperbilirubinemia.
- Imaging modalities for assessing the right upper quadrant include ultrasound (right upper quadrant and endoscopic), magnetic resonance cholangiopancreatogram (MRCP), endoscopic retrograde cholangiopancreatogram (ERCP, both diagnostic and therapeutic), and computed tomography (CT) scan with intravenous contrast specifically timed for examining the liver and pancreas.
- CA19-9 is the tumor marker used most frequently for surveillance in pancreatic cancer, though it should not be used as a diagnostic marker.
- Resectability in pancreatic cancer is dependent on a tumor's relationship to major arteries and veins that surround the pancreas. Additionally, any metastatic disease precludes primary resection of pancreatic cancer.
- Tumors of the head of the pancreas are treated with pancreaticoduodenectomy (Whipple), and those of the body and tail are treated with a distal pancreatectomy with or without splenectomy.
- Adjuvant chemotherapy is an important part of the treatment for pancreatic cancer.
- Pancreatic cancer, although improving, has an overall poor prognosis with 1-year survival being approximately 20% and 5-year survival being approximately 5% with all stages combined.

Suggested Readings

Allen, P. J., Kuk, D., Catillo, C. F., et al. (2017). Multi-institutional validation study of the American Joint Commission on Cancer changes for T and N staging in patients with pancreatic adenocarcinoma. *Ann Surg, 265*, 185.

Brand, R. (2001). The diagnosis of pancreatic cancer. *Cancer J, 7*, 287.

DeWitt, J., Devereaux, B., Chriswell, M., et al. (2004). Comparison of endoscopic ultrasonography and multidetector computed tomography for detecting and staging pancreatic cancer. *Ann Intern Med, 141*, 753.

Liao, W. C., Chien, K. L., Lin, Y. L., et al. (2013). Adjuvant treatments for resected pancreatic adenocarcinoma: A systematic review and network meta-analysis. *Lancet Oncol, 14*, 1095.

CHAPTER 27

Splenomegaly in a 40-Year-Old Female

Elizabeth Ann Jackson Carlson ■ Adnan Alseidi

A 40-year-old female presents to her primary care physician with a complaint of abdominal fullness. She describes a nontender mass in the left upper quadrant of her abdomenm which she first noticed approximately 2 months ago. She reports that she had previously been feeling well, but over the last several weeks she has noted some worsening fatigue, weight loss, and chills at night that she has attributed to increased stress at work. On physical examination, the patient's abdomen is soft and nontender with a firm, palpable mass in the LUQ that extends 8 cm below the costal margin. Her examination is otherwise unremarkable.

What is the Differential Diagnosis of Splenomegaly?

The most common etiology for a left upper quadrant mass is splenomegaly. There are multiple etiologies of splenomegaly, many of which do not require surgical treatment. They can be categorized based on their underlying pathophysiology (Table 27.1). Frequently, splenomegaly is the result of pathology outside the spleen itself, and as such, interventions on the spleen provide only symptomatic relief rather than a cure. Acute surgical problems related to splenomegaly are relatively few but include rupture, hemorrhage, and refractory cytopenias. Surgery may at times be appropriate for management of symptoms of splenomegaly, including abdominal pain, early satiety, and chronic transfusion requirements.

How Is Splenomegaly Evaluated on Physical Examination?

Physical examination for splenomegaly follows all tenets of a good abdominal examination and includes inspection, auscultation, palpation, and percussion. Splenomegaly is rarely visible on inspection, particularly given the average body habitus of the modern Western patient population, but the inferior tip may be seen as it traverses the costal margin with the respiratory cycle. Auscultation is rarely helpful, but a splenic rub may indicate splenic infarction. Dullness to percussion in the LUQ can identify the spleen if it is enlarged but not palpable; the percussed dullness should shift down toward the costal margin in accordance with splenic movement during inspiration. Palpation under the costal margin can identify the splenic tip. The spleen size is typically measured on physical examination in the number of centimeters of spleen palpable below the left costal margin in the midclavicular line. Under normal circumstances, the spleen is not palpable.

What Workup Should Be Included in the Evaluation of the Spleen?

Splenomegaly is most frequently a reflection of an underlying disease not directly related to the spleen itself, and workup should therefore be directed toward identifying the underlying pathophysiology. Workup of splenomegaly should include a detailed history and physical examination to uncover findings suggestive of an etiology—for example, a history of alcohol use that may contribute to cirrhosis and resulting portal hypertension. Laboratory studies, particularly a complete blood count and a peripheral

TABLE 27.1 ■ Differential Diagnosis of Splenomegaly

Etiology	Examples
Congestive	Cirrhosis Portal vein malformations Thrombosis or compression of the portal or splenic vein systems
Storage Diseases	Lipoid (e.g., Niemann-Pick disease, Gaucher disease) Nonlipoid (e.g., Letterer-Siwe disease)
Myelo- and Lymphoproliferative	Polycythemia vera, other myelodysplastic disorders Leukemia Lymphoma
Chronic hemolytic anemias	Thalassaemias Sickle cell anemia
Structural	Red cell abnormalities (e.g., hereditary spherocytosis, elliptocytosis)
Infectious or inflammatory	Systemic lupus Rheumatoid arthritis Immune thrombocytopenic purpura Autoimmune hemolytic anemia

smear, may be helpful in identifying both splenic function and cytologic abnormalities. Ultrasound is a useful adjunct that can accurately report splenic size as well as evaluate other abdominal organs, particularly the liver, for possible etiologies of splenomegaly. Abdominal computed tomography (CT) can identify structural abnormalities or masses in the spleen as well as providing detailed information about the other abdominal organs and vasculature, particularly the portal vein. In rare cases, PET scan can be used to evaluate splenic lesions. Splenic biopsy is rarely performed given the risk of bleeding.

CLINICAL PEARL (STEPS 2/3)

Splenomegaly is the result of an underlying pathophysiologic process rather than that of primary splenic origin. Management of splenomegaly should start with identification of the underlying cause of splenomegaly rather than intervention on the spleen itself—unless, of course, there is an acute splenic issue such as uncontrolled hemorrhage.

BASIC SCIENCE PEARL (STEP 1)

The spleen is located in the left upper quadrant of the abdomen, closely associated with a number of vascular structures and organs (Fig. 27.1). Superiorly and posteriorly, the spleen is bounded by the diaphragm and suspended by the splenophrenic ligaments. The greater curve of the stomach is medial with the short gastric vessels and left gastroepiploic artery contained in the splenogastric ligament. Anteriorly is the splenic flexure of the colon with the associated splenocolic ligament. The left kidney is inferior to the spleen, and the splenic vessels and the tail of the pancreas reside in the splenorenal ligament. The splenic artery has two common branching patterns: a) distributed, with branches arising distant from the splenic hilum; and b) magistral or bundled, with branches arising close to the hilum only.

The patient undergoes a full set of laboratory analyses. A complete blood count (CBC) and peripheral blood smear are notable for leukocytosis to 35×10^9 cells/L, mild anemia, with a left shift and 2% blast cells. Due to the leukocytosis and blasts present in the peripheral smear, the patient undergoes a bone marrow biopsy. Analysis of her bone marrow reveals hypercellularity with increased myelocytes and 4% blasts, and genetic testing confirms BCR-ABL1 fusion gene. She is diagnosed with chronic myelogenous leukemia.

Spleen in Situ

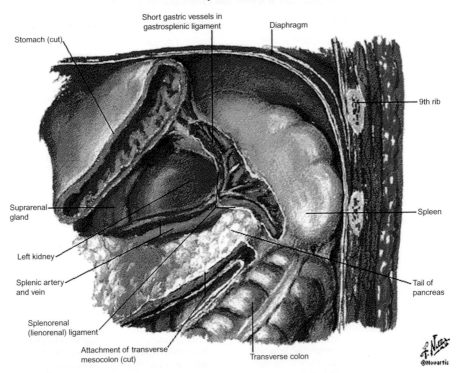

Fig. 27.1 Splenic anatomy. (Redrawn from Netter FH: *Atlas of Human Anatomy,* ed 4, Philadelphia, 2019, Elsevier.) (Plate 289 in Netter)

What Is the Differential Diagnosis for Myeloproliferative Disorders Causing Splenomegaly?
A number of myeloproliferative disorders cause splenomegaly (Table 27.2). They have similar underlying pathology relating to abnormal gene regulation of hematopoietic stem cells. Many of these diseases involve mutations in the JAK-STAT signal transduction pathways leading to abnormal myeloproliferation. Lymphoproliferative disorders, specifically B and T cell leukemias and lymphomas which constitute an extremely heterogeneous group of disorders, can also cause splenomegaly and can occur rapidly. Splenomegaly caused by these myeloproliferative disorders is usually gradually progressive, but in some cases, such as blast crises, splenic enlargement can occur relatively quickly, potentially leading to spontaneous splenic rupture.

Over the next 2 weeks, the patient experiences rapid increase in splenomegaly and begins to have left upper quadrant pain. She has met with a hematologist, and initiation of treatment is planned but not yet initiated. She presents to the emergency department (ED) early in the morning with severe left upper quadrant pain and reports that she has been feeling increasingly fatigued and lightheaded since the evening prior. Her vital signs on presentation include a heart rate of 124 bpm and a blood pressure of 98/70 mm Hg; she appears pale. A CBC is notable for leukocytosis to 80×10^9 cells/L, hematocrit of 25% (down from 38% on previous outpatient visits), and 21% blasts. She receives 2 L crystalloid in the ED with improvement in heart rate to 106 bpm, and she is typed and crossed for blood products. A CT of the abdomen and pelvis with contrast is obtained and shows hemoperitoneum with a grade 3 splenic laceration and a small amount of contrast extravasation from the laceration. She is diagnosed with blast crisis and is evaluated by the surgical team for splenectomy.

TABLE 27.2 ■ Differential Diagnosis of Myelo- and Lymphoproliferative Disorders

Disorder	Diagnosis[a]	Pathophysiology	Treatment
Primary myelofibrosis	JAK2, CALR, or MPL mutation with megakaryocytic proliferation	Abnormal regulation of growth factors and cytokines	Based on disease characteristics
Peripheral T-cell lymphomas	Diagnosis based on cytopathologic, genetic, immunologic, and clinical factors; many variants	Frequently involve activation of tyrosine kinases with downstream activation of JAK-STAT paths; some subtypes are associated with viral infections, such as HTLV-1 retrovirus	Frequently CHOP[b] or CHOP-like therapies, but varies with subtype
B-cell lymphomas	Diagnosis based on cytopathologic, genetic, immunologic, and clinical factors; many variants	Multiple factors, including defects in BCL6 regulation of survival and cell cycle progression and in nuclear factor kappa-B (NFk-B) regulation of differentiation	Chemotherapy often first line; varies by subtype
B- and T-cell leukemias	Based on blood and bone marrow smears with immunohistochemical staining with genetic testing in some cases	Upregulation of lymphoblastic production; specific pathway depends on subtype	Chemotherapy as first-line treatment; consideration of bone marrow transplant if refractory
Chronic neutrophilic leukemia	Diagnosis of exclusion based on WHO criteria, often with CSF3R mutation	Constitutive activation of colony-stimulating factor 3 receptor with activation of JAK-STAT pathway	Based on disease characteristics
Chronic myeloid leukemia	BCR-ABL1 fusion gene; Philadelphia chromosome	BCR-ABL1 oncogene activation of tyrosine kinase signal pathways	Targeted tyrosine kinase pathway inhibition (tyrosine kinase inhibitors include imatinib, erlotinib, sorafenib, sunitinib, dasatinib, gefitinib)
Essential thrombocythemia	JAK2, CALR, or MPL mutation with megakaryocyte proliferation and platelets > 450 x 10⁹/L	Upregulation or megakaryocyte lineages	Hydroxyurea

TABLE 27.2 ■ **Differential Diagnosis of Myelo- and Lymphoproliferative Disorders** (Continued)

Disorder	Diagnosis	Pathophysiology	Treatment
Polycythemia vera	Gain of function JAK2 mutation with elevated hgb/hct and bone marrow trilinear hypercellularity	JAK2 kinase activation of EPO receptors	Aspirin, therapeutic phlebotomy
Unclassifiable myeloproliferative neoplasms	Any myeloproliferative disorder not meeting criteria for a defined entity	Upregulation of myeloid lineages	Based on disease characteristics

[a]Diagnosis criteria simplified here; see WHO guidelines for diagnosis for complete criteria of these diseases.
[b]CHOP is a chemotherapy regimen: cyclophosphamide, hydroxydaunomycin, vincristine (brand name Oncovin), and prednisone.

What Are the Indications for Splenectomy?

Splenectomy is indicated for splenic rupture (traumatic or spontaneous) with hemorrhage, typically corresponding to injuries grade III to V (see Chapter 39). Splenomegaly is also indicated for treatment of neoplasm, abscess, and splenic vascular malformations such as aneurysm with high risk of hemorrhage. It may also be indicated for diagnostic purposes in some hematological malignancies, for management of refractory hypersplenism, or for symptomatic relief of splenomegaly.

What Approaches Are Available for Splenectomy?

The decision for approach depends on the indications and urgency of splenectomy. In general practice, the most common indication for splenectomy is traumatic rupture that warrants exploratory laparotomy. Laparoscopic splenectomy is a viable option for nontraumatic cases. To be removed laparoscopically, the spleen must be morcellated in a bag while still in the abdominal cavity and then delivered via a trocar or enlarged laparoscopic portsite. In cases in which morcellation and delivery of the spleen via a trocar is inadvisable or infeasible, the specimen can be extracted through a small Pfannenstiel incision. In selected cases, embolization by interventional radiology can provide a functional splenectomy with slow involution of the devitalized spleen over time. The surgical approaches will be discussed here.

Laparoscopic Splenectomy

1. Position the patient in either a lateral (right side down) or supine position, depending on the degree of splenomegaly and other exposure that may be necessary.
2. Trochar placement—technique is based on surgeon's preference and the positioning being used.
3. Explore the abdomen to assess for accessory spleens. From most to least frequent, common locations include the splenic hilum, gastrosplenic and splenorenal ligaments, and greater omentum.
4. Mobilize the spleen by taking down the gastrosplenic ligament, the splenic flexure of the colon, and the splenorenal and phrenicosplenic ligaments. Mobilize the tail of the pancreas off the splenic hilum as needed. (Note that injury to the tail of the pancreas is a common and bothersome complication.)
5. Divide the splenic vessels at the hilum with a linear stapler or surgical clips.
6. Remove the spleen either through a trochar as a fractured specimen in an endocatch bag or whole through a separate minilaparotomy incision.

Open Splenectomy

1. Position the patient supine or with hips tilted to 45 degrees with the left side up.
2. Make a left subcostal incision or midline laparotomy (preferred in the setting of severe splenomegaly).
3. Explore for accessory spleens.
4. Mobilize the spleen and ligate the splenic vessels separately (there is increased risk of AV fistula formation when the artery and vein are ligated together). In the case of a friable spleen prone to fracture, it is often advisable to ligate the splenic artery through the lesser sac before splenic mobilization.
5. Remove the spleen and close. A drain can be left in place to assess for bleeding or pancreatic disruption (check drain fluid amylase).

CLINICAL PEARL

Careful dissection during splenectomy is critical to avoid injury to the extensive vasculature and to avoid damage to the overlying pancreatic tail.

What Are the Major Complications of Splenectomy?

The major complication of splenectomy is intraoperative and postoperative hemorrhage. Open splenectomy is associated with higher rates of intraoperative transfusion. This risk can be reduced by meticulous dissection intraoperatively and aggressive hemostasis. Postoperatively, patients frequently experience thrombocytosis and leukocytosis with counts peaking around postoperative day 10 that can lead to thrombotic events—most frequently, splenic or portal vein thrombosis.

Loss of splenic activity against encapsulated organisms increases the risk of overwhelming postoperative infection (OPSI) that typically is related to pneumococcal infection and, less commonly, *H. influenza* type B or *Neisseria meningitides*. For planned splenectomy, patient should receive pneumococcal, *H. influenzae* B, and meningococcal vaccines 2 weeks before the operation. For emergent splenectomy, these vaccines should be given postoperatively, with timing of vaccination varying with the indication for splenectomy (e.g., trauma versus hematologic malignancy) and immune status.

CLINICAL PEARL

All splenectomy patients should receive vaccines against encapsulated organisms (*Haemophilus influenzae*, *Streptococcus pneumoniae*, and *Neisseria meningitidis*) to reduce the risk of overwhelming postsplenectomy infection.

The patient undergoes emergent open splenectomy without complication and initiates treatment for her blast crisis with allopurinol and hydroxyurea. She receives pneumococcal, *H. influenzae* B, and meningococcal vaccinations and is discharged from the hospital after 5 days. She returns for follow-up 2 weeks later. She is doing well without any signs or symptoms of complications.

BEYOND THE PEARLS

- Splenomegaly is almost always secondary to extrasplenic pathology.
- Workup of splenectomy should be directed at identifying the underlying cause.
- Splenomegaly itself is not an indication for surgical intervention.
- Both laparoscopic and open techniques are appropriate for splenectomy, with open splenectomy preferred for traumatic rupture or massive splenomegaly.
- The most common complication of splenectomy is hemorrhage.
- All patients with splenectomy should receive vaccination against encapsulated organisms.

Suggested Readings

Cervantes, F., Dupriez, B., Pereira, A., et al. (2009). New prognostic scoring system for primary myelofibrosis based on a study of the International Working Group for Myelofibrosis Research and Treatment. *Blood, 113*, 2895–2901. https://doi.org/10.1182/blood-2008-07-170449.

Crary, S. E., & Buchanan, G. R. (2009). Vascular complications after splenectomy for hematologic disorders. *Blood, 114*(14), 2861–2868.

Musallam, K. M., Khalife, M., Sfeir, P. M., et al. (2013). Postoperative outcomes after laparoscopic splenectomy compared with open splenectomy. *Ann Sur, 257*(6), 1116–1123.

Patel, N. Y., et al. (2012). Outcomes and complications after splenectomy for hematologic disorders. *American Journal of Surgery, 204*(6), 1014–1020.

Rialon, K. L., Speicher, P. J., Ceppa, E. P., et al. (2015). Outcomes following splenectomy in patients with myeloid neoplasms. *J Surg Oncol, 111*(4), 389–395. https://doi.org/10.1002/jso.23846. Epub 2014 Dec 9.

Weledji, E. P. (2014). Benefits and risks of splenectomy. *International Journal of Surgery, 12*(2), 113–119. https://doi.org/10.1016/j.ijsu.2013.11.017.

Vascular Surgery

CHAPTER 28

Leg Pain in a 55-Year-Old Male

Julia Glaser ■ Venkat Kalapatapu

A 55-year-old man with a history of type 2 diabetes, hypertension, and hyperlipidemia presents to his physician with a complaint of calf pain, left worse than right. He states the pain is worse when he walks and will stop a few minutes after he stops walking. He is able to walk approximately one block before the pain causes him to stop walking. The pain ceases when he stops and rests. The pain has been present for 2 years and has appeared at progressively shorter distances over that time. He is hindered in his job as a mail carrier due to the pain. Currently, he smokes one pack of cigarettes per day, although he previously smoked two packs per day.

What Is the Differential Diagnosis for Leg Pain?

Leg pain can be caused by many etiologies. The most common cause for this history of intermittent pain is due to peripheral arterial disease (PAD), but there are musculoskeletal, rheumatologic, neurogenic, and other etiologies as well. Of special consideration is the length of time the leg pain has been occurring because it can help inform the differential diagnosis. Specifically, the acute onset of pain can point to acute arterial insufficiency, which, whether embolic or thrombotic in nature, may constitute a surgical emergency.

The classic presentation of claudication is pain that starts with a predictable distance of ambulation and stops at rest. However, many patients with PAD present with atypical symptoms rather than textbook claudication. Patients with severe PAD may present with rest pain and may describe dangling their foot over the side of the bed at night to relieve the pain. Those who develop a diabetic wound in the setting of PAD may not experience pain at all due to advanced diabetic neuropathy, and they may complain only of a wound that has been slow to heal or progressively worsening.

Who Is at Risk for Peripheral Arterial Disease and How Is the Severity Graded?

Peripheral vascular disease is the lack of sufficient blood flow due to atherosclerotic plaque causing either stenosis or occlusion of the peripheral vessels. Risk factors for PAD include atherosclerosis, diabetes, hypertension, hyperlipidemia, and a history of smoking—are at risk for peripheral vascular disease. The severity ranges from asymptomatic (patients who only have evidence of PAD on imaging but have no symptoms) to patients with critical limb ischemia (rest pain, tissue loss, or gangrene). The most commonly used system for grading the severity of PAD is the Rutherford System (Table 28.1).

BASIC SCIENCE PEARL (STEP 1)

An understanding of the anatomy of the arterial system of the lower extremities is fundamental to the appreciation of the physical examination findings and therapies for peripheral vascular disease (Fig. 28.1).

TABLE 28.1 ■ Rutherford Classification System for Peripheral Artery Disease

Grade	Category	Clinical description	Objective criteria
0	0	Asymptomatic—no hemodynamically significant occlusive disease	Normal treadmill or reactive hyperemia test
	1	Mild claudication	Completes treadmill exercise[b]; AP after exercise > 50 mm Hg but at least 20 mm Hg lower than resting value
I	2	Moderate claudication	Between categories 1 and 3
	3	Severe claudication	Cannot complete standard treadmill exercise[b] *and* AP after exercise < 50 mm Hg
II[a]	4	Ischemic rest pain	Resting AP < 40 mm Hg, flat or barely pulsatile ankle or metatarsal PVR; TP < 30 mm Hg
III[a]	5	Minor tissue loss—nonhealing ulcer, focal gangrene with diffuse pedal ischemia	Resting AP < 60 mm Hg, ankle or metatarsal PVR flat or barely pulsatile; TP < 40 mm Hg
	6	Major tissue loss—extending higher than TM level, functional foot no longer salvageable	Same as category 5

AP, Ankle pressure; *PVR,* pulse volume recording; *TP,* toe pressure; *TM,* transmetatarsal.
[a]Grades II and III, categories 4, 5, and 6, are embraced by the term chronic *critical* ischemia.

[b]Five minutes at 2 mph on a 12% incline.
Reprinted with permission from Elsevier: Rutherford, et al: Recommended standards for reports dealing with lower extremity ischemia: revised version, *J Vasc Surg* Sep;26(3):517–538, 1997.

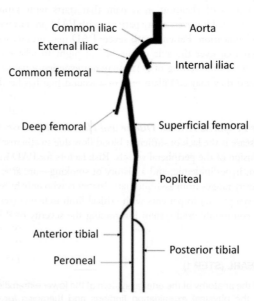

Fig. 28.1 Schematic of the arterial supply of the right lower extremity. (Modified from Kwon, JH, Shin, JH: Hypoplastic superficial femoral artery combined with connection of the deep femoral artery to the popliteal artery, *Radiol Case Rep* Feb;13(1):39–42, 2018.)

What Are the Expected Physical Examination Findings in Peripheral Vascular Disease?

As with many disease processes, vascular disease has a spectrum of physical findings which reflects disease severity. Patients who are claudicants, for example, may have a diminished or absent peripheral pulse and an otherwise normal extremity examination. Patients who have more severe vascular disease, on the other hand, are likely to have dependent rubor (redness), loss of hair on the shins, and slow-to-heal or nonhealing wounds in addition to diminished or absent peripheral pulses.

On physical examination, the patient's vital signs are within normal limits. His heart has a regular rate and rhythm, and his lungs are clear to auscultation bilaterally. His abdomen is soft, nontender, and nondistended. His peripheral reflexes and tone are normal bilaterally. He has no pain on palpation of his knees, ankles, or calves, and he has no peripheral edema or knee effusions. He has palpable femoral pulses but popliteal, dorsalis pedis, and posterior tibial pulses are absent bilaterally. There are no wounds on his feet.

CLINICAL PEARL (STEPS 2/3)

The most common peripheral pulses that are assessed on physical examination are femoral, popliteal, dorsalis pedis, and posterior tibial. These pulses are easily palpable in patients who do not have peripheral vascular disease, but a handheld Doppler ultrasound may be required to assess flow in patients whose pulses are diminished.

What Studies Are Useful in the Diagnosis of Peripheral Arterial Disease?

Several studies can help establish the presence and extent of PAD. Ankle-brachial indices (ABIs) and pulse volume recordings (PVRs) are noninvasive vascular laboratory tests that can help establish the presence of vascular disease without the risk of radiation or an invasive procedure; these are often the first-line test to determine the presence of PAD. In these tests, blood pressure cuffs are placed at several locations on the lower extremities. The blood pressure at each location is recorded, as well as the pressure at both brachial arteries. The ratio of the highest blood pressure (dorsalis pedis or posterior tibial) to the highest brachial pressure is the ankle-brachial index. An ABI of 0.9 to 1.4 is considered normal. An ABI of 0.4 to 0.9 is associated with claudication, and an ABI of less than 0.4 is associated with critical limb ischemia (rest pain, tissue loss, or gangrene). The ABI cutoffs are not absolute, and a patient with a low ABI may not have symptoms. A high ABI (> 1.4) suggests the presence of noncompressible vessels, which can often be seen in diabetes. Pulse volume recordings examine the waveform across the cardiac cycle in the peripheral vasculature. As stenoses develop and become more severe, the normal waveform becomes dampened. This can also be seen when listening to pulses with a handheld Doppler. A normal Doppler signal has a crisp, triphasic sound. This sound transitions to biphasic then to monophasic as the degree of proximal stenosis increases.

Computed tomography angiograms (CTA) and magnetic resonance angiograms (MRA) provide a noninvasive method to more accurately assess vascular disease. These studies can be useful to evaluate for other pathology in addition to assessing the burden of vascular disease. However, unlike an angiogram, CTA and MRA do not allow the opportunity to intervene simultaneously.

An angiogram is the traditional, gold-standard test to assess the degree of PAD and is often performed in conjunction with angioplasty or stents, two modalities frequently used to treat atherosclerotic lesions causing stenoses. Note that angiography is invasive and carries the risks both of radiation and potential nephrotoxicity of contrast dye.

What Are the Treatment Options for Patients With Peripheral Vascular Disease?
In patients who have claudication that is not lifestyle-limiting as the only manifestation of their peripheral vascular disease, the primary treatment is medical management and walking. Patients are counseled to walk as far as they can until they start to experience leg pain and then keep going if they are able. Patients who are on a walking program can experience significant improvement in their symptoms over time. The other critical portion of the treatment of such patients is risk reduction. PAD is a marker of advanced atherosclerotic disease, and, therefore, PAD is a risk factor equivalent for coronary artery disease. Thus all patients with PAD should be counseled about coronary artery disease, have their comorbidities (such as diabetes and hypertension) adequately managed, and should all be placed on a statin. Patients with PAD and diabetes should be educated about protecting their feet, as they are particularly at risk for the development of nonhealing ulcers.

CLINICAL PEARL

Patients with claudication that is not lifestyle-limiting can be managed medically. Patients with more advanced PAD (rest pain, tissue loss, or gangrene) should undergo endovascular or surgical revascularization if the risk of the procedure is not prohibitive.

What Interventions Are Performed for Patients With Peripheral Arterial Disease?
Patients who have lifestyle-limiting claudication or critical limb ischemia warrant an intervention. Interventions for PAD may be endovascular or open surgical procedures. Through the use of endovascular therapies continues to evolve, a consensus has been reached among several societies about which anatomic lesions should be treated with endovascular methods vs open surgery, The TASC classification. Norgren et al, J Vasc Surg. 2007 Jan;45 Suppl S:S5–67.

Endovascular interventions involve balloon angioplasty (balloon dilation of a lesion), stenting, and atherectomy (endovascular removal of atherosclerotic plaque). These are accomplished through percutaneous access at the groin or, occasionally, brachial artery. After stenting or atherectomy, patients are frequently placed on dual antiplatelet therapy (aspirin and Plavix) in order to preserve the patency of interventions.

Some lesions are not amenable to endovascular therapy and are best treated by open interventions. Isolated common femoral disease can be treated by a common femoral endarterectomy, in which occlusive plaque is removed from the common femoral artery. Occlusions in the distal leg can be treated with open surgical bypass. The proximal and distal targets of the bypass depend upon the location of the obstructing lesion.

The patient undergoes a diagnostic angiogram of his left leg and is found to have a total occlusion of his superficial femoral artery (SFA) for almost its entire length. His circulation reconstitutes at his popliteal artery above the knee via collateral vessels, and he has intact three-vessel runoff (dorsalis pedis, posterior tibial, and peroneal arteries) distally. The lesion is not amenable to endovascular repair, and the physician recommends a bypass procedure.

What Preoperative Workup Is Necessary Before a Peripheral Bypass?
All patients with PAD are at risk for coronary atherosclerosis, therefore, evaluation for cardiac disease is essential. Treadmill stress tests often cannot be performed in these patients secondary to the physical limitations of their PAD; nuclear stress test and/or consultation with a cardiologist are recommended for risk stratification. Screening for carotid disease with carotid duplex ultrasound is also usually performed for patients undergoing elective vascular surgery.

What Types of Peripheral Bypass Are Possible?

Peripheral bypasses are planned based on the location of the lesion (see Fig. 28.1). Many bypasses start at the common femoral artery; the locations for the distal anastomoses for peripheral bypasses vary but can utilize the popliteal artery above the knee, the popliteal artery below the knee, the posterior tibial artery, the anterior tibial artery, or the peroneal artery. Though uncommon, bypasses can also be performed that reach to the dorsalis pedis artery or posterior tibial artery in the foot.

What Are the Considerations in Planning a Bypass?

In bypass procedures for peripheral vascular disease, there are three important considerations: (1) inflow, (2) outflow, and (3) type of conduit. All three issues must both immediate and long-term flow and patency of the bypass.

Inflow refers to the quality of flow proximal to the intended bypass. If a patient has a significant iliac stenosis, for example, then this stenosis should be treated before a bypass which starts at the common femoral artery in order to maximize the inflow into the bypass.

Outflow refers to the capacity of the vessels of the distal anastomosis to receive improved inflow. The receiving vessel should be free of significant disease for optimal results. For example, in a patient who has an occluded SFA that reconstitutes briefly at the above-knee popliteal but has no patent tibial vessels, the bypass is likely to have limited patency.

The type of conduit refers to what the bypass itself is made of. Large studies show that a patient's own vein is the best conduit for a bypass in terms of long-term patency. The vein that is used in bypasses for PAD is most commonly the greater saphenous vein, although other veins (including the small saphenous, basilic, and cephalic) may also be used. In the absence of suitable vein, prosthetic conduit made of polyethylene terephthalate or polytetrafluoroethylene (PTFE) can be used.

CLINICAL PEARL

A greater saphenous vein that is larger than 3 mm in diameter is the preferred conduit for all lower extremity bypass procedures.

Femoral to Above-Knee Popliteal Bypass

1. Mark skin overlying the vein intended for use as conduit. This can either be performed preoperatively as part of the assessment for suitability of the vein, or in the operating room after the induction of general anesthesia.
2. Expose the common femoral artery for the proximal anastomosis via a vertical incision in the groin, centered over the femoral artery (see Fig. 28.2). Gain proximal control at the common femoral artery at the level of the inguinal ligament as well as control of the superficial femoral artery and profunda.
3. Expose the above-knee popliteal artery via an incision just above the knee just anterior to the border of the sartorius (Fig. 28.3). Avoid the deep femoral veins, and gain control of the above-knee popliteal artery proximally and distally.
4. If a vein conduit is to be used, expose the greater saphenous vein along its length, and ligate all side branches. Remove the required amount of vein, and flush to check for holes. Prepare the graft material if a graft will be used.
5. Create a tunnel from the common femoral artery to the above-knee popliteal artery (Fig. 28.3). Pass the conduit (vein or graft) through the tunnel, ensuring it does not get twisted. The vein should be reversed in order to have flow in the correct direction related to valves.
6. Systemically heparinize the patient and clamp the common femoral artery, profunda, and SFA.
7. Perform the proximal anastomosis. Flush the graft, and then perform the distal anastomosis.
8. Ensure an adequate pulse within and distal to the graft and close the incisions.

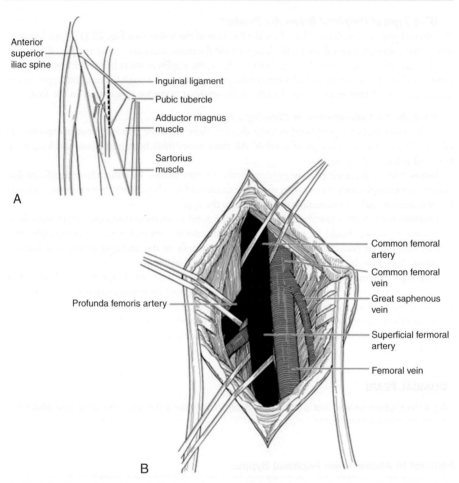

Fig. 28.2 Exposure of the right common femoral artery and vein. Incision is made at the dotted line (A) and dissection through soft tissue reveals underlying anatomy (B). Note that the left side of the image is lateral. (Reprinted with permission from Elsevier from: Chaikof E, Cambria R: *Atlas of vascular surgery and endovascular therapy: anatomy and technique*, 2014.)

CLINICAL PEARL

Bypasses can be performed with reversed greater saphenous vein (as described previously) or with vein that is left *in situ*. For *in situ* bypasses, the valves are lysed with a valvulotome and the major side branches ligated. Evidence is equivocal as far as which approach is better.

What Are the Potential Complications of Lower Extremity Bypass for Peripheral Arterial Disease?

Pulses in the bypass and distal to it must be checked frequently in the immediate postoperative period to monitor for graft thrombosis. Graft thrombosis that occurs within the first 24 hours after surgery is thought to be due to a technical problem and warrants immediate return to the operating room. Thrombosis that presents later can be associated with progression of disease proximal or distal to the bypass or with intimal hyperplasia leading to stenosis within the bypass. As with any

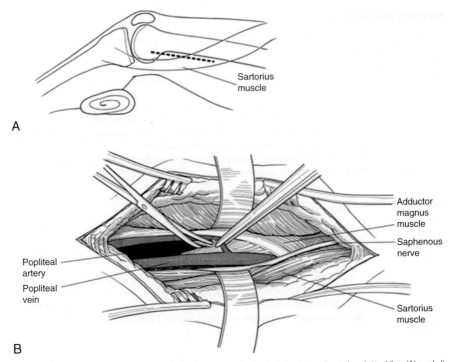

Fig. 28.3 Exposure of the above knee popliteal artery and vein. Incision is made at the dotted line (A) and dissection through soft tissue reveals underlying anatomy (B). (Reprinted with permission from Elsevier from: Chaikof E, Cambria R: *Atlas of vascular surgery and endovascular therapy: anatomy and technique*, 2014.)

surgery involving heparinization, bleeding is a potential complication after bypass, and incisions over anastomoses should be monitored for hematoma development. Wound infection can also occur and is of special concern due to the possibility of synthetic graft infection necessitating graft removal. Injury to the vessels, either from a clamp injury or due to anastomotic technique, is also possible. If the bypass is performed with *in situ* vein, a retained valve can limit patency.

How Are Patients Who Undergo a Peripheral Bypass Followed Postoperatively?

It is important to remember that patients who have developed clinically significant PAD at one site are likely to develop evidence of advanced atherosclerosis at other sites. Patients should be followed for the development of other manifestations of atherosclerosis, including PAD in the contralateral limb and carotid atherosclerotic disease. After a peripheral bypass, patients are typically followed with a graft duplex ultrasound. Intimal hyperplasia can limit the patency of bypass grafts; surveillance by ultrasound is of value as progressive lesion will often appear as an elevated velocity on ultrasound before the stenosis is significant enough to cause bypass graft occlusion or symptoms.

The patient undergoes a left femoral to above-knee popliteal artery bypass. Distal arterial pulse signals are obtained by Doppler signal postoperatively. The patient is referred for physical therapy and is discharged home on the third postoperative day. He returns to work 2 weeks later and has no pain with ambulating on his mail route.

BEYOND THE PEARLS

- Peripheral artery disease (PAD) can be asymptomatic or can present with claudication, rest pain, tissue loss, or gangrene.
- Patients with PAD often have concurrent coronary artery disease.
- Interventions for PAD are indicated for lifestyle-limiting claudication, rest pain, tissue loss, or gangrene.
- A variety of endovascular interventions can be performed for peripheral vascular disease. Some anatomic distributions of disease are better served by open bypass.
- Vein is always the preferred conduit for lower extremity bypass. Synthetic graft materials are appropriate when a patient's native vein is deemed unsuitable.
- After a procedure for PAD, patients are surveilled for their lifetime for progression of their disease and the durability of the intervention.

Suggested Readings

Gerhard-Herman, M. D., Gornik, H. L., Barrett, C., Barshes, N. R., Corriere, M. A., Drachman, D. E., et al. (2017). 2016 AHA/ACC guideline on the management of patients with lower extremity peripheral artery disease: A report of the American College of Cardiology/American Heart Association Task Force on Clinical Practice Guidelines. *J Am Coll Cardiol*, *69*(11), e71–e126.

McGrae McDermott, M., Mehta, S., & Greenland, P. (1999). Exertional leg symptoms other than intermittent claudication are common in peripheral arterial disease. *Arch Intern Med*, *159*(4), 387.

Norgren, L., Hiatt, W. R., Dormandy, J. A., Nehler, M. R., Harris, K. A., & Fowkes, F. G. R. (2007). Intersociety consensus for the management of peripheral arterial disease (TASC II). *J Vasc Surg Jan*, *45*(Suppl 1), S5–S67.

CHAPTER 29

66- and 68-Year-Old Sisters with Lower Extremity Swelling

Michael J. Qaqish ■ Robert Meisner

A 68-year-old-female is referred to your office by her primary care physician for evaluation of her left lower extremity swelling. The woman states the swelling has been progressive over the past week after her flight home from Europe. The swelling began in her ankle and has progressed up her leg to about her midcalf. She is on amlodipine 5mg daily for her blood pressure and denies any other medications or medical problems. She is aware of the mild swelling the amlodipine has caused since she began taking it, but there is an obvious discrepancy between her two legs now. On examination, her lungs are clear bilaterally, her heart sounds are within normal limits without murmurs, gallops, or rubs. Her abdomen is soft, nontender, nondistended, and has no rebound or guarding. The right lower extremity has +1 pitting edema to 5 cm above the ankle. On the left lower extremity, she has +2 pitting edema from her foot to 3 cm below the tibial tuberosity. No skin changes are noted, and there is no tenderness or erythema. She has a +2 palpable dorsalis pedis and posterior tibialis pulses bilaterally.

What Is the Differential Diagnosis of Leg Swelling?

The differential diagnosis for leg swelling is broad and most commonly includes venous insufficiency, outflow obstruction, lymphatic obstruction, and systemic cardiovascular disease. Important factors to consider in the initial evaluation of leg edema is whether this is an acute or chronic problem and whether the edema is present in one or both lower extremities (Table 29.1). When considering the causes of acute leg swelling, a consideration of the pathophysiology should guide the work up. The various pathologies to consider are those that result in more fluid in the interstitial space: increased intracapillary hydrostatic pressure (i.e., increase in blood volume in the venous system or poor venous outflow); or increased vascular permeability (i.e., inflammation).

BASIC SCIENCE PEARL (STEPS 1/2/3)

Starling's law describes principles that relate to how fluid is distributed between the intravascular and interstitial space. The law has four key components: intracapillary hydrostatic pressure, intracapillary oncotic pressure, interstitial hydrostatic pressure, and interstitial oncotic pressure.

Hydrostatic pressure tends to force fluid from the capillary to the interstitial space whereas the oncotic pressure, typically exerted by proteins, tends to draw fluid into or keep fluid within the capillary (Fig. 29.1). Lymphatic drainage is also an important component of drainage of the interstitial space. Any alteration in these factors can lead to accumulation of fluid in the interstitial space and manifest as edema.

TABLE 29.1 ■ Causes for Lower Extremity Edema

Bilateral Lower Extremity	Unilateral Lower Extremity
• Congestive heart failure • Sodium/Water retention; increased intravascular volume • Low oncotic pressure (i.e., cirrhosis, nephrotic syndrome) • Lymphedema • Drug-induced (i.e., calcium channel blockers)	• Deep venous thrombosis (DVT) • Venous outflow obstruction other than DVT • Ruptured Baker's cyst • Trauma • Cellulitis • Lymphedema

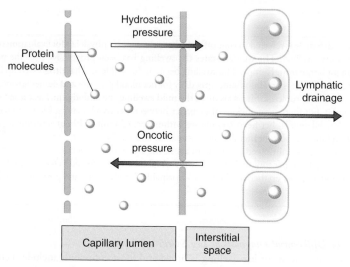

Fig. 29.1 Determinants of intravascular and interstitial fluid distribution. (Redrawn from Yaqoob MM, McCafferty K: Water, electrolytes and acid-base balance. In Kumar P, Clark M, editors: *Kumar and Clark's Clinical Medicine*, ed 9, Edinburgh, 2017, Elsevier, pp 149–181.)

CLINICAL PEARL (STEPS 2/3)

The manifestations of edema can help elucidate the etiology, so it is important to distinguish between pitting and nonpitting edema. This is established by applying pressure with one finger over the edematous limb for 3 to 5 seconds. If an impression is left in the leg, then this is considered pitting edema and is caused by an increase of fluid in the interstitium. Additionally, if there is discoloration of the edematous leg, known as lipodermatosclerosis, the chronicity of the edema of months or even years is established. This is due to hemosiderin deposition from red blood cells that have broken down after extravasating through damaged capillaries. In our patient, she has only had this swelling for a week and we would not expect to find lipodermatosclerosis. On physical examination, one should evaluate for warmth, tenderness, and erythema as inflammation is a possible cause.

What Is the Workup of a Patient Who Presents with Lower Extremity Edema?

The workup of lower extremity edema should be dictated by the most likely diagnoses given the patient's history and physical examination. A complete blood count (CBC) and a comprehensive metabolic profile (CMP) are good starting points as assessment of electrolyte abnormalities.

D-Dimer, which is typically sent off with initial labs, functions as a screening test that is highly sensitive but not specific to venous thrombosis. Alterations in liver function tests (especially albumin) can help to assess potential alterations in oncotic pressure within the vascular system, and elevations in the white blood cell count can help to detect the presence of inflammation or infection. Erythrocyte sedimentation rate (ESR) and C-reactive protein can also useful in consideration of inflammatory diseases. Brain natriuretic peptide (BNP) is also an important laboratory value in the evaluation of patients with congestive heart failure.

Radiographic studies are important in the workup of patients with lower extremity edema. Typically, the first radiographic study used to assess venous structures in the affected leg is a Doppler venous ultrasound. The benefits of a Doppler ultrasound include the fact that it is noninvasive, inexpensive, is not associated with radiation exposure, and is both highly sensitive and specific (95% for both). For these reasons, Doppler venous ultrasound is a very common first study for a wide range of complaints affecting the lower extremities.

Doppler ultrasound is technologist dependent but is largely reproducible between vascular labs; there are some limitations, however, including visualization of the veins in the pelvis (that is, lack of the vein compressibility used as the principle ultrasound determination for thrombosis of the vein). Duplex ultrasound can also help determine the acuity or chronicity of a thrombus identified (Fig. 29.2). When evaluating outflow obstruction in the iliac veins, duplex ultrasound is often helpful but not always definitive. In normal anatomy, the waveforms at the common femoral vein will have respiratory variation; in the setting of iliac vein obstruction, however, one can often demonstrate dampened monophasic waveforms.

If abnormalities are suspected within the pelvic veins, a computed tomography (CT) venogram or MRV is useful. Although also noninvasive, a CT venogram requires the administration of intravenous contrast, so one needs to consider the patient's kidney function.

Laboratory analyses acquired for the patient show no signs of systemic inflammation with an erythrocyte sedimentation rate and C-reactive protein within normal limits. She has a brain natriuretic peptide (BNP) that is within normal limits and rules out congestive heart failure. D-Dimer was elevated. A Duplex ultrasound of the left lower extremity is ordered and shows a noncompressible common femoral vein suggestive of an acute deep vein thrombosis.

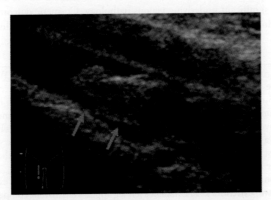

Fig. 29.2 Ultrasound of the right femoral vein demonstrating lack of compressibility and flow. A thrombus is seen obstructing the vein *(arrows)*. (Redrawn from Watanabe C, Ichiba T, Naito H: Left subclavian and right femoral vein thrombosis in a pregnant patient with antithrombin deficiency, *J Cardiol Cases* 18(4): 149–151, 2018.)

What Are the Therapeutic Options for Patients with Lower Extremity Edema?
The therapeutic options for patients with lower extremity edema depend largely on the etiology.

MEDICAL/SYSTEMIC CAUSES

Lower extremity edema that is the manifestation of a more systemic cause such as heart or liver disease should be treated by managing the primary disease process. Compression of the affected lower extremities may help to manage symptoms.

DEEP VENOUS THROMBOSIS

The usual and standard treatment option for deep venous thrombosis (DVT) is systemic anticoagulation using oral anticoagulation therapy. Only in a small percentage of cases will insertion of an inferior vena cava filter be necessary (such as if the patient is bleeding or has other contraindication to anticoagulation therapy). The goals of treatment with anticoagulants are to prevent propagation of the thrombus and to prevent the development of a pulmonary embolus.

Systemic thrombolytic therapy with tPA is not routinely administered for DVT due to the high risk of bleeding. Catheter-directed thrombolysis is an invasive option for clot dissolution that can be used to rapidly lyse a clot and limits the systemic dose of tPA required for clot lysis. This invasive treatment is usually reserved for the patient with very large clot burden (including IVC or iliac vein thrombus) and for those who are highly symptomatic, including those rare patients with phlegmasia of the affected limb. For patients with their first clinical DVT, anticoagulation is used for 3 months.

If there is a family history of thrombosis or there is an absence of routine risk factors, a more intense hypercoagulable profile would be appropriate, including a prothrombin time, international normalized ratio (INR), Factor V Leiden, Protein C and S levels, prothrombin gene mutation, anticardiolipin antibody, and beta2-glycoprotein I antibody.

CHRONIC VENOUS INSUFFICENCY

The therapeutic options for the many manifestations of chronic venous insufficiency (CVI) range from simple compression garments to more invasive venous valvuloplasty or vein stripping and ligation. Although treatment may be difficult, removal of incompetent superficial veins may help control bothersome symptoms. Varicose veins, which are often treated due to their appearance, are often signs of more significant underlying venous pathology. Cosmetic outcomes can be managed with laser and ablation therapies, but full assessment for underlying venous disease should also be undertaken.

The patient is diagnosed with a left common femoral deep vein thrombosis (DVT) with her long flight from Europe as a risk factor for the development of DVT.

Interestingly, 5 months later, the patient's sister, a 66-year-old-female with no significant past medical history, comes to the office with similar left leg swelling, cramping, and discomfort. She states, "I think I have the same problem my sister had some months ago." She has become concerned she may also have a DVT. She states she has noticed her leg has become more swollen and heavy feeling over the past 5 to 8 months and reports it is typically worse at the end of the day. She has also noticed a rash over her left lower leg over the past 2 weeks.

On examination, the patient's vital signs are normal as is her general physical examination—with exception of her lower extremities. The patient's left leg appears edematous compared with her right leg. There is overlying brownish-red color in the distal lower extremity, and the right leg has pitting edema from her foot to midthigh. Both lower extremities have palpable dorsalis pedis and posterior tibial arteries. She has full sensation and full range of motion of both lower extremities with no tenderness to palpation.

The patient's laboratory analyses show no abnormalities in CBC or CMP. Brain natriuretic peptide is less than 100, erythrocyte sedimentation rate is 12, C-reactive protein is 5, and her D-dimer is negative—all within normal limits. On physical examination she has signs of lipodermatosclerosis that suggest this swelling is a chronic issue. A Doppler ultrasound of the left lower extremity shows patent and compressible superficial and deep veins. It is noted, however, that the common femoral vein is nonphasic (blunted waveform) and shows no respiratory variations. A CT scan of the abdomen, pelvis, and lower extremities with intravenous contrast is ordered for further evaluation. The CT scan shows engorged left lower extremity veins and moderate compression of the left common iliac vein by the right common iliac artery (Fig. 29.3). She is diagnosed with iliac vein compression syndrome, commonly referred to as May-Thurner syndrome.

What Are Additional Causes of Venous Outflow Obstruction?

There are numerous potential causes of venous outflow obstruction, iliac vein compression syndrome (May-Thurner syndrome) being one of them. Often patients will require both a diagnostic and therapeutic venogram in the operating room or interventional suite, with which the surgical team endeavors to identify the exact location of obstruction or stenosis. In addition to traditional venography, a more sophisticated intravascular ultrasound (IVUS), more sensitive than a venogram, can help to more thoroughly assess the point of venous obstruction. The IVUS is a catheter-based device that is inserted intravenously during endovascular surgery. It is capable of yielding real time, 360-degree ultrasound imaging, which gives more detail regarding the area and etiology of the stenosis. The layers of the vein wall and the extravascular structures that surround the vein can be seen. Venous stents can be placed in areas of venous stenosis or compression to maximize venous outflow.

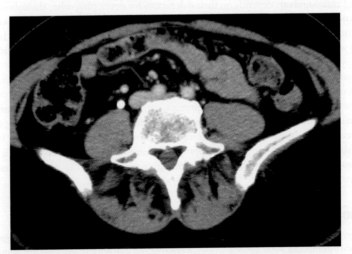

Fig. 29.3   Axial CT showing compression of the left common iliac artery (LCIV) *(arrow)* by the overlying right iliac artery. The LCIV at the point of maximal compression measures 4 mm. (Redrawn from Ahmed O, Ng J, Patel M, et al: Endovascular stent placement for May-Thurner syndrome in the absence of acute deep vein thrombosis, *J Vasc Intervent Radiol* 27(2):167–173, 2016.)

The patient is consented for a left lower extremity venogram. A wire followed by a catheter is advanced into the inferior vena cava via access from both the right and left common femoral veins. Both sides are evaluated to ensure that no pathology is missed on the unaffected side. Contrast is injected that shows patent bilateral iliac veins. An intravascular ultrasound (IVUS) probe is inserted into the left femoral vein and significant compression is seen at the proximal end of the left common iliac vein where the right common iliac artery crosses over the vein. The IVUS is then used on the right side which shows no compression or pathology of the right iliac or femoral veins. A self-expanding stent is placed in the left iliac vein and balloon dilation of the stent is performed to profile the stent to the appropriate size of the vein. The IVUS is used one last time to evaluate the left iliac vein with the new stent in place. A completion venogram is performed at the end of the case showing widely patent common iliac veins. The catheter and the sheaths are removed, and pressure is held over the puncture sites for hemostasis.

CLINICAL PEARL (STEPS 2/3)

The Seldinger technique is a method of percutaneous insertion of a catheter into a blood vessel or other space. A needle is used to puncture the structure, and a guide wire is threaded through the needle. When the needle is withdrawn, a catheter is threaded over the wire; the wire is then withdrawn, leaving the catheter in place. Several important procedures are performed using this technique, including angiography, central line insertion, and percutaneous tracheostomy.

What Are the Long-term Strategies for Treatment and Follow-up in Patients with Lower Extremity Venous Disease?

In addition to surgical therapy, patients with lower extremity venous disease often need prolonged medical therapy. For patients with DVT, the course of therapeutic anticoagulation with warfarin or newer novel anticoagulants depends on their risk factors for developing other thromboses, but normally the course of treatment is limited to 6 months. Patients with no underlying hypercoagulable state require therapy for 3 months only. Patients with anatomic compression (e.g., May-Thurner syndrome) who have undergone stenting require treatment with 3 months of clopidogrel and indefinite therapy with aspirin to decrease the risk of stent thrombosis.

Many patients with venous insufficiency will, in addition to edema, present with skin ulcers that result from venous stasis. Wound care must be part of the long-term treatment plan for patients who have venous stasis ulcers in order to prevent progression, superinfection, or the more rare malignant transformation. Unfortunately, lower extremity venous disease is a progressive disease; despite initial treatment successes, patients often require subsequent therapies, and recurrence is common. Repeat imaging with ultrasound with appropriate long-term clinical follow up is necessary. Adjuncts such as compression therapies, including compression socks and pneumatic pumps, are beneficial as well.

BASIC SCIENCE PEARL (STEPS 1/2/3)

Clopidogrel works at the level of the endothelial cells to prevent platelet aggregation and subsequent stent thrombosis. After several weeks, it is expected that endothelial cells will migrate to line the newly placed stent, a process called reendothelialization. Aspirin works at the level of the platelets to help prevent thrombus formation within the stent.

After recovery in the postanesthesia care unit, the patient is discharged home with prescriptions for clopidogrel 75 mg and aspirin 81 mg. She is also instructed to continue wearing compression stockings to help resolve the edema. She follows up 2 weeks postoperatively and reports she has noticed less pain both at rest and with ambulation. She feels there has also been a decrease in the swelling. She is given instructions to follow up again in 3 months with a repeat Doppler ultrasound and to call the office if she notes any increases in lower extremity pain.

BEYOND THE PEARLS

- There are medical and surgical causes for lower extremity edema. Systemic causes will more frequently present with bilateral edema.
- Peripheral vascular disease is very common, and it is important to assess whether a patient's presentation is consistent with venous disease, arterial disease, or both. See Chapter 28 for a discussion of peripheral artery disease.
- Venous ulcers require wound care in addition to the treatment of venous disease.
- Varicose veins, although potentially only a cosmetic problem, should prompt evaluation for more significant underlying venous disease.
- Compression is a very important component in the management of lower extremity edema.

Suggested Readings

Kearon C, Ageno W, Cannegieter SC, et al: Categorization of patients as having provoked or unprovoked venous thromboembolism: guidance from the SSC of ISTH, *J Thromb Haemost* 14:1480, 2016.

Neglet, P., & Raju, S. (2002). Proximal lower extremity chronic venous outflow obstruction: recognition and treatment. *Semin Vasc Surg, 15*(1), 57–64.

O'Donnell, T. F., Jr., Passman, M. A., Marston, W. A., et al. (2014). Management of venous leg ulcers: clinical practice guidelines of the Society for Vascular Surgery and the American Venous Forum. *J Vasc Surg, 3S*, 60.

O'Sullivan, G. J., et al. (2000). Endovascular management of iliac vein compression (May-Thurner) syndrome. *J Vasc Intervent Rad, 11*(7), 823–836.

CHAPTER 30

Transient Vision Loss in a 74-Year-Old Female

Daniel Choi ■ Vincent DiGiovanni

A 74-year-old female with a medical history of hypercholesterolemia, hypertension, and type 2 diabetes presents to the office with a chief complaint of a prior episode of vision loss in her left eye 1 week ago. The vision loss occurred gradually and resolved spontaneously after 20 minutes. The patient reports that this is her first time experiencing vision loss. The patient recalls no pain associated with the incident. On further history, she recalls an episode of temporary difficulty using her right hand 6 months prior that lasted for roughly 30 minutes. The patient is currently taking a statin, an ACE inhibitor, and metformin.

What Is the Differential Diagnosis for Vision Loss?

When considering vision loss, it is useful to group potential etiologies by whether it is monocular or binocular, as well as considering the onset and duration.

Whether a single eye or both eyes are involved in vision loss provides clues into the anatomic location of the problem. Generally, monocular vision loss suggests pathology along the optic pathway starting from the eye to the optic chiasm. Binocular vision loss suggests an issue between the optic chiasm and the occipital lobes. In practice, patients may have difficulty distinguishing between monocular and binocular vision loss, and therefore it may be useful for physicians to keep the differential diagnosis broad.

The onset and duration of vision loss often provide more insight into the cause. Gradual onset of symptoms is often a result of chronic conditions such as diabetic retinopathy, glaucoma, cataracts, or slow tumor growth along the neural pathways. Acute onset points toward ischemia due to vascular compromise. Ischemic strokes are a potential etiology that themselves can be either embolic or thrombotic. Ischemic strokes that do not result in acute infarction of tissue are categorized as transient ischemic attacks (TIA); previously, TIAs were defined as strokes with neural deficits lasting less than 24 hours. Thrombotic strokes arise from the rupture of an atherosclerotic plaque, with carotid plaques being the most common variety. Embolic strokes occur when an embolus from a distant source finds its way into the cerebral vasculature causing a thromboembolism, and the potential sources are numerous. A common source to consider is the heart in patients with atrial fibrillation, ventricular dysfunction post myocardial infarction, or bacterial endocarditis. Less commonly, deep vein thrombosis in patients with an atrial septal defect can create emboli that have the potential to reach the brain. Lastly, patients may experience vision loss from general lack of perfusion to the structures of the optic pathway. The retina in particular has high metabolic demand. Hypoperfusion from cardiac dysfunction or arterial stenosis can cause temporary losses in vision. Some other causes of hypoperfusion include papilledema and migraine auras. Papilledema results in increased intracranial pressures, and the consequent vision loss usually lasts seconds. Auras preceding migraines, although not completely understood, are thought to cause vision loss due to arterial vasospasms, and symptoms may last up to an hour.

TABLE 30.1 ■ Etiologies of Cerebrovascular Disease

Type	Subtype	Etiology	Symptoms
Hemorrhagic	Intracerebral	Rupture of Charcot-Bouchard microaneurysm in lenticulostriate vessels (caused by hypertension and hyaline arteriolosclerosis)	Nausea, severe headache, vomiting, may lead to coma
	Subarachnoid	Rupture of berry aneurysms that most commonly form at branch points of the circle of Willis (branch points lack a media layer are inherently weak)	Thunderclap headache, nuchal rigidity, yellow tinge on lumbar puncture
Ischemic	Thrombotic	Rupture of atherosclerotic plaques, most commonly a bifurcation of carotid arteries	Focal neurologic deficits, result in pale infarcts
	Embolic	Thromboemboli most commonly from the heart (atrial fibrillation, poor ventricular function post myocardial infarction)	Focal neurologic deficits, result in hemorrhagic infarcts
	Lacunar	Small noncortical infarcts due to complete occlusion of small branching arteries, most commonly involves lenticulostriate vessels from the middle cerebral artery affecting areas of basal ganglia	Focal neurologic deficits, results in cystic areas of infarction called lacunes

Acute onset, transient, monocular vision loss is known as *amaurosis fugax*. A complete history of other neurologic symptoms and of any known cardiovascular disease is important in determining the etiology and likely location of the lesion responsible for the symptoms. Retinal artery stenosis is more likely in patients who have only ocular complaints, whereas carotid stenosis is more likely in patients in whom other more global neurologic symptoms are identified.

Other causes for cerebrovascular symptoms are outlined in Table 30.1.

CLINICAL PEARL (STEPS 2/3)

Giant cell temporal arteritis is a large vessel vasculitis that is usually seen in elderly females. This vasculitis affects the branches of carotid artery. Common symptoms include unilateral headache, jaw claudication, and monocular vision loss. Left untreated, this condition will eventually lead to irreversible blindness due to occlusion of the ophthalmic artery. High clinical suspicion may warrant initiation of treatment with high-dose corticosteroids to prevent vision loss. Although the gold standard to confirm diagnosis is temporal artery biopsy, the procedure takes time, and a negative result does not necessary rule out the condition.

BASIC SCIENCE PEARL (STEPS 1/2)

Atherosclerosis is the pathologic thickening of the intimal wall layer of medium to large arterial vessels. The abdominal aorta, coronary, popliteal, and internal carotid arteries are most commonly involved. Pathogenesis begins with damage to the endothelium that allows lipids, mostly low-density lipoproteins (LDL), to enter the intima. These lipids oxidize, triggering chronic inflammation and recruiting leukocytes. As inflammation continues, extracellular matrix remodeling takes place. LDLs and the macrophages consuming them continue to accumulate, narrowing the blood vessel. The initial formations of this buildup are known as fatty streaks. This plaque is eventually covered by a fibromuscular cap consisting of smooth muscle. These streaks stay indolent for many years until the plaque eventually ruptures, causing thrombosis. The cause of the rupturing is not yet fully understood. Modifiable risk factors include: hypertension, hypercholesterolemia, cigarette smoking, and diabetes. Nonmodifiable risks factors include: age, male, postmenopausal females (estrogen increases HDL and decreases LDL, thus having a cardiovascular protective effect), and genetics.

What Are the Primary Physical Examination Techniques to Evaluate Potential Carotid Stenosis?

A thorough cardiac examination can help rule out cardiac sources of emboli. Atrial fibrillation presents with tachycardia along with irregular rhythm. Left-sided heart murmurs, indicating pathologies such as mitral stenosis, mitral valve prolapse, and mitral regurgitation, may also increase risk for emboli that could result in this patient's symptoms. An atrial septal defect will result in a fixed splitting of the second heart sound.

A vascular examination with emphasis on the carotids is critical in patients with presumed cerebrovascular disease. This begins with the auscultation of the carotid arteries. This is best heard posterior to the angle of the mandible while the patient is holding her breath, so as to eliminate background noise. The presence of a bruit indicates turbulent flow as a result of vessel stenosis. The next step is palpation: decreased pulses in the carotids may indicate that the stenosis is proximal to this location. Atherosclerosis most commonly affects the abdominal aorta, and it is important to auscultate and palpate this structure. The iliac bifurcation occurs roughly at the level of the umbilicus. Palpation proximal to the umbilicus can reveal an abdominal aortic aneurysm, which is a long-term complication of atherosclerosis. Moving distally, palpation of peripheral pulses is important to asses for the presence of peripheral arterial disease. Examination of the radial, femoral, popliteal, posterior tibial, and dorsalis pedis arterial pulses should be conducted both by palpation and, if needed, by portable Doppler ultrasound. Evidence of hair growth, healthy epidermis/toenails, and capillary refill are all indicators of good vascular perfusion.

Additionally, a neurologic evaluation should be undertaken in order to detect any residual deficits from current or previous cerebrovascular insults.

BASIC SCIENCE PEARL (STEP 1)

Recall that turbulent flow is determined by the Reynold's number. This number is directly proportional to the velocity of blood flowing through a vessel. As the carotid artery becomes stenosed, the cross-sectional area dramatically decreases. Flow rate always remains conserved through a vessel, causing increased blood flow velocities in narrow portions of an artery. This, along with other factors, is responsible for the conversion of laminar flow to pathologic turbulent flow.

Upon physical examination, the patient's temperature is 99.1°F, pulse is 88 bpm and regular, blood pressure is 135/78 mm Hg, and respirations are 15/min. No evidence of abnormal cardiac murmurs or clicks is found. The carotid pulse is strong bilaterally. On auscultation, bruits are heard in both carotids. The remainder of the vascular examination was found to be normal. Muscle strength is 5/5 bilaterally on all extremities. No sensory deficits were discovered.

What Is the Next Step in Evaluating Carotid Stenosis?

After history and physical examination reveal a suspicion for carotid artery disease, the next step is to order imaging of the carotid artery vasculature. There are several options. In the past, the gold standard has been conventional cerebral angiography (CCA). CCA provides the greatest amount of information to the clinician, as it can visualize the entire carotid artery system, plaque morphology, and the atherosclerotic state of nearby vessels. However, it is a high-cost, invasive procedure with a 1% chance of serious stroke complication. The risk and invasive nature of CCA have largely rendered it unsuitable for screening purposes.

Carotid duplex ultrasound (CDUS) is a completely noninvasive study that has become a first-line screening modality for carotid artery disease (Fig. 30.1). CDUS combines B-mode ultrasound and Doppler ultrasound, providing both imaging of the vasculature and velocity of blood flow. Unfortunately, CDUS may be limited by carotid bifurcation anatomy and is partially dependent on technician skill level. It is also unable to provide insight into plaque morphology. Some studies

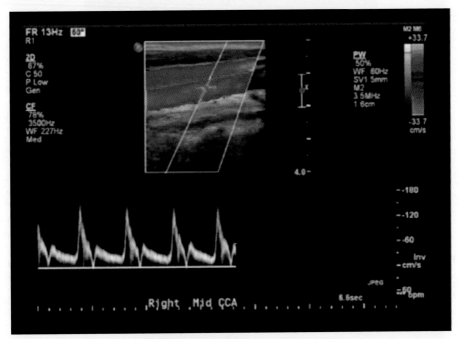

Fig. 30.1 Duplex color sonography of the carotid artery. (From Herring W: Duplex color sonography of the carotid artery. In *Learning radiology: recognizing the basics,* ed 3, Philadelphia, 2015, Elsevier.)

have shown its limited ability in distinguishing very high-grade stenosis from complete occlusion. This is relevant, as other studies have shown limited therapeutic benefit in treating complete carotid artery occlusions. CDUS is also limited in its ability to provide information regarding nearby cranial vessels. However, it may be coupled with transcranial Doppler, which provides information regarding collateral flows and reversal of flows. This aids in determining the role and significance of a patient's carotid stenosis in his or her disease state, which is critical in making the decision to intervene surgically.

Magnetic resonance angiography (MRA) is another noninvasive procedure that is highly sensitive and specific for severe carotid stenosis. Although expensive, it is less operator-dependent and provides information on the plaque morphology (such as fibrous cap rupture and intraplaque hemorrhage). In addition to high cost, MRA is also a more time-consuming option.

Computed tomography angiography (CTA) is the final noninvasive option (Fig. 30.3). CTA provides an accurate 3D reconstruction of the carotid arteries in addition to information about the nearby tissues and vessels. Some limitations include cost and necessity of contrast, which may not be suitable for patients with kidney dysfunction.

BASIC SCIENCE PEARL (STEPS 1/2/3)

Evaluating imaging studies of the carotid arteries requires a good knowledge of the anatomy of the cerebrovascular system (Fig. 30.3). The right and left common carotid arteries arise from the innominate artery and aortic arch, respectively. These vessels branch into the internal and external carotid arteries. The internal carotid artery gives rise to many branches, including the ophthalmic artery and the arteries that make up the circle of Willis that supply the brain. The external carotid artery gives rise to facial, maxillary, and meningeal branches.

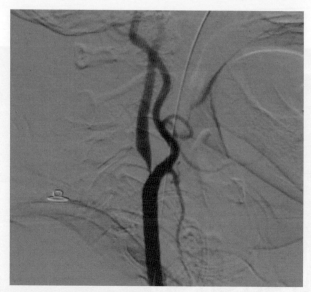

Fig. 30.2 Computed tomography angiogram (CTA) of the neck demonstrating severe stenosis of the left internal carotid artery. (From Adamczyk P, Liebeskind DS: Vascular imaging: computed tomographic angiography, magnetic resonance angiography, and ultrasound. In Daroff RB, Jancovic J, Mazziotta JC, Pomeroy SL, editors: *Bradley's neurology in clinical practice,* ed 7, London, 2016, Elsevier, pp 459–485.)

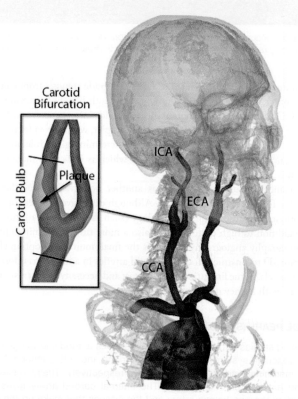

Fig. 30.3 Anatomy of the carotid artery system in which the common carotid artery (CCA) gives rise to the internal (ICA) and external carotid arteries (ECA). The carotid bulb is shown in the inset and is the most common location for atherosclerotic disease in the carotid. (From Kamenskiy AV, Pipinos II, Carson JS, MacTaggart JN, Baxter BT: Age and disease-related geometric and structural remodeling of the carotid artery, *Journal of Vascular Surgery* 62(6):1521–1528, 2015.)

The patient endorses an allergy to contrast dye, and a carotid duplex ultrasound study is ordered. Study results report 80% stenosis in the left internal carotid artery and 40% stenosis in the right internal carotid artery coupled with high velocities in both vessels. The patient is seen by a vascular surgeon to discuss options regarding the treatment of these stenoses.

What Are the Options and Recommendations for the Management of Carotid Stenosis?

Carotid stenosis can be managed by either medical or surgical intervention. The use of aspirin and statins is typically discussed with patients who are diagnosed with low-grade stenoses. Blood pressure control is also important.

Although surgical intervention includes options such as angioplasty and stenting, carotid endarterectomy is the preferred procedure. Angioplasty and stenting are generally reserved for patients deemed to be poor surgical candidates. Other indications for angioplasty and stenting include: stenosis due to radiation, anatomic limitations of the carotid bifurcation, and restenosis after a prior CEA procedure. The clinical determination to perform a carotid endarterectomy is largely driven by two factors: the patient's symptoms and degree of stenosis. The following are some landmark studies that have helped shape treatment guidelines.

Endarterectomy for Asymptomatic Carotid Artery Stenosis (ACAS)

This study looked at outcomes from 1167 asymptomatic patients from 1987 to 1993. Results from this study found that asymptomatic patients with 60% or greater stenosis benefited from CEA with decreased 5-year risk for ipsilateral stroke. Surgical intervention provided a 53% risk reduction.

North American Symptomatic Carotid Endarterectomy Trial (NASCET)

This study looked at outcomes from 659 symptomatic patients with stenosis ranging from 70% to 99% and found significant reduction in absolute risk by 17% for ipsilateral stroke at 2 years ($p < 0.001$) in the CEA group compared with the medical therapy group. The evidence was so overwhelming that this trial was ended early (sample size of 659 includes all eligible data before trial ending).

Randomized Trial of Endarterectomy for Recently Symptomatic Carotid Stenosis: final results of the MRC European Carotid Surgery Trial (ECST)

This study looked at outcomes from 3024 symptomatic patients from 1981 to 1994. Results from this study found that symptomatic patients with 80% or greater stenosis benefited from CEA. The risk of death or major stroke at 3 years was 26.5% without surgery and 14.9% with a CEA procedure.

There are other considerations in determining surgical candidates. A major factor may be the presence of concomitant disease of the cerebral vasculature. Patients with extensive arteriosclerosis of the cerebral arteries may receive modest to no therapeutic benefit from CEA. In such cases, the physician may determine that the benefits of the procedure do not outweigh the potential risks and elect to treat with medication instead. In patients with severe bilateral stenosis, CEA poses increased risks of hypoperfusion to the brain as a result of decreased collateral perfusion.

In addition to CEA, carotid stenting is another option for treating carotid stenosis. Patients for whom stenting is indicated are those who have restenosis after CEA, a history of neck radiation, previous ipsilateral neck surgery, and an inability to tolerate anesthesia (though local anesthesia for CEA is an option; see later in this chapter).

The patient and vascular surgeon have a discussion about the risks and benefits of surgical intervention. With neurologic symptoms and greater than 70% stenosis in the left internal carotid artery, the decision to perform a left carotid endarterectomy is made. The surgeon discusses that the 40% stenosis of the right internal carotid artery does not at this time meet criteria for surgical intervention. A plan is made for the right-sided stenosis to be monitored with surveillance imaging and treated with medical therapy. A computed tomography angiography (with a prestudy dye preparation in order to avoid allergic reaction) is ordered to confirm CDUS findings and aid in presurgical planning.

Carotid Endarterectomy

1. Incise along the anterior border of sternocleidomastoid muscle.
2. Divide and open platysma along incision line to reveal the deep cervical fascia.
3. Open deep cervical fascia to enter the carotid sheath, which encases carotid arteries, internal jugular vein, and the vagus nerve.
4. Common facial vein is dissected and divided with ties to provide visualization of the carotid bifurcation. (The facial vein may be safely sacrificed.)
5. Dissect internal, external, and common carotid and control with vessel loops.
6. Clamp the following vessels (in specific order so as to prevent migration of emboli into the cerebral vasculature):
   a. Internal carotid artery
   b. External carotid artery
   c. Superior thyroid artery
   d. Common carotid artery
7. Incise the common carotid superiorly along the vessel into the internal carotid to reveal plaque.
8. Bluntly dissect the plaque beginning from the inferior border. This dissection plane is within the media layer of the vessel.
9. Close the arteriotomy using a patch. Near the completion of the patch repair, back bleed the vessels from the internal and external carotid arteries and then forward flush from the common carotid artery.
10. Remove vascular clamps in reverse order.
11. Close the soft tissue and skin.

What Are the Potential Complications of Carotid Endarterectomy?

Although generally a safe and effective procedure, CEAs are not without risk. Studies have shown 0.5% to 3% risk of mortality from this procedure. There is also potential for postoperative neurologic deficits, which may be caused by low intraoperative perfusion to the brain. Intraoperative monitoring using nerve-monitoring devices, transcranial Doppler, or performing the procedure under local anesthesia and having the patient perform simple neurologic functions are common. Using a carotid shunt allows the procedure to be performed with continued cerebrovascular flow.

Poor technique during closure of the vessel may result in embolic and thrombotic complications. These complications are indications for reexploration and revision of the original repair. Hemorrhage and resultant hematoma at the site of repair may cause increased intracervical pressures. The neck compartment is a limited space, and increased pressures may quickly lead to airway compromise that must be emergently addressed in the operating room.

There are numerous cranial nerves that course through the area of surgical repair. Stretching of or incidental damage to any of these structures may result in temporary or even permanent deficits. The vagus nerve runs posteriorly and along the common carotid artery. As the vagus nerve gives rise to the recurrent laryngeal nerve, unilateral damage to this nerve will manifest with hoarseness. Bilateral damage to the recurrent laryngeal nerves will lead to airway compromise. The hypoglossal nerve runs across the anterior of both internal and external carotid arteries superior to the bifurcation. Damage to this nerve will cause deficits in motor control to the tongue. Although the glossopharyngeal nerve runs even more cranially, it too can be damaged and would manifest as difficulty swallowing.

The patient does well postoperatively and has no bleeding or neurovascular complications. She is discharged home the next day. On her follow-up appointment 3 weeks later, the patient's incision is found to be healing well. She describes no continued neurologic symptoms and has gone back to performing all her activities of daily living independently.

BEYOND THE PEARLS

- Carotid duplex ultrasound and computed tomography (CT) of the neck are the imaging techniques used to evaluate the degree of carotid stenosis.
- Carotid stenosis can be managed with surveillance, carotid endarterectomy, or carotid stenting depending on the degree of stenosis, symptomatology, and other patient factors.
- It is largely accepted that the carotid endarterectomy procedure with patch closure reduces the risk of restenosis by increasing the lumen diameter of the repaired artery.
- Carotid endarterectomies are generally durable and effective procedures; however, carotid arteries may undergo restenosis, and surveillance using carotid ultrasound is typically performed at 6 months and yearly afterward.
- It is important to encourage patients to optimally manage underlying conditions such as hypertension, hyperlipidemia, and diabetes to lower risk of carotid restenosis and other sequelae, such as cardiac ischemia, related to these medical comorbidities.

Suggested Readings

European Carotid Surgery Trialists' Collaborative Group. (1998). Randomised trial of endarterectomy for recently symptomatic carotid stenosis: Final results of the MRC European Carotid Surgery Trial (ECST). *Lancet*, *351*(9113), 1379–1387.

Falk, E. (2006). Pathogenesis of atherosclerosis. *J Am Coll Cardiol*, *47*(8 Suppl), C7–12.

Ferguson, G. G., et al. (1999). The North American symptomatic carotid endarterectomy trial: Surgical results in 1415 patients. *Stroke*, *30*(9), 1751–1758.

Walker, M. D., et al. (1995). Endarterectomy for asymptomatic carotid artery stenosis. *JAMA*, *273*(18), 1421–1428.

CHAPTER 31

Abdominal Pain in a 55-Year-Old Male

Erin Kenning ■ Christopher Greenleaf ■ Alexander Uribe

A 55-year-old male with past medical history significant for poorly controlled hypertension and social history consistent with a 40 pack-year tobacco use presents to the emergency department with complaint of acute onset of abdominal pain. He notes that his pain woke him from sleep. He describes it as an "11 out of 10," tearing pain that radiates to his left flank. He took over-the-counter nonsteroidal antiinflammatory medication, but the pain is persistent.

What Is the Differential Diagnosis for Acute, Severe Abdominal Pain?

Patients presenting with acute onset, severe abdominal pain may have one of several etiologies for their pain (Table 31.1); diagnosis can often be gleaned from detailed history-taking and physical examination. Although acute surgical emergencies usually present suddenly, patients may have already had some antecedent pain. It should be noted, though, that hemodynamic instability accompanying abdominal pain necessitates a more expeditious approach to diagnosis and management.

What Are the Primary Physical Examination Techniques to Evaluate Acute Abdominal Pain?

Although various diagnoses of acute abdominal pathology may be suspected from a detailed history, no diagnosis can be confirmed or treatment strategy initiated without a physical examination. Physical examination using techniques of visualization and palpation may reveal the location, radiation, and severity of pain. The abdominal wall and bilateral groins should be assessed for surgical scars and palpated for bulges, both at rest and when straining. Auscultation over the abdomen will reveal a pattern of bowel sounds and possibly bruits. When evaluating abdominal pain in the lower quadrant(s), a pelvic examination should be performed in female patients and a genital examination should be performed in male patients. A pulsatile mass should be identified, if it exists, and bimanually approximated in size. If a pulsatile abdominal mass is palpated, with or without auscultation of a bruit, a pulse examination of the lower extremities is warranted.

On physical examination, the vital signs reveal that the patient is afebrile; his systolic blood pressure is 94/44 mm Hg in the left upper arm. His heart rate is 105 bpm. On palpation of the abdomen, there is a pulsatile, tender abdominal mass that measures approximately 7 cm. His upper and lower extremity pulses are 2 +, and Doppler signals of these peripheral vessels are biphasic. The patient undergoes bedside ultrasound with Doppler flow (Fig. 31.1A), which reveals flow outside the wall of an aneurysmal aorta, consistent with a ruptured abdominal aortic aneurysm (AAA). The vascular surgeon on call is called to see the patient.

TABLE 31.1 ■ **Differential Diagnosis for Acute Onset Severe Abdominal Pain**

	Pathology	Signs and Symptoms
Gastrointestinal	Perforated diverticulitis	Left lower quadrant pain, fevers, change in bowel habits
	Perforated peptic ulcer	"Gnawing," epigastric pain and tenderness
	Closed-loop bowel obstruction	Colicky pain, nausea, vomiting and obstipation, tympanitic abdomen
	Appendicitis	Periumbilical pain migrating to the right lower quadrant, fever, tenderness in the right or bilateral lower quadrants
Vascular	Acute mesenteric ischemia	Pain out of proportion to examination
	AAA	Pulsatile abdominal mass
Abdominal Wall	Strangulated Hernia	Lack of bowel function, nonreducible abdominal bulge
Genitourinary	Ovarian Torsion	Female, severe pelvic pain, adnexal mass

BASIC SCIENCE PEARL (STEP 1)

The abdominal aorta is a retroperitoneal structure that enters the abdominal cavity through the aortic hiatus at the level of T12. The branches-off of it include (in descending order) the two phrenic arteries, celiac axis, superior mesenteric artery, renal arteries, inferior mesenteric artery, and bilateral common iliac arteries. The location of an AAA is generally referred to in relation to the renal vessels.

CLINICAL PEARL (STEPS 1/2/3)

An aneurysm is defined as an increase in arterial diameter to 1.5 times the normal diameter of the vessel. The absolute risk of rupture of an aneurysm, such as with the abdominal aorta, is directly proportional to the diameter of the aneurysmal segment. For example, a 6-cm aneurysm has a 20% lifetime risk of rupture whereas an 8-cm aneurysm has a 50% lifetime risk of rupture. The threshold for intervention on an asymptomatic aneurysm is surpassed when the risk of rupture is greater than the risk associated with surgical repair. Therefore the 5.5-cm aneurysm size is used as a cutoff to intervene on an asymptomatic aneurysm. It is rare, albeit not impossible, that a small aneurysm will rupture. In addition, other indications for surgery are growth greater than 1 cm per year and presence of clinical symptoms.

CLINICAL PEARL (STEP 3)

In the presence of an AAA, associated aneurysms of the peripheral vasculature are a well-known phenomenon. For example, synchronous popliteal aneurysms occur with a prevalence of 14% in patients presenting with an AAA. Any physical examination concerning for a pulsatile abdominal mass is not complete without palpation of the popliteal fossae to evaluate for concomitant aneurysmal disease.

What Are the Imaging Modalities That Can Be Used for Abdominal Aortic Aneurysms?

AAAs can be assessed either by abdominal ultrasound or computed tomography (CT) scan. Abdominal ultrasound is inexpensive and has a sensitivity of nearly 100% and specificity of 96% in the detection of AAAs, but it is highly user dependent. Abdominal CT, though also nearly 100% sensitive, is more expensive and exposes patients to both radiation and intravenous contrast.

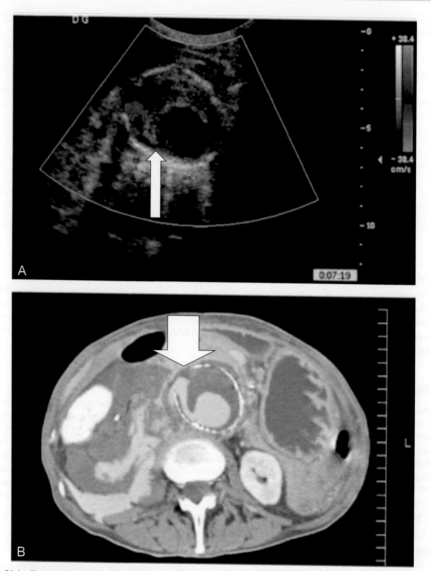

Fig. 31.1 Ruptured abdominal aortic aneursm seen on ultrasound with Doppler flow (A) and computed tomography (CT) scan with intravenous contrast (B). The extravasation of blood at the site of rupture is identified by the arrow in each image. (The Retroperitoneum Diagnostic Ultrasound. Bertino, Raymond E.; Mustafaraj, Elton... Published January 1, 2018. Pages 432–469. © 2018.)

CT does have the added benefit of 3D imaging that is essential in operative planning for patients who are undergoing elective AAA repair.

Asymptomatic patients with AAAs should undergo surveillance imaging to assess aneurysm expansion and, ultimately, indications for elective repair. Typically, surveillance imaging is performed using abdominal ultrasound, given its lack of patient exposure to radiation and intravenous contrast. Table 31.2 outlines surveillance imaging intervals based on aneurysm size, though a shorter interval may be indicated for other features such as high rate of increase in aneurysm diameter.

TABLE 31.2 ■ **Surveillance Recommendations for Patients With Asymptomatic Abdominal Aortic Aneurysms**

Aneurysm Size	Surveillance Imaging Interval
3.0–3.9 cm	3 years
4.0–4.9 cm	1 year
5.0–5.4 cm	6 months

CLINICAL PEARL (STEPS 2/3)

The US Preventive Services Task Force recommends screening for AAAs in men aged 65 to 75 years who have smoked.

What Are the Clinical Findings of Aortic Aneurysm Rupture?

Many patients with a ruptured AAA do not survive to medical evaluation due to hemodynamic compromise. Of those that survive, presentation is notable for acute onset of abdominal, back, or flank pain and hypotension in a patient with a pulsatile abdominal mass. The patient may appear pale and diaphoretic, with or without evidence of peripheral ischemia. Imaging will often confirm aneurysm rupture. When imaging does not demonstrate rupture, acute onset of abdominal or back pain in association with an AAA must be considered an impending rupture.

CLINICAL PEARL (STEP 2/3)

Permissive hypotension is important in the initial management of the patient with ruptured AAA. Lower blood pressures limit the extravasation of blood and can maintain a patient in a relatively stable hemodynamic situation. Systolic blood pressures between 80 and 99 mm Hg may be appropriate as long as end organ function is maintained, including cognition. Inappropriate fluid administration, transfusion, and the use of vasopressors to regain "normal," physiologic blood pressures may actually exacerbate the rupture.

What Are the Types of Surgery for Repair of Abdominal Aortic Aneurysms?

AAAs have historically been repaired in an open fashion. Open surgical repairs were approached from either a midline laparotomy or with a retroperitoneal approach. As of the early 1990s, however, endovascular techniques have been increasingly employed to repair AAAs and are currently the prevailing technique used by contemporary vascular surgeons. Whereas open repairs are generally thought to be more durable and do not necessitate aggressive surveillance postrepair, endovascular repairs require yearly imaging to ensure that patients do not develop complications of the device or the repair. Still, endovascular repairs entail much less morbidity in the immediate perioperative period for an otherwise highly comorbid patient population.

The patient is taken urgently to the hybrid operating room. An angiogram confirms your suspicion of an AAA. It extends 1 cm below the renal arteries to 1 cm above the iliac artery bifurcation. There is a small amount of extravasation from the left side of the aneurysm. An endovascular stent graft is placed without complication, and a completion angiogram shows no flow of contrast outside the stent graft into the aneurysm sac.

Endovascular Aortic Aneurysm Repair

1. Access the femoral arteries bilaterally and position sheaths for ongoing access.
2. Inject contrast dye to perform an angiogram.
3. Identify the neck of the aneurysm and an appropriate proximal landing zone, the orientation of the aneurysm relative to the renal arteries, the distal landing zone, and biiliac anatomy/topography.
4. Deploy the stent graft with proximal and distal ends within each landing zone.
5. Balloon dilate the stent graft to seal it against the landing zones.
6. Remove the sheaths and repair the arteries.

BASIC SCIENCE PEARL (STEPS 1/2/3)

When accessing the femoral artery percutaneously, it is always important to remember the orientation of the surrounding structures. The mnemonic "N-A-V-E-L" can be used to remember this orientation. From lateral to medial in the groin the orientation is femoral **n**erve, femoral **a**rtery, femoral **v**ein, **e**mpty space, and then **l**ymphatics.

Open Abdominal Aortic Aneurysm Replacement

1. Incise along the midline abdomen.
2. Obtain supraceliac control of the abdominal aorta by occluding it.
3. Eviscerate the small bowel to the patient's right side.
4. Lift the transverse colon cephalad.
5. Open the retroperitoneum over the aneurysm, initiating this opening at the ligament of Treitz.
6. Obtain proximal and distal control at the level of the infrarenal aorta and iliac arteries, respectively.
7. Open the aneurysm and remove the thrombus.
8. Suture a stent graft in place to exclude the aneurysm.
9. Remove the clamps placed for proximal and distal control, first with the distal clamps and then with the proximal clamp.
10. Close the aneurysm sac over the stent graft.
11. Suture the retroperitoneal lining over the aneurysm repair.
12. Close the laparotomy incision.

CLINICAL PEARL (STEPS 2/3)

There are multiple ways to approach an AAA. The most common open technique uses an intraabdominal approach. In an effort to obtain proximal control of the AAA, the supraceliac aorta is often dissected before exposing the aneurysm. The supraceliac aorta is exposed through the gastrohepatic ligament. The distal esophagus and proximal stomach are retracted laterally. The gastrohepatic ligament is divided. One should be mindful of a replaced left hepatic artery within this ligament so that it will be identified and preserved. The right crus of the diaphragm is sharply divided. Blunt dissection is used to get around both sides of the aorta. The aorta should not be circumferentially dissected to prevent any posterior arterial branches from being avulsed.

What Are the Potential Complications of Endovascular Aortic Aneurysm Repair?

Perioperative Complications arising in the perioperative period include infection at access sites, bleeding, pseudoaneurysm, and cardiopulmonary morbidity. The groin incisions can be

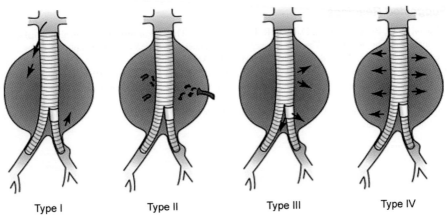

Type I   Type II   Type III   Type IV

Fig. 31.2 Endoleaks after an endovascular aneurysm repair (EVAR). The arrows represent blood flow into the aneurysm sac. (Redrawn from Fairman RM, Wang GJ: Aortoiliac aneurysms: endovascular treatment. In Sidawy AN, Perler BA, editors: *Rutherford's vascular surgery and endovascular therapy,* ed 9, Philadelphia, 2019, Elsevier, pp 910–928.)

troublesome to heal and are prone to infection. Bleeding and pseudoaneurysms can occur on a spectrum from small and asymptomatic to clinically significant and potentially fatal. Moreover, given that risk factors for AAA are consistent with risk factors for cardiac atherosclerotic disease, the most frequent cause of morbidity and mortality after coverage or replacement of an AAA is cardiac in origin.

Long Term The most common long-term complication of endovascular AAA repair is an endoleak. There are five types of endoleaks, each defined by persistent blood flow into the aneurysm sac via a specific route as outlined here and shown in Fig. 31.2.

Type I: Flow via the proximal or distal attachment sites
Type II: Flow from backbleeding lumbar or inferior mesenteric arteries
Type III: Flow through a defect in the graft fabric or disunion between modular components of the graft
Type IV: Flow due to graft fabric porosity
Type V: Increased pressure within the aneurysm sac without overt evidence of an endoleak

The patient does well postoperatively and is discharged home 4 days after endovascular aneurysm repair (EVAR). He returns to the office 1 month after discharge and has no complaints. He states that he has returned to all his normal activities and hobbies. A routine CT angiogram shows a fully excluded aneurysm that has thrombosed, with no endoleak identified. He is counseled about the need for ongoing endograft surveillance and is scheduled for a follow-up in 1 year.

BEYOND THE PEARLS

- An aneurysm larger than 5.5 cm, symptomatic, or growing more than 1 cm per year should be considered for surgical intervention.
- Hypotension should be permitted to limit extravasation during the initial care of a patient presenting with a ruptured aortic aneurysm.
- Endovascular aortic aneurysm repair decreases your risk of mortality in the first year but is balanced by greater risk of subsequent reinterventions.
- Endoleaks are the most common late complication after endovascular aortic aneurysm repair.

Suggested Readings

Chaikof, E. L., Brewster, D. C., Dalman, R. L., et al. (2009). The care of patients with an abdominal aortic aneurysm: The Society for Vascular Surgery practice guidelines. *J Vasc Surg, 50*(4 Suppl), S2–S49.

De Bruin, J. L., Baas, A. F., Buth, J., et al. (2005). DREAM study group. *N Engl J Med, 352,* 2398–2405.

Lederle, F. A., Freischlag, J. A., Kyriakides, T. C., et al. (2012). OVER Veterans Affairs Cooperative Study Group. Long-term comparison of endovascular and open repair of abdominal aortic aneurysm. *N Engl J Med, 367,* 1988–1997.

Sidawy, A. N., & Perler, B. A. (Eds.). (2019). *Rutherford's vascular surgery and endovascular therapy (9th ed.).* Philadelphia: Elsevier.

Trauma

Trauma

CHAPTER 32

The Trauma Patient: An Introduction

Andrea L. Lubitz ■ Lars Ola Sjoholm ■ Amy J. Goldberg

Background

HISTORY

The history of trauma care in the United States began during the Civil War from 1861 to 1865, during which the first systems for injury management were established. President Abraham Lincoln was credited with establishing the first trauma manual during this time period. During World War II, researchers began going onto the battlefields to directly study trauma systems and outcomes. After World War II came the development of emergency rooms, which further led to the development of emergency medical services (EMS) systems. After the US interstate highway system's creation in the 1950s came paramount reports outlining the increase in traumatic injuries. In 1966, the National Academy of the Sciences came out with the report, "Accidental Death and Disability: The Neglected Disease of Modern Society," which deemed traumatic injuries to be a national epidemic. This report led to efforts to establish paramedic training programs and the creation of regional EMS and 911 programs. At the same time the American College of Surgeons (ACS) Committee on Trauma worked toward developing standards for trauma centers and creating a national database. Legislation progressed, and eventually all states were required to develop EMS systems. Around this time, the ACS released the Optimal Hospital Resources for the Injured Patient manual, which was the first report to try to establish standards for optimal care at all stages of trauma, from prehospital to rehabilitation and research. After this, ACS followed with establishing levels of care for hospitals and establishing guidelines for designating trauma centers.

One of the defining moments in establishing trauma care came in February 1976 when Dr. Jim Styner, an orthopedic surgeon, crashed his plane in rural Nebraska, killing his wife on impact and seriously injuring himself and his four children. In response to the care he and his family received, Dr. Styner said, "When I can provide better care in the field with limited resources than what my children and I received at the primary care facility, there is something wrong with the system, and the system has to be changed." In 1978, Advanced Trauma Life Support (ATLS) debuted and later spread around the United States and Canada in 1980. ATLS provides physicians with the skills to quickly assess a patient's condition, resuscitate and stabilize patients based on their needs, triage patients to determine whether they can meet their needs at their facility, or determine and arrange for the patient to be appropriately transferred to a facility that has the capacity to treat the patient's needs.

EPIDEMIOLOGY

Traumatic injuries cause significant morbidity and mortality in the United States. Injury and violence are the leading cause of death in people aged 1 to 44. The mortality rate for traumatic injuries is roughly 4.4%. In 2014, approximately one person died from a traumatic injury every 3 minutes, 2.5 million people were hospitalized due to their injuries, and 26.9 million were treated in an emergency department for their injuries. These injuries come not only with physical consequences but also emotional and financial costs—in 2013, the cost of injuries totaled roughly $671 billion. In terms of injury patterns, falls and motor vehicle accidents account for the majority of traumas in the United States, 44% and 26%, respectively. Penetrating injuries such as cuts or firearm injuries account for only 4% of traumatic injuries. Although firearm injuries occur infrequently, they have the highest case fatality rates, along with suffocations and drownings. The largest number of deaths is caused by fall-related injuries, motor vehicle injuries, and firearm injuries.

Care of the Trauma Patient

The care of the trauma patient is paradoxical in that each patient presents under a different set of circumstances and often with different injuries, but is triaged and initially assessed in the same way regardless of injury. This systematic method (described later in this chapter) allows the trauma team to provide optimal care to the patient without being distracted by other injuries or circumstances surrounding the patient's presentation. Importantly, all findings on the assessment of a trauma (including normal findings) must be correctly and accurately documented by the trauma team, as there is a possibility that the patient may deteriorate after the initial assessment, and it is imperative to be able to accurately compare findings.

IDENTIFICATION OF INJURY PATTERNS

The initial triage of patients occurs through fire rescue or emergency department physicians. They are responsible for identifying specific injury patterns, which ultimately determine the level of trauma that is activated. This initial triage is important, as it mobilizes different resources in an appropriate manner depending on the level of severity of the patient's injuries. Each institution's criteria differ and are not finite or all-inclusive but are meant to be used as guidelines for triaging alerts and can be modified at the discretion of the emergency department (ED) physician or trauma physicians.

UNIVERSAL PRECAUTIONS

In order to protect providers and patients from the exposure of bodily fluids in the trauma bay, the practice of universal precautions should be used. All providers involved in the patient's care should wear a surgical cap, a mask with protective eye shield, a gown, gloves, and shoe covers when caring for a patient in the trauma bay. These items should be worn during all activations with no exceptions. Personal protective equipment should be removed before leaving the trauma bay.

PRIMARY SURVEY

The primary survey in trauma was developed to quickly assess and identify threats to life in a systematic fashion. These steps are known as the ABCDEs of trauma and are identified as follows: **A**irway maintenance and cervical spine protection; **B**reathing and ventilation; **C**irculation with hemorrhage control; **D**isability—neurologic status; and **E**xposure/Environmental control. This sequence allows clinicians to identify injuries and prioritize them by the degree to which they pose a threat to life. By adhering to this algorithm, the most life-threatening injuries are identified and managed first. In busy trauma centers that serve a high penetrating trauma population, patients may be quickly rolled (for posterior exposure) before beginning the primary survey in order to determine trajectory and injury pattern.

   Airway Maintenance With Cervical Spine Protection. The airway should first be assessed for patency. Many patients can simply be asked to verbalize their name; if a patient is able to verbally communicate, the airway is likely patent. In order to further assess patency, the airway may need to be suctioned or inspected for foreign bodies and/or fractures. Additionally, maneuvers may need to be employed, such as the chin lift or jaw thrust, in order to maintain airway patency. Patients who are neurologically impaired, typically with a Glasgow Coma Score (GCS, see later in this chapter) of 8 or less, may also require placement of a definitive airway. If the clinician identifies the airway as unstable or that the patient cannot maintain his or her airway, measures should be taken to immediately address this problem. Orotracheal intubation is usually the preferred method of controlling the airway. A surgical airway such as a cricothyroidotomy can be performed to secure an airway. It is important to note that airway assessment is a continuous and dynamic process, and it should be repeatedly evaluated and managed if needed.

Along with airway assessment, the patient's head and neck should be handled with care in order to avoid hyperextension, hyperflexion, or rotation that could potentially exacerbate a cervical spine injury. The threat of cervical spinal cord injury should be assessed based on the mechanism of injury, and if necessary, the cervical spine should be immobilized. Mechanisms of injury that are concerning for cervical spine injury include blunt multisystem traumas, in particular if there is neurologic impairment or a direct blow above the clavicle. If immobilization devices need to be removed for further assessment or intervention, it is important that a team member hold inline immobilization by stabilizing the patient's head and neck.

Breathing and Ventilation. In order for a patient to adequately ventilate, they must have a patent airway and good gas exchange, which requires the lungs, chest wall, and diaphragm to all be functioning appropriately. Breathing is rapidly assessed by first observing the patient and looking for effort of breathing, tracheal position, and chest wall motion. Next, auscultation can be performed to evaluate the lungs. The chest wall can be palpated to determine whether any chest wall abnormalities are present that could lead to respiratory compromise, such as flail chest or crepitus. Lastly, the chest wall can be percussed to ascertain dullness or resonance. Potential immediate threats to breathing include pneumothorax or hemothorax, tension pneumothorax, open pneumothorax, and flail chest with pulmonary contusion. Tension pneumothorax is life threatening and should be managed immediately (see Chapter 37). Other conditions requiring immediate chest tube placement are hemothorax and simple pneumothorax. Table 32.1 outlines the common signs of different lung pathology that can be found on primary survey.

TABLE 32.1 ■ **Lung Pathology Presentation and Management**[a]

Pathology	Tracheal Deviation	Expansion	Breath Sounds	Percussion	Management
Tension Pneumothorax	Away	Decreased, may have fixed hyperexpansion	Diminished or absent	Hyper-resonant	Needle decompression, then chest tube
Simple Pneumothorax	Midline	Decreased	Diminished or normal	Normal, may be hyper-resonant	Chest tube
Hemothorax	Midline	Decreased	Large volume—diminished Small volume—normal	Dull	Chest tube
Pulmonary Contusion	Midline	Normal	Normal, crackles	Normal	Supportive care
Lung collapse	Towards	Decreased	Reduced	Normal	Chest tube

[a]Adapted from the Temple University Hospital Trauma Manual

Circulation With Hemorrhage Control. In trauma, hemorrhage is the cause of hypotension and shock until proven otherwise; thus it must be rapidly assessed and corrected. There are three components of the physical examination that allow for rapid assessment of a patient's hemodynamic status: level of consciousness, skin color, and pulse examination. Decreased circulating blood volume leads to decreased cerebral perfusion and altered consciousness. This is not absolute, as patients who have lost significant amounts of blood can remain conscious. Next, a patient's skin color should be assessed. Signs of hypovolemia include ashen, gray facial skin and pale, cool extremities. Lastly, central pulses such as the carotids or femoral pulses should be assessed for quality, rate, and regularity. A patient who is hypovolemic may have a rapid and thready pulse, whereas a normovolemic patient may have a strong and regular pulse. At this point, signs of bleeding should be identified and managed if needed. External bleeding can be managed by direct digital pressure or tourniquet in an extremity if needed. If internal bleeding is suspected, it can be managed by placement of pelvic binders or splints and surgical intervention if needed. Circulatory access also needs to be established. Upon arrival in the trauma bay, patients should have two large-bore intravenous (IVs) lines placed. If there is difficulty placing these IVs, then central access should be considered via the femoral or subclavian approach. If these methods fail, one can turn to intraosseous access (IO) or direct cut down on the femoral or saphenous vein. Initial fluid resuscitation for adults should be 1 to 2 L of warmed isotonic electrolyte solutions. If massive blood loss is suspected, uncrossmatched blood can be given in the trauma bay. Additionally, a massive transfusion protocol, which allows for the quick preparation and release of blood products to meet hemorrhagic demands, can be activated. Data has shown that matching transfusion of packed red blood cells, fresh frozen plasma, and platelets in a 1:1:1 fashion and administering it early on has improved survival in some patients.

Disability (Neurologic Evaluation). Neurologic examination should be performed as part of the primary survey. This evaluation is comprised of determining a patient's level of consciousness, pupillary size and response, presence of lateralizing signs, or spinal cord injury. Consciousness can be quantified using the Glasgow Coma Scale (GCS), which is outlined in Table 32.2. A patient's eye, motor, and verbal responses to stimuli are graded during the course of the examination. The best possible score on GCS is a 15; the worst possible score is a 3.

TABLE 32.2 ■ **Glasgow Coma Scale**

Assessment Area	Score
Eye Opening (E)	
Spontaneous	4
To speech	3
To pain	2
None	1
Verbal Response (V)	
Oriented	5
Confused conversation	4
Inappropriate words	3
Incomprehensible sounds	2
None	1
Best Motor Response (M)	
Obeys commands	6
Localizes to pain	5
Flexion withdrawal to pain	4
Abnormal Flexion (decorticate)	3
Extension (decerebrate)	2
None (flaccid)	1

Exposure and Environmental Control. In order to appropriately examine the patient, all clothing should be removed, which sometimes requires that garments be cut off. This often is performed by other team members simultaneously to other parts of the primary survey. Additionally, the patient should be kept warm using warm blankets, warm fluids, and warm ambient temperature in order to preserve a patient's metabolic and clotting functions.

SECONDARY SURVEY

The secondary survey is completed after the primary survey and all deficits discovered on the primary survey have been addressed. The secondary survey includes an inclusive, head-to-toe examination to further evaluate all organ systems and any potential injuries. The secondary survey also includes a patient history component and examination adjuncts, such as radiography and the Focused Assessment with Sonography for Trauma (FAST) examination.

The history component of the examination can be elucidated by using the mnemonic AMPLE: allergies, medications, past illnesses/pregnancy, last meal, and events/environment related to injury. All of these aspects of the patient history are crucial to the care of an injured patient.

The examination portion of the secondary survey begins with the head, including examination of the eyes, ears, and maxillofacial structures. The examination then progresses to the cervical spine and neck. The trachea and vascular structures of the neck should be examined thoroughly, and the cervical spine should be palpated for tenderness or step-offs. This progresses to a full evaluation of the spine, palpating the thoracic and lumbar spines for tenderness and step-offs. The patient is often log-rolled for this portion of the examination with inline immobilization of the neck. During this portion of the examination the perineum is also examined visually, and a rectal examination is performed to evaluate for blood, gross tone, and prostate position in males. Once the patient is returned to the supine position, the examination progresses to the chest, where the chest wall is again visually inspected and palpated for possible defects. The lungs should also be reexamined at this time. The abdomen is then examined for tenderness or distention as well as external signs of injury. The musculoskeletal examination is then assessed, which includes evaluating the pelvis for stability by placing anterior to posterior pressure to the anterior superior iliac spines. The upper extremities and lower extremities are then assessed for gross defects or fractures. Lastly, a complete neurologic examination is completed, assessing gross motor strength and sensation in all extremities. The secondary survey then progresses with radiographic examinations and the FAST examination.

Use of Radiographs in the Trauma Bay

Chest radiography is usually the first adjunct performed in the trauma bay as part of the secondary survey and is used to identify fracture patterns, pneumothorax, and hemothorax. Abdominal radiography is typically only used to verify missile trajectory or location. Pneumoperitoneum, if present, can be visualized on x-ray. Pelvic radiography is typically used to verify presence of pelvic fracture, which may be the source of hemorrhage in a blunt trauma patient, or missile trajectory in penetrating trauma.

Use of Ultrasound in the Trauma Bay

The use of ultrasound as an adjunct in the trauma bay began in the 1990s, and although extremely useful, the results are user-dependent. The FAST examination by nature is a limited ultrasound examination with the goal of assessing the abdomen and pericardium for free intraperitoneal and pericardial fluid. In the hands of an experienced provider, as little as 200 mL of fluid can be detected in less than 1 minute. The FAST examination focuses specifically on four areas for free fluid: the perihepatic and hepatorenal space (also known as Morison's pouch and the most dependent space in the upper peritoneal cavity); the perisplenic space; the pelvis (the pouch of Douglas in females and the rectovesical pouch in males); and the pericardium. The interface between organs and investing mem-branes is examined for the presence of blood, which appears as hypoechoic (black) on ultrasound.

The expanded FAST (e-FAST) utilizes ultrasound to include views of the thoracic cavity to assess for pneumothorax or hemothorax. The e-FAST obtains a view perpendicular to the ribs, looking at the pleural interface.

Patient Disposition

It is critically important that the trauma team begin thinking about a patient's disposition early in the assessment and care of the patient. Specifically, if the team identifies injuries that their particular institution is not able to effectively treat, the goal should be for stabilization of the patient and trans-fer to a facility with the capability to provide effective and appropriate treatment. Similarly, although the trauma bay is equipped with all the tools and materials needed to assess and stabilize a patient, the team must determine whether the patient requires formal imaging in radiology, surgical inter-vention in the operating room, a procedure in interventional radiology, or hospital admission to the intensive care unit or general medical/surgical floor. The patient should be transported swiftly to the location of their definitive treatment once stabilized.

References

Advanced trauma life support: student course manual (9th ed.). (2017). Chicago, IL: American College of Surgeons.

American College of Surgeons. Part 1: A brief history of trauma systems. https://facs.org/quality-programs/trauma/trauma-series-part-I. Updated 2017.

Centers for Disease Control and Prevention (CDC), *Key injury and violence data. https://www.cdc.gov/injury/wisquars/overview/key_data.html.*

Montoya, J., Stawicki, S. P., Evans, D. C., et al. From FAST to E-FAST: An overview of the evolution of ultrasound-based traumatic injury assessment. *Eur J Trauma Emerg Surg, 42*(2), 119–126.

Pieper, A., Thony, F., Brun, J., et al. (2018). Resuscitative endovascular balloon occlusion of the aorta for pelvic blunt trauma and life-threatening hemorrhage: A 20-year experience in a level-I trauma center. *J Trauma Acute Care Surg, 84*(3), 449–453.

CHAPTER 33

Fall From Standing in an 88-Year-Old Female

Drew A. Spencer ■ George R. Cybulski

An 88-year-old female presents to the emergency department with primary complaints of a headache and intermittent dizziness for the past 4 days. The headache is right-sided, constantly 4/10, and can get up to 7/10 with strenuous activity. Acetaminophen and ibuprofen provide temporary headache relief, but the pain never gets lower than 2/10. The dizziness is described as an unsteady feeling on standing, as if the floor is moving as she tries to gather herself. She reports a fall from standing when cleaning her home about 10 days ago. Past medical history is significant for a seizure disorder, well-controlled on carbamazepine. The patient is a retired teacher who does not smoke or use illicit drugs and has an occasional glass of wine. She denies loss of consciousness, vertigo, seizure, nausea/vomiting, vision change, extremity weakness, numbness, or tingling. She has no gait or bowel/bladder disturbance.

What Is the Differential Diagnosis of Headache and Dizziness After a Fall?

Headache and dizziness after a fall in the absence of other pathology is worrisome for a traumatic brain injury. Intracranial hemorrhage is the most common of traumatic brain injury, which includes subdural hematoma (SDH), epidural hematoma (EDH), and subarachnoid hemorrhage. Other possibilities include ruptured aneurysm, stroke, and neoplastic disease.

The history of even minor trauma in an elderly patient is key to narrowing the differential diagnosis to SDH. Often, the traumatic event is subtle and may either be considered insignificant or not remembered at all. In an elderly patient, the periosteal dura is adherent to the skull, stretching the bridging veins and predisposing this age group to subdural versus epidural hematoma. The initial injury can and often does cause a hematoma that is small to moderate and often is asymptomatic or causes nonspecific complaints. The hematoma then progressively increases in size due to its intrinsic pathology and repetitive minor trauma.

Sudden loss of consciousness or onset of a severe headache is typically associated with subarachnoid hemorrhage, whereas a subdural hematoma is classically associated with a lucid interval between the initial traumatic event and neurologic deterioration. Ruptured aneurysm typically occurs as a first event in nonelderly patients. Stroke remains a relevant concern in the elderly patient, and the workup must be completed with this in mind, including a search for localizing signs on physical examination. Neoplastic disease—whether primary or metastatic—is a legitimate concern in patients who present with complaints of subacute headache and neurologic signs and should prompt questions for other cancer diagnoses in the history and inform the physical examination and choice of imaging studies.

Anterior communicating a.

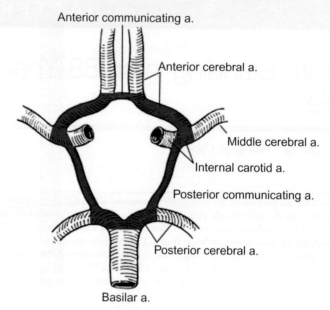

Anterior cerebral a.

Middle cerebral a.

Internal carotid a.

Posterior communicating a.

Posterior cerebral a.

Basilar a.

Fig. 33.1   Circle of Willis.

BASIC SCIENCE PEARL (STEP 1)

The brain requires oxygen and glucose to maintain homeostasis. Blood supply to the brain is derived from the internal carotid arteries and the vertebral arteries, which branch from the sub-clavian arteries. The internal carotid arteries branch to form the anterior and middle cerebral arter-ies, which form the anterior circulation and serve the forebrain. The vertebral arteries join to form a singular basilar artery and form the basis of the posterior circulation. The circle of Willis (Fig. 33.1) is the confluence of these arteries and permits collateralization.

   What Is the Evaluation for a Patient Who Presents With Acute or Subacute Neurologic Symptoms?
As with any traumatic injury, patients presenting with a history of recent traumatic events should be assessed using the ABCDE method. If stable, a thorough secondary examination with a focus on the musculoskeletal and neurologic examinations should be undertaken to assess for subtle findings that may inform the differential diagnosis. Neuroimaging, typically using computed tomography (CT), is also performed once the patient is stabilized.

On physical examination, the patient's temperature is 98.6°F, pulse is 72 bpm, blood pressure is 132/68 mm Hg, respiratory rate is 14/min, and oxygen saturation is 98% on room air. She is awake and in no acute distress, with lungs clear to auscultation and normal heart sounds. The head and rest of her body are without obvious signs of trauma. On neurologic examination, she is alert and ori-ented x 3 with fluent speech. Her cranial nerves are intact. Strength in her left arm is 4 +, and she is otherwise motor and sensory intact. She has intact coordination on finger-nose-finger testing, and gait is slow but steady. Her reflexes are diffusely 1 + without pathologic reflexes. She undergoes a noncontrast CT of the head, which reveals a right-sided 2.6-cm, crescent-shaped, extraaxial sub-dural collection. A midline shift from right to left of 7 mm is noted (Fig. 33.2).

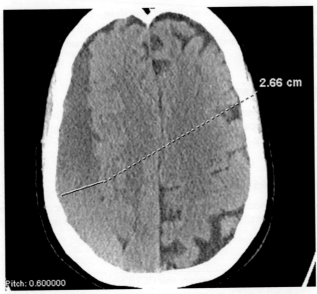

Fig. 33.2 Preoperative noncontrast CT of the head shows a mixed density subdural hematoma, 2.6 cm in maximal thickness with 7 mm of midline shift.

What Are the Common Historical Keys and Examination Findings Consistent With Subdural Hematoma?

The key positives in most patients presenting with SDH are advanced age, chronicity of symptoms, and a confirmed trauma. Headache is a common but nonspecific complaint and may be due to either a postconcussive state or dural irritation from the hematoma itself. Dizziness is a nonspecific finding. Contralateral weakness, mainly in the face and arm, are the most common deficits noted on neurologic examination. Only in rare instances of acute trauma, with rapid development of midline shift, is the so-called Kernohan's notch phenomenon observed, with ipsilateral weakness and typically profound impairment in level of consciousness.

CLINICAL PEARL (STEPS 2/3)

SDH is increasingly a disease of the elderly as the population ages in general. In recent series, over 40% of patients with SDH are over the age of 80.

What Are the Indications for Treatment of an Intracranial Hematoma?

Both EDH and SDH can be managed operatively or nonoperatively based on patient and imaging characteristics. For SDH the indications for operative management are well established: surgery via drainage or evacuation of the hematoma is recommended for any hematoma over 1 cm with greater than 0.5 cm of midline shift with localizing signs on neurologic examination. Smaller hematomas with less mass effect may resolve or stabilize spontaneously or with the assistance of medical therapies. The decision for surgical management also requires careful assessment of the fine details to determine the correct combination of strategies for the individual case. Burr hole drainage offers a relatively quick and safe method of drainage that is tolerated well by a majority of patients.

Since at least the 1990s, sporadic reports have surfaced advocating for treatment of chronic SDH with corticosteroids that results in shrinkage, resolution, or decreased recurrence of the hemorrhage.

Other treatments with sporadic reports of efficacy have shown tranexamic acid to arrest growth of SDH and lower rates of recurrence when given perioperatively. All medical therapies have contraindications and adverse effects and have demonstrated a significant cohort of partial or nonresponders who ultimately progress to surgery.

CLINICAL PEARL (STEPS 2/3)

Acute and chronic SDH present in very different patterns. Acute SDH follows high-speed impact and can affect all age groups. Chronic SDH follows trivial or often silent trauma and is largely a process seen in the elderly.

CLINICAL PEARL (STEPS 2/3)

SDH has varied appearances on CT based on the age of the blood. Acute hematoma is hyperdense to brain tissue, whereas subacute and chronic hematomas are isodense and hypodense, respectively.

The patient is admitted to the intensive care unit (ICU) with hourly neurologic assessments. She is kept nothing by mouth (NPO) and started on maintenance intravenous fluids. Her home dose of carbamazepine is continued for seizure prophylaxis. The neurosurgical team discusses with the patient and her family that, based on the history and appearance of the hematoma on CT, burr hole drainage is indicated and that purely medical therapy is unlikely to treat her condition. After informed consent is obtained, burr hole drainage is performed the next day. Postoperative CT head shows evacuation of the hematoma, with a subdural drain in good position. On postoperative day 3, after a repeat head CT confirmed a marked decrease in the size of the subdural hematoma, the subdural drain was removed. After being cleared for discharge by physical and occupational therapy, she was discharged home neurologically intact, with follow-up scheduled 2 weeks after surgery.

What Are the Potential Complications of Surgical Evacuation of Intracranial Hematomas?
Drainage of intracranial hematomas using burr hole and craniotomy is associated several potential complications such as recurrence, seizure, stroke, acute hemorrhage, postoperative infection, and medical complications. The overall complication rates are approximately 9% and 50% in burr hole and craniotomy, respectively. Overall, chronic SDH recurs in as many as 30% of cases. Risk factors for recurrence include age, limited evacuation, preoperative midline shift greater than 1 cm, and septated or separated hematoma. Recurrence requires reoperation in up to 15% of cases.

CLINICAL PEARL (STEPS 2/3)

Chronic SDH has a substantial risk of recurrence (overall approximately 30%), with reports in the literature varying between 12% and 30%.

The patient returns to clinic 2 weeks after surgery. She reports improved headaches and dizziness and is doing all of her activities of daily living with some light walking. On examination the patient is neurologically intact with incisions that are healing well. She is continued on carbamazepine with planned follow-up and is to begin outpatient physical therapy in 6 weeks.

BEYOND THE PEARLS

- Subdural hematoma affects 1 to 5 in 100,000 people, mainly in the elderly age group.
- Subdural hematoma recurs in 30% of cases, with bilateral hematoma, increasing age, septated hematoma, and greater than 1 cm of preoperative midline shift as independent risk factors.
- Medical therapy for chronic SDH is variably effective and unproven at best. Surgical evacuation is the only definitive therapy with a favorable long-term course.
- Overall mortality in subdural hematoma is currently 15%, improved from prior studies.
- Factors shown to increase the success of treatment for SDH include irrigation of the subdural space, duration of subdural drainage, and postoperative activity restriction.
- Surgical treatment for subdural hematoma, although largely successful (80%), is still plagued by significant complications, recurrence, and overall mortality.
- Each case of subdural hematoma requires careful patient assessment, interpretation of imaging studies, and technically sound surgical intervention to maximize the possibility of a successful outcome.

References

Brennan, P. M., Kolias, A. G., Joannides, A. J., et al. (2017). The management and outcome for patients with chronic subdural hematoma: A prospective, multicenter, observational cohort study in the United Kingdom. *J Neurosurg* ***, 1–8.

Ohba, S., Kinoshita, Y., Nakagawa, T., & Murakami, H. (2013). The risk factors for recurrence of chronic subdural hematoma. *Neurosurg Rev*, 36(1), 145–149, discussion 149–150.

Ryan, C. G., Thompson, R. E., Temkin, N. R., Crane, P. K., Ellenbogen, R. G., & Elmore, J. G. (2012). Acute traumatic subdural hematoma: Current mortality and functional outcomes in adult patients at a Level I trauma center. *J Trauma Acute Care Surg*, 73(5), 1348–1354.

Won, S. Y., Dubinski, D., Brawanski, N., et al. (2017). Significant increase in acute subdural hematoma in octo- and nonagenarians: Surgical treatment, functional outcome, and predictors in this patient cohort. *Neurosurg Focus*, 43(5), E10.

CHAPTER 34

Stab Wound to the Neck in a 33-Year-Old Male

Shane Morris ■ Austin D. Williams ■ Joshua A. Marks

A 33-year-old male is brought to the emergency department (ED) by his wife with a bleeding neck wound. He is able to speak, is in only mild distress and is holding a blood-soaked t-shirt on the wound. The patient states that his wife was in the kitchen making dinner and, because the floor was wet, he slipped and knocked them both to ground causing him to fall onto the knife she was holding. On initial evaluation, the patient is cooperative, and vital signs are: heart rate 128 beats per minute, blood pressure 120/74 mm Hg, respirations 20 per minute, and oxygen saturation of 99% on room air.

What Is This Initial Assessment for a Patient Who Presents With a Traumatic Neck Injury?
A penetrating neck injury has access to a variety of critical structures. Therefore, a high index of suspicion must be maintained with even what might appear to be superficial neck injuries.

As with any trauma evaluation, it is imperative to begin with an assessment of the patient's **A**irway, **B**reathing, and **C**irculation as outlined in Chapter 32. Specifically, patients with neck trauma are at risk of having injured the trachea or carotid arteries, so the primary survey should be undertaken with care. In a stab wound of the neck with its potential for major vessel or tracheal injury, it should be kept in mind that compression due to an expanding hematoma may also be the source of circulatory or respiratory compromise.

The primary survey reveals a grossly intact airway with normal breath sounds bilaterally and 2+ carotid, radial, and femoral pulses bilaterally. The patient has a Glasgow Coma Scale (GCS) score of 15. Secondary survey reveals a single neck laceration 2 cm in length just anterior to the sterno-cleidomastoid at the level of the superior aspect of the thyroid cartilage. There is minimal overt bleeding from the wound; no bubbling is present, and no hematoma is noted. The trachea is mid-line, there is no crepitus on palpation of the neck, and there is no hoarseness of his voice.

BASIC SCIENCE PEARL (STEP 1)

The neck is anatomically complex due to the number of vital structures it contains (Fig. 34.1). Vital structures in the neck include the trachea, esophagus, carotid arteries, jugular veins, and the thyroid. Depending on the level of neck penetration (both how deep and how cephalad or caudad), different underlying soft tissue and neurovascular structures are most at risk for injury (see later in this chapter). The platysma is the most superficial muscular structure, and its penetration gives access to the other vital structures. A "superficial neck injury" is defined as that superficial to the platysma. A "penetrating neck injury" is defined as one deep to the platysma.

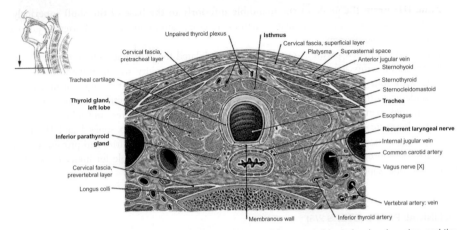

Fig. 34.1 Vital structures in the neck include the trachea, esophagus, carotid arteries, jugular veins, and thyroid. (From Paulsen F: Neck. In Sobotta J: *Atlas of human anatomy*, vol 3, ed 15, Munich, 2013, Elsevier GmbH, pp 161–210.)

How Are Injuries to the Neck Categorized Anatomically?

Categorization of traumatic neck injuries based on anatomic landmarks is important in understanding the structures that may be injured and the workup to determine whether an injury has occurred (Fig. 34.2). It should be noted that injury to one specific zone does not preclude injury in another zone.

Zone I: From the thoracic outlet, as defined by the clavicles inferiorly to the cricoid cartilage superiorly. Structures at risk: major vascular structures (great vessels, carotid and vertebral arteries, internal jugular veins), the apices of the lungs, esophagus, thoracic duct, and cervical nerve trunks.

Zone II: From the cricoid cartilage inferiorly to the angle of the mandible superiorly. Structures at risk: major vascular structures (carotid and vertebral arteries, jugular veins), the esophagus and major airway structures (pharynx, trachea, larynx).

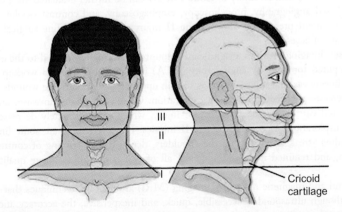

Fig. 34.2 Categorization of traumatic neck injuries based on anatomic landmarks is important in understanding the structures that may be injured and the workup to determine whether an injury has occurred. Zone I is below the cricoid cartilage and Zone II is above the mandible. (From Rathlev NK, Medzon R: Penetrating neck trauma. In Adams JG, editor: *Emergency medicine,* ed 2, Philadelphia, 2013, Elsevier, pp 673–680.)

Zone III: From the angle of the mandible inferiorly to the base of the skull superiorly.
Structures at risk: major vascular structures (internal carotid and vertebral arteries, jugular veins) and the pharynx.

Classically, all patients with a zone II injury that violated the platysma underwent mandatory neck exploration; this led to many operations in which no injury was identified. Currently, patients with zone II injuries who are stable and have no hard definitive signs of underlying injury undergo further evaluation (CT angiography of the neck) and selective management based on the injuries identified. Zones I and II are bounded by bony structures, and injuries to these areas can be more difficult to access. Stable patients with an injury to zones I and II should undergo diagnostic studies (CT angiography of the neck) to identify injuries and provide a "road map" for the appropriate operative intervention. Remember: it is possible for injury to occur in more than one zone.

CLINICAL PEARL (STEPS 2/3)

Despite not meeting other criteria for intubation, patients with penetrating neck wounds may require intubation in order to complete the diagnostic workup. Specifically, patients undergoing endoscopic evaluation require sedation. While the presence of an endotracheal tube enables performing bronchoscopy through the tube, one must be sure that the presence of the endotracheal tube does not obscure an injury.

What Are the Next Steps in Management After an Injury to a Neck Structure Is Suspected or Diagnosed?

Similar to traumatic injuries in other body locations, unstable patients with traumatic neck injuries require surgical exploration. Patients with hemodynamic instability who present with clinically detectable signs of injury, such as expanding hematomas, active hemorrhage, neurologic symptoms, bruit, thrill, hematemesis, hemoptysis, stridor, or air leak, undergo immediate surgical exploration.

Management of neck injuries in stable patients is dictated by which neck zone is affected. A patient presenting with an injury to **Zone I or III** can be further evaluated via a combination of catheter-based angiography, bronchoscopy, esophagoscopy, and contrast swallow evaluation. Classically, a patient presenting with a **Zone II** injury underwent routine surgical exploration because of ease of access.

In all cases, imaging provides a significant amount of information related to the extent of the injury. Computed tomography angiography (CTA) is increasingly used in workup due to the ability to delineate vascular injury, which is seen in up to 25% of penetrating wounds. Utilization of CTA decreases the need for surgical exploration. CTA is rapid, noninvasive, and relatively inexpensive and can clarify the trajectory of injury, which may ultimately decreases the need for surgical exploration, especially in Zone II injuries. However, there are some limitations to CTA, including streak artifacts from the shoulders, dental fillings, timing of contrast or failed IV injection, and retained metallic fragments, all of which can affect image quality and read accuracy.

Ultrasound and magnetic resonance imaging (MRI) are imaging techniques that can also be utilized. Although ultrasound is accessible, quick, and inexpensive, the accuracy and technique is very operator dependent, and there may be several limiting factors in evaluation of vital structures. MRI is great for soft tissue evaluation, vascular injury, and spinal and cerebral evaluation but is time consuming. Note that retained metallic bodies may contraindicate MRI.

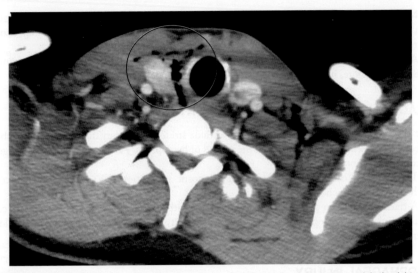

Fig. 34.3 Computed tomography (CT) scan of the head and neck revealing subcutaneous air in the right neck *(red circle)*.

A chest radiograph in the trauma bay is normal. The patient undergoes laboratory tests that are normal except for a urine drug screen positive for cannabis. A computed tomography (CT) scan of the head and neck is performed (Fig. 34.3) and reveals subcutaneous air in the right neck. There is no extravasation of contrast or hematoma to suggest a vascular injury. The patient is taken to the operating room and undergoes bronchoscopy and esophagogastroscopy. There is no blood or injury seen on any of the studies. His neck wounds are then irrigated and repaired with absorbable suture.

What Are the Most Common Injuries Resulting from Penetrating Neck Trauma and What Are the Appropriate Steps in Management?

CAROTID ARTERY INJURY

An injury to the carotid artery may be partial (laceration) or complete (transection). Clinical findings may include active arterial bleeding, expanding hematoma, a bruit, hemodynamic instability, or a new hemiparesis.

The diagnosis can be made clinically or by angiography (which would be expected to demonstrate extravasation of IV contrast or abrupt vessel cut-off).

If the patient is neurologically intact, every effort should be made to repair the carotid.

JUGULAR VEIN INJURY

An injury to the jugular vein may be partial (laceration) or complete (transection). Clinical findings are usually bleeding and hematoma.

The specific diagnosis of Internal Jugular vein injury is usually made during formal neck exploration.

Note that the external jugular vein can be ligated without adverse effect. The internal jugular vein should be repaired if the patient's condition permits; otherwise, this structure may also be ligated.

As indicated previously, injury to a major venous structure in the neck can lead to death from air embolus. Therefore, be sure to cover all open wounds, applying pressure as necessary.

TRACHEAL INJURY/LARYNGEAL INJURY

The clinical findings of an airway injury may include stridor, respiratory distress, crepitus, subcutaneous emphysema, air bubbling from the wound or hemoptysis. Patients may report a change in voice, dysphagia or odynophagia.

The diagnosis can be made with visual diagnostic modalities such as direct laryngoscopy, tracheoscopy or bronchoscopy.

A tracheal laceration can be repaired in one layer with an absorbable suture. If there is a concomitant injury to the esophagus or an artery in the vicinity, a vascularized flap of muscle should be interposed between the two structures to prevent fistulizaiton.

ESOPHAGEAL INJURY

The key to the patient with an esophageal injury is to identify the injury early. Significant morbidity and mortality are associate with delayed diagnosis and treatment of esophageal injuries.

Clinical findings may include air and saliva coming from the wound, dysphagia, odynophagia and hematemesis.

The diagnosis can be made with pharyngoscopy and esophagoscopy (with which a hematoma, bleeding or laceration may be identified), and barium swallow (which may demonstrate extravasation of oral contrast).

An esophageal injury should be debrided and repaired in two layers placing a flap of muscle over the repair to help prevent fistula formation.

Postoperatively the patient is admitted for overnight observation due to the possibility of an occult injury that was not identified during diagnostic workup. When the surgeon is updating the patient's wife on the operative findings, he notes that she has bruising around her right eye. Due to strong suspicions that both individuals' injuries are secondary to domestic violence, the surgeon calls the social worker to assist with evaluation. In one-on-one discussions with both the patient and his wife they both initially deny that their injuries were non-accidental, ultimately, however, admit during a group discussion that the patient had hit his wife during an argument and she subsequently stabbed him.

The next day the patient is medically stable for discharge. With consent, the social worker involves the families of both individuals and creates a safety plan which includes the patient being discharged to his parents' home. Follow up with a marriage counselor is arranged for the next week and both individuals are given print and community-based resources related to the prevention of domestic violence.

BEYOND THE PEARLS

- The neck contains more vital structures in a small space than any other area of the body.
- Both blunt and penetrating neck trauma can produce life-threatening injuries.
- Although rare, tracheal injuries must be addressed immediately, as they have the likelihood of resulting in significant morbidity and mortality.
- Patients who are unstable require urgent operative intervention.

- The location of neck injuries determines which structures are most at risk and therefore dictates the management of the patient.
- The trauma team should involve social workers and case managers to aid in the care and discharge planning of trauma patients, especially when domestic abuse is suspected.

Suggested Readings

LeBlang, S. D., & Nunez, D. B., Jr. (2000). Noninvasive imaging of cervical vascular injuries. *AJR Am J Roentgenol, 174*, 1269–1278.

Núñez, D. B., Jr., Torres-León, M., & Múnera, F. (2004). Vascular injuries of the neck and thoracic inlet: Helical CT-angiographic correlation. *Radiographics, 24*, 1087–1098, discussion 1099–1100.

Pathak, A. S., & Trankiem, C. T. (2009). Penetrating Neck Injury. In Mann, *SURGERY-A Competency-Based Companion* (pp. 396–402). Elsevier.

Saito, N., et al. *Penetrating head and neck injuries in the US.* https://www.ncbi.nlm.nih.gov/pubmed/24965876.

Woo, K., Magner, D. P., & Wilson, M. T. (2005). Margulies DR: CT angiography in penetrating neck trauma reduces the need for operative neck exploration. *Am Surg, 71*, 754–758.

CHAPTER 35

Gunshot Wound to the Chest in a 23-Year-Old Male

Michael Martyak ■ L.D. Britt

A 23-year-old male presents to the emergency department after having sustained a gunshot wound to the left chest. He is sitting up on the stretcher and is able to speak. He has diminished breath sounds on the left. His blood pressure is 100/50 mm Hg, his heart rate is 115 bpm, his respiratory rate is 27/min, and his oxygen saturation is 96% on a nonrebreather mask. Patient denies any allergies to medications, denies taking any medications, and has no notable past medical history. A single gunshot wound was noted in the left anterolateral chest wall in the fourth intercostal space. The patient refuses to lay flat and is incredibly anxious. Two large-bore intravenous lines are inserted, and one liter of crystalloid is given with no improvement in his heart rate or blood pressure. He has palpable and equal radial pulses. At this point, the transfusion of two units of packed red blood cells is initiated.

What Are the Initial Steps in the Management of Patients With Penetrating Thoracic Trauma?
As in all trauma patients, the evaluation should begin with the primary survey. During this initial assessment the first priority should be assessing for adequacy of **airway** protection. The second priority should be **breathing:** assess the adequacy of the patient's ability to ventilate. In chest trauma this should be a serious concern. Often in patients who develop hemothorax, pneumothorax, or even just significant injury to the chest wall, mechanical ventilation is required in order to achieve optimal oxygenation and ventilation. Interventions to treat the hemothorax or pneumothorax should be performed, but securing a definitive airway is often necessary initially. Also, in the primary survey, **circulation** is assessed. Pulses are evaluated, blood pressure and heart rate are monitored, and adequate intravascular access is established. Completion of the primary survey necessitates an expeditious assessment of **disability** and implementation of **exposure** and environmental control.

CLINICAL PEARL (STEPS 2/3)

Patients presenting with pericardial tamponade may be able to maintain a perfusing blood pressure initially. Upon establishing a definitive airway, however, the medications used for rapid-sequence intubation may reduce preload to the heart sufficiently to render the heart's compensatory measures inadequate, causing the patient to arrest. Preparations must be made, therefore, to quickly intervene in the event the patient sustains cardiac arrest after induction of anesthesia, having the surgical instruments ready and available and possibly even having the patient prepped before proceeding.

What Is the Differential Diagnosis for Penetrating Thoracic Injuries?

Table 32.1 outlines the lung pathologies that may be encountered in the trauma bay. In patients who present with hemodynamic instability after sustaining penetrating chest trauma, three diagnoses must be considered, as prompt recognition and immediate intervention can be lifesaving. These diagnoses are pericardial tamponade, tension pneumothorax, and massive hemothorax with hemorrhage from great vessels, the pulmonary hilum, the lung parenchyma, or intercostal arteries. Many of these injuries prove fatal in the field, so it is of utmost importance to make an expedient diagnosis and intervention upon arrival of the patient to the hospital. In stable patients who do not exhibit signs and symptoms of a life-threatening injury, further history and physical examination may prove useful as may additional radiographic studies.

What Are the Primary Physical Examination Techniques and Adjunctive Tests That Can Be Used to Evaluate the Patient With Penetrating Chest Trauma?

"Classic" physical examination findings are often difficult to fully assess in the noisy environment of the trauma bay. Attempting to diagnose a pericardial effusion by relying on auscultation of muffled heart sounds is often not realistic. Jugular venous distension may also be absent in the setting of a hypovolemic, bleeding patient who also has pericardial tamponade. However, the use of adjunctive radiography and ultrasound in the trauma bay allows for a more accurate assessment.

Chest radiography can be suggestive of a pericardial effusion if an enlarged cardiac silhouette is identified. However, in most trauma patients, only a small volume of pericardial blood is needed to cause tamponade, so the size of the cardiac silhouette is very nonspecific for a cardiac injury. Radiography is also helpful for identifying the location of retained missiles and diagnosing a pneumothorax or hemothorax.

For chest trauma, the **FAST (focused assessment with sonography in trauma)** examination can identify a pericardial effusion with great precision. The cardiac window is achieved by placing the transducer probe in the subxiphoid position and directing the probe toward the patient's left shoulder. If the cardiac view cannot be obtained from this maneuver either because the patient is obese or has significant abdominal discomfort, a parasternal long-axis view can be attempted. A pericardial effusion can be identified as a black stripe between the cardiac chambers and the pericardium (Fig. 35.1). Tamponade physiology may even be identified with compression of the right atrium or right ventricle. One must be cautious, as a cardiac injury cannot be completely ruled out with a negative ultrasound examination for pericardial effusion. Especially in a penetrating cardiac injury, the pericardium can decompress into the thoracic cavity if there is a communication from the missile tract.

The E-FAST (extended FAST) has been adopted to expand the diagnostic reach of the sonographic examination in trauma to further assess thoracic pathology. The high-frequency linear probe is used to assess the patient for a pneumothorax. With the indicator toward the patient's head in a long-axis orientation, the probe is initially placed just below the clavicles in the midclavicular line. The presence of sliding between the visceral and parietal pleura indicates the absence of a pneumothorax in the area being scanned. The ultrasound can even be helpful in attempting to diagnose a hemothorax. When performing the hepatorenal and splenorenal views on the FAST, the probe can be moved just slightly cephalad to now gain a view of the junction between the diaphragm and the chest cavity. With this view, the presence of a hemothorax can potentially be identified.

On physical examination, a single wound is identified in the left lateral chest at the level of the fourth intercostal space with some blood draining from it. A chest radiograph is obtained and reveals a moderate hemothorax and small pneumothorax on the left as well as a retained missile along the left lateral aspect of the cardiac silhouette.

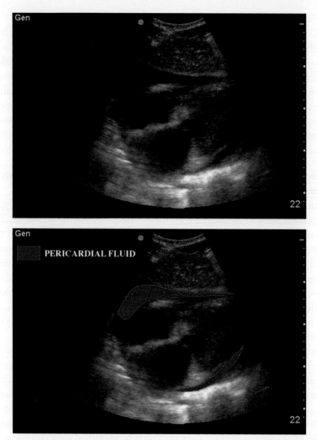

Fig. 35.1 Pericardial effusion is shown with blood seen adjacent to the right and left ventricles. Note: the lower figure is a repeat of the upper figure, marking the peridardial effusion in red. (From Rippey JCR, Royse AG: Ultrasound in trauma, *Best Pract Res Clin Anaesthesiol* 23(3):343–362.)

What Is the Treatment for Tension Pneumothorax, Pneumothorax, and Hemothorax?

Tension pneumothorax should be suspected and treated even before a chest radiograph is obtained by noting the findings of decreased or absent breath sounds in one hemothorax with tracheal deviation away from the affected side. Needle thoracostomy is a simple, temporizing maneuver that can be lifesaving in a patient presenting with a tension pneumothorax. Pneumothorax and hemothorax are typically diagnosed on chest radiography and should be treated by thoracostomy tube placement.

Needle Thoracostomy

1. Prep the second intercostal space in the midclavicular line.
2. Insert a 14-gauge needle catheter or angiocatheter at this site. A rush of air should be encountered.
3. Remove the needle, leaving the catheter in place and secure it.
4. Insert a formal thoracostomy tube to evacuate the residual simple pneumothorax.

Thoracostomy Tube Placement

1. Position the patient with the ipsilateral arm above the head and identify the interspace between the fourth and fifth ribs. (This typically corresponds to the nipple line in men and the inframammary crease in women.)
2. Prep the site and, if time permits, infiltrate local anesthetic in the skin and subcutaneous tissues along the planned tract.
3. Make a 3- to 4-cm incision just below the fourth rib.
4. Tunnel in the subcutaneous tissues to the superior edge of the fifth rib with a Kelly clamp.
5. Advance the clamp through the pleura over the superior border of the fifth rib, in order to avoid the intercostal neurovascular bundle lying just below the fourth rib. A rush of air, blood, or fluid should be encountered depending on the indication for the chest tube.
6. Spread the clamp along the direction of the fifth rib and insert a finger into the pleural space to ensure the lung or empty space is palpated and not liver or spleen and to ensure no pulmonary adhesions.
7. Insert the chest tube using a Kelly clamp, and advance, directing it posteriorly and toward the apex of the thoracic cavity.
8. Attach the chest tube to the pleurovac and place to suction.

CLINICAL PEARL (STEPS 2/3)

When determining the indication for thoracotomy to control ongoing bleeding, the recognized indication is a chest tube output of 1500 mL or more upon insertion of the chest tube or 250 mL/hour or more over 3 consecutive hours after tube thoracostomy placement.

A left chest tube is placed with 750 mL of blood evacuated. The patient then becomes more hypoxic with oxygen saturation of 80% on the nonrebreather. A FAST examination is performed and a pericardial effusion is identified. The patient is intubated for airway protection, and as the patient is being intubated, the patient becomes severely hypotensive, and no femoral or carotid pulse can be palpated.

What Is the Treatment for the Hypotensive Patient With Hemothorax or Traumatic Pericardial Tamponade?

RESUSCITATIVE THORACOTOMY

The resuscitative thoracotomy can be used to address a few life-threatening injuries in the patient presenting with profound refractory shock or recent loss of vital signs. By means of a resuscitative thoracotomy, the following can be accomplished: a pericardiotomy can be made to relieve pericardial tamponade; temporary control of bleeding from a cardiac laceration with manual compression can be achieved; control of intrathoracic bleeding vessels or bleeding lung parenchyma can be obtained; and cross-clamping of the aorta to limit continued blood loss from hemorrhage originating below the diaphragm can be performed. The Western Trauma Association guidelines indicate that a resuscitative thoracotomy should be considered in the patient presenting with no signs of life and undergoing cardiopulmonary resuscitation less than 10 minutes in blunt trauma and less than 15 minutes in penetrating trauma or in patients presenting in profound refractory shock.

The resuscitative thoracotomy is a left anterolateral thoracotomy. The patient is positioned in the supine position with the arms extended. An incision is made in the fourth intercostal space just superior to the fifth rib, which is located just below the nipple or the inframammary fold. The incision is extended from the edge of the sternum to the posterior axillary line. The chest should ideally be entered with bold strokes of the scalpel, first dividing the skin and subcutaneous tissues, and then through the intercostal muscles; finally, the pleura is incised, gaining entry to the thoracic cavity. Care should be made to avoid the intercostal neurovascular bundle. The rib spreader is then inserted with the handle toward the bed and in the axilla so as to ensure an unobstructed field in the event of needing to convert to a clamshell thoracotomy (Fig. 35.2). As the left thoracotomy is being

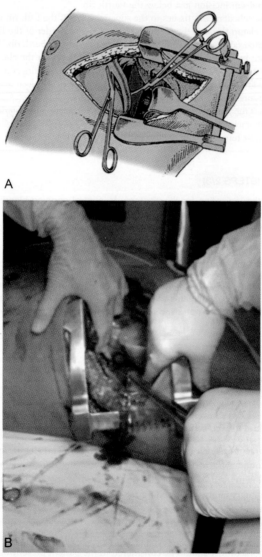

Fig. 35.2 Illustration (A) and photograph (B) of a resuscitative thoracotomy with pericardiotomy and thoracic aortic cross-clamping. The pericardium should be opened longitudinally and anterior to the phrenic nerve. (A: From Raja AS: Thoracic trauma. In Walls RM, editor: *Rosen's emergency medicine: concepts and clinical practice*, ed 9, Philadelphia, 2018, Elsevier, pp 382–403. B: from Menaker J, Scalea TM: Emergency department thoracotomy. In Cameron JL, Cameron AM, editors: *Current surgical therapy*, Philadelphia, 2017, Elsevier, pp 1141–1145.)

performed, a right chest tube should be placed by another provider simultaneously to assess for bleeding in the right chest, potentially identifying the need to convert to a clamshell thoracotomy.

Once in the chest, the pericardium should be inspected first. A small incision is made in the pericardium with care taken to remain anterior to the left phrenic nerve to avoid injury. The tense pericardium in pericardial tamponade is not easily incised with scissors, so the use of a scalpel can assist with initially opening the pericardium. The scissors are then used to complete the pericardiotomy longitudinally. The next step is to mobilize the lung by dividing the inferior pulmonary ligament. Then the lung should be retracted anteriorly, and the descending thoracic aorta should be identified in preparation to cross-clamp. Large blunt scissors should be used to dissect the pleura overlying the aorta ensuring that the clamp will not slip. The vascular clamp should be placed across the aorta and if a nasogastric or orogastric tube has been placed, it can assist with identifying the esophagus and avoiding injury. At this point, if a bleeding lung injury is identified, it can be addressed with various maneuvers such as performing a tractotomy or, in desperate circumstances, performing a hilar twist.

MEDIAN STERNOTOMY

In the somewhat rare instance that a patient presents with a traumatic hemopericardium but has not yet developed significant tamponade physiology and hence is able to maintain a perfusing blood pressure, the median sternotomy is an excellent surgical approach. If tamponade is encountered, the pericardium is incised with a scalpel and the remainder of the pericardium opened with scissors. The phrenic nerve is posterior so should be avoided in the median sternotomy approach. With the heart exposed, a cardiac injury can be identified and repaired. Care should be taken to ensure there is no concomitant posterior cardiac injury as well.

CLINICAL PEARL

The median sternotomy provides excellent exposure for identification and repair of a cardiac injury. If the luxury of time is available in the trauma patient with hemopericardium, rapidly transporting the patient to the operative suite for a median sternotomy certainly provides the best operative exposure for the cardiac injury. However, the patient's hemodynamic instability often will not allow any delays and certainly the anterolateral thoracotomy is the most expeditious maneuver to gain access to the chest cavity to relieve the cardiac tamponade and gain control of bleeding.

The patient undergoes an emergency room thoracotomy. The pericardium is opened and an injury to the left ventricle is identified, which is initially controlled with the surgeon's finger. The patient regains a perfusing rhythm and the ventricular injury is primarily repaired with pledgeted sutures. He is transferred to the operating room for further exploration and then to the trauma intensive care unit for further resuscitation.

Suggested Readings

Burlew, C. C., Moore, E. E., Moore, F. A., et al. (2012). Western Trauma Association critical decisions in trauma: Resuscitative thoracotomy. *J Trauma Acute Care Surg, 73*, 1359–1363.

Menaker, J., & Scalea, T. M. (2017). Emergency department thoracotomy. In J. L. Cameron, & A. M. Cameron (Eds.), *Current surgical therapy* (pp. 1141–1145). Philadelphia: Elsevier.

Raja, A. S. (2018). Thoracic trauma. In R. M. Walls (Ed.), *Rosen's emergency medicine: Concepts and clinical practice* (9th ed., pp. 382–403). Philadelphia: Elsevier.

Rippey, J. C. R., & Royse, A. G. (2009). Ultrasound in trauma. *Best Pract Res Clin Anaesthesiol, 23*(3), 343–362.

CHAPTER 36

Bicycle Crash Involving a 37-Year-Old Male

Amanda Lee ■ Steven R. Allen

A 37-year-old male bicyclist, who is otherwise healthy, was struck by a motor vehicle. He was thrown approximately 10 feet into the air and landed on his left side with his chest striking the ground first. At the scene he was complaining of severe left-sided chest pain and difficulty breathing. He was brought to the trauma center by emergency medical services (EMS). Upon his arrival, the primary survey (described in previous chapters) is as follows: Airway is patent; he is noted to have absent breath sounds on the left side with a respiratory rate of 35 bpm and an oxygen saturation of 88% on nonrebreather face mask. His heart rate is 130 beats per minute and blood pressure is 90/40 mm Hg; his Glasgow coma score is 14 (eyes: 4; verbal: 4 [he is confused]; motor: 6), and he is moving all four extremities.

What Injuries Are Most likely in Victims of Blunt Chest Injury and What Are the Steps in Diagnosis and Management?

Patients who suffer from severe chest trauma have the potential to have significant injuries that can ultimately translate into significant morbidity or mortality. Chapter 37 describes the assessment of patients who present with chest trauma and their workup. In patients with blunt chest trauma specifically, the care team must be vigilant to diagnose either a tension pneumothorax or tension hemothorax based on absent breath sounds and hemodynamic instability. Other associated injuries that one must consider are rib fractures and pulmonary contusions, as well as blunt great vessel or aortic injury due to the high energy and sudden deceleration by striking the ground with this chest.

Given the pathognomonic signs and symptoms of tension pneumothorax or tension hemothorax with hemodynamic instability, one must treat a patient immediately with needle decompression of the chest cavity with needle decompression to alleviate the tension physiology followed by and tube thoracostomy with a formal chest tube to definitively drain any hemothorax.

CLINICAL PEARL

Tension pneumothorax is a clinical diagnosis. The clinical findings consistent with tension pneumothorax are: absent breath sounds, tachycardia, hypotension, distended neck veins, trachea deviated away from the affected side, and dyspnea. **Tension pneumothorax is a clinical diagnosis**. When tension pneumothorax is diagnosed, one should perform needle decompression or definitive tube thoracostomy (chest tube placement). One should not delay treatment by obtaining a chest radiograph to confirm the diagnosis.

The patient undergoes immediate needle decompression of his left chest with a 16-guage angiocath in the midclavicular line at the second intercostal space. There is a significant rush of air from the angiocath upon insertion. His vital signs normalize, and his work of breathing improves significantly. A definitive left-sided tube thoracostomy is placed in sixth intercostal space and placed to -20 cm H_20 suction. Approximately 200 mL of blood is drained from the chest tube. Now that his vital signs have normalized with this intervention, the primary survey is repeated and adjuncts to the primary survey (chest radiograph (CXR)) are obtained.

When Is a Chest Radiograph Indicated?

A chest radiograph (CXR) should be obtained in nearly all trauma situations to rule out chest injury and to identify injuries that could later evolve into life-threatening situations such as a simple pneumothorax or hemothorax which could later lead to tension physiology. The CXR can also help identify other potentially significant injuries such as rib fractures, pulmonary contusions, a widened mediastinum, diaphragmatic rupture, etc. As discussed above, when tension physiology is diagnosed, a CXR for confirmation of the diagnosis is contraindicated prior to needle or tube decompression of the chest cavity.

What Are Common Findings of Severe Chest Injury on CXR?

The vast majority of CXRs in the acute trauma patient are performed in the supine position for trauma. Accordingly, one will not see the typical meniscus of a hemothorax or pleural effusion that one would see on an upright CXR. Instead the side of the chest with the hemothorax may demonstrate a "haziness" or opacification compared with the uninjured side. One may also see a widened mediastinum as well as other signs suggestive of aortic or other great vessel injury (Box 36.1). Pulmonary contusions may appear as patchy opacifications or infiltrates within the lung fields, but may be difficult to differentiate from hemothorax in the case of extensive pulmonary injury. Rib fractures may be identified on CXR. Diaphragmatic ruptures can also be visualized, especially on the left side, as elevations of the hemidiaphragm or the appearance of a gastric bubble in the chest cavity.

BOX 36.1 ■ Radiographic Signs of Blunt Aortic Injury

- Widened mediastinum (> 8 cm when supine or > 6 cm when upright)
- Indistinct or abnormal aortic contour
- Deviation of trachea or nasogastric tube to the right
- Depression of the left main bronchus
- Loss of the aortopulmonary window
- Widened paraspinal stripe
- Widened paratracheal stripe
- Left apical pleural cap
- Large left hemothorax

Modified from: Sharma R, D'Souza D: Thoracic aortic injury, Radiopaedia. *https://radiopaedia.org/articles/ thoracic-aortic-injury. Accessed June 26, 2018.*

The patient's CXR demonstrates that his trachea is midline, and his lungs are expanded bilaterally, although he has patchy opacification of the left lung concerning for pulmonary contusion. His mediastinum is widened, measuring 9 cm, and there is loss of the aortic knob. Both diaphragms appear intact. The left-sided chest tube is in good position. There are multiple displaced left-sided rib fractures (Fig. 36.1). A focused assessment with sonography for trauma (FAST) examination is performed and is negative in all four views of the study. Upon further inspection, it is noted that the patient has approximately 350 mL of blood in the chest tube canister over the past 20 minutes. He remains slightly tachycardic (heart rate 110), but his blood pressure remains normal (125/76); his respiratory rate is 20, and oxygen saturation is 99% on 2 liters nasal cannula. Based on his current clinical status and to rule out additional injury to his torso, he is taken to the computed tomography (CT) scanner for further evaluation.

The CT scan of the abdomen and pelvis demonstrates no acute traumatic abnormality, but the chest CT scan demonstrates a significant left-sided pulmonary contusion. In addition, multiple ribs on the left side are fractured in multiple areas consistent with a diagnosis of flail chest (Fig. 36.2).

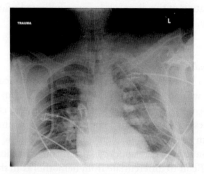

Fig. 36.1   CT chest demonstrates initial CXR with left-sided chest tube and wide mediastinum.

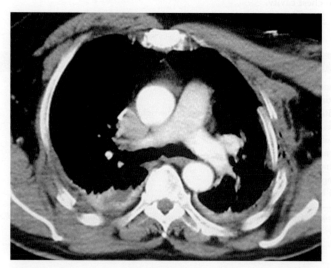

Fig. 36.2   CT scan of the chest that demonstrates a left-sided flail chest.

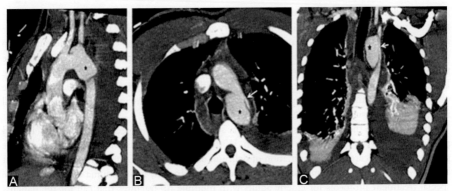

Fig. 36.3   CT scan demonstrating a grade III aortic injury *(arrow)* in sagittal (A), axial (B), and coronal (C) views.

Several of the rib fractures are significantly displaced. The patient is also noted to have a grade III aortic injury just distal to the take-off of the left subclavian artery with a periaortic hematoma (Fig. 36.3).

The lungs are surrounded by visceral (attached to the lungs) and parietal (attached to the thoracic cavity) pleura. The pleura secretes a lubricating fluid which allows the pleural layers to slide on one another during respiration and also has adhesive properties lung expansion in the chest cavity during inspiration. Air (pneumothorax) or fluid (hemothorax or chylothorax) accumulating between the pleural surfaces interferes with these respiratory mechanics.

There are several criteria that are used to determine whether operative intervention is required in the face of chest trauma and the presence of a hemothorax: (1) drainage of 1500 mL of blood immediately from the chest tube; (2) drainage of a moderate amount of blood (750 mL to 1000 mL) from the chest tube with a significant amount of undrained blood noted on imaging of the chest; (3) drainage of 250 mL per hour for 3 hours. Each of the above criteria are indications for surgical intervention with thoracotomy to identify and control the ongoing bleeding.

What Are the Management Options for Rib Fractures?

Rib fractures vary in severity based on their number, location, and whether they are displaced. A nondisplaced solitary rib fracture, for example, may be managed with analgesia only and may potentially be managed in the outpatient setting. At the other extreme, a flail chest, defined as two or more consecutive ribs broken in two or more locations, disrupts respiratory mechanics—the flail segment moves inward during inspiration. Flail chest, therefore,must be managed by immobilization of the flail segment and analgesia in the inpatient setting.

Rib fractures often result in severe pain, especially with deep breathing and coughing. Therefore adequate pain control is paramount in order to optimize the patient's pulmonary status. Pain control usually requires a combination of acetaminophen, nonsteroidal antiinflammatory drugs (NSAIDs), and opioids is required. To minimize the need for opioid pain medication, one may consider thoracic epidurals or regional blocks with pain catheters. Setting realistic expectations with the patient that the pain will not be eliminated is essential. The goal is to reduce the pain sufficiently to allow the patient to breathe deeply and to cough in order to clear their secretions. Careful attention to the patient's pulmonary status is essential. The patient must be encouraged to cough, breathe deeply, and to utilize the incentive spirometer. These measures help mitigate the risk of a subsequent pneumonia. For those with poor pain control and ineffective pulmonary mechanics despite aggressive pain control methods, rib fixation may prove beneficial. Rib fixation has been shown to benefit a subset of patients with severe chest trauma; however the exact indications and patient population for whom this treatment modality will be beneficial remains controversial.

Rib fractures in the elderly must be taken very seriously due to the preexisting frailty and limited physiologic reserve of the geriatric population. With regard to analgesia, one must ensure adequate pain control with care to avoid initiation of delirium or oversedation. Aggressive pulmonary toilet and close monitoring of pulmonary effort is paramount. In fact, many trauma centers now have special treatment protocols for elderly adults with multiple rib fractures that call for the patients to be placed in the intensive care unit to allow for close monitoring, adequate pain control, and optimal pulmonary care by trained respiratory therapists.

The patient is admitted to the intensive care unit (ICU) because of the need for a chest tube, grade III aortic injury, and persistent tachycardia and to ensure adequate pain control in the face of multiple rib fractures and severe pulmonary contusions. In the ICU, he is noted to remain tachycardic. Due to his persistent tachycardia in the setting of a blunt aortic injury, he is started on an esmolol drip. The esmolol drip is successful in controlling his heart rate, with his most recent heart rate of 75 and his blood pressure 110/45. The vascular surgery team is consulted to evaluate the need for intervention for the aortic injury. He is taken to the OR urgently for endovascular stenting of the aortic injury. The stent is placed without incident (Fig. 36.4). He is transferred back to the ICU for further monitoring. His pulmonary status and analgesic requirement are monitored carefully postoperatively.

What Are the Grades of Blunt Aortic Injury and What Are the Indications for Repair of Aortic Injuries?
Blunt chest trauma can lead to a range of aortic injuries, most of which are diagnosed on an angiogram of the chest. The severity of the injury informs the treatment options, which are outlined in Table 36.1.

TABLE 36.1 ■ **Aortic Injuries: Grading System and Treatment Options**

Grade of Blunt Aortic Injury	Description of Injury	Treatment Options
Grade I	Intimal tear: no aortic external contour abnormality; tear or associated thrombus < 10 mm	Medical management with antiplatelet therapy
Grade II	Large intimal flap: no aortic external contour abnormality; tear or associated thrombus > 10 mm	TEVAR
Grade III	Pseudoaneurysm: aortic external contour abnormality but contained	TEVAR
Grade IV	Rupture: aortic external contour abnormality; not contained, free rupture	TEVAR/OR (emergent)

TEVAR: Thoracic endovascular aortic repair.
Modified from: Starnes, BW, Lundgren, RS, et al: A new classification scheme for treating blunt aortic injury, *J Vasc Surg* 55:47–54, 2012.

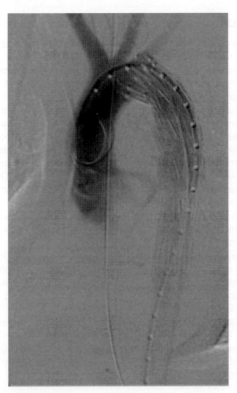

Fig. 36.4 Intraoperative angiographic image demonstrating a well-positioned aortic stent graft originating just distal to the left subclavian artery.

CLINICAL PEARL

Hemothorax is usually a result of fractured ribs with adjacent lung laceration or intercostal artery, great vessel, pulmonary hilar, or cardiac injuries. A hemothorax may also occur if the patient has intraabdominal bleeding and a concomitant diaphragm injury. A hemothorax can lead to tension physiology. The minimum amount of blood needed to produce CXR findings is 200 mL to 500 mL but may require a larger amount of blood if the CXR is performed in the supine or semierect positions. CT scans are more sensitive than CXR, with as many as 80% of hemothoraces detected on CT but not seen on CXR.

Over the subsequent two days the chest tube output decreases to less than 150 mL and is sequentially removed without incident. The CXR demonstrates, no evidence of retained hemothorax, and a well-positioned aortic stent graft. His oxygen requirement resolves; he is able to cough and has adequate pulmonary toilet and is able to obtain 1500 mL on the incentive spirometer. He is discharged from the hospital on postinjury day 10 with instructions for follow-up in 1 week.

BEYOND THE PEARLS

- Thoracic trauma is a major source of morbidity and mortality, second only to head injury as cause of death in injured patients.
- Life-threatening injuries to the chest include: tension/open pneumothorax, massive hemothorax, flail chest and pulmonary contusion, air embolism, great vessel and aortic transection, and pericardial tamponade.
- Pericardial tamponade may result from a cardiac injury (most often from penetrating trauma). Accumulation of even a small amount of blood is enough to result in tamponade. Beck's triad (muffled heart tones, distended neck veins, and hypotension) are pathognomonic for pericardial tamponade. Pericardial tamponade requires immediate decompression of the pericardial sac by median sternotomy or, in the case of cardiovascular collapse, a resuscitative thoracotomy. It should be noted that pericardiocentesis is no longer advised in the trauma setting.
- Resuscitative thoracotomy (see Chapter 35), a left anterolateral thoracotomy, is a potentially life-saving procedure when used in the appropriate patient population. This procedure should be used in patients who are in extremis or pulseless. It should not be performed in a patient who lost vital signs for more than 10 minutes in the case of blunt trauma or more than 15 minutes in the case of penetrating trauma.
- Occult pneumothorax can usually be observed; however, there are several situations in which non-interventional management is likely to fail: (1) the rim of air in the chest is greater than 7 mm; (2) the presence of co-exisiting hemothorax (3) the patient is likely to require positive pressure ventilation; (4) the presence of respiratory distress; (5) and increasing size of the pneumothorax on serial CXR.
- Due to the low sensitivity of CXR in the identification of pneumothorax (sensitivity for pneumothorax 28% to 75%), there is now a tendency to utilize a modified version of the FAST (called the "extended" FAST) in which one uses the vascular probe of the ultrasound machine to look for a lack of lung sliding along the pleural interface (sensitivity to identify a pneumothorax: 86% to 98%).

Suggested Readings

Bellister, S. A., Dennis, B. M., & Guillamondegui, O. D. (2017). Blunt and penetrating cardiac trauma. *Surg Clin North Am*, *97*(5), 1065–1076.

Clancy, K., Velopulos, C., Bilaniuk, J. W., et al. (2012). Screening for blunt cardiac injury. *J Trauma*, *73*(5), S301–S306.

DuBose, J., Inaba, K., Demetriades, D., et al. (2012). Management of post-traumatic retained hemothorax: A prospective, observational, multicenter AAST study. *J Trauma Acute Care Surg*, *72*(1), 11–22.

Kasotakis, G., Hasenboehler, E. A., Streib, E. W., et al. (2017). Operative fixation of rib fractures after blunt trauma: A practice management guideline for the Eastern Association for the Surgery of Trauma. *J Trauma Acute Care Surg*, *82*(3), 618–626.

Trust, M. D., & Teixeir, P. G. R. (2017). Blunt trauma of the aorta, current guidelines. *Cardiol Clin*, *35*(3), 441–451.

CHAPTER 37

Stab Wound to the Right Upper Quadrant in a 20-Year-Old Male

Kaitlyn Kennard ■ George Koenig

A 20-year-old male with an unknown past medical history is found lying on the sidewalk by police after a 911 call from a bystander. The patient states that he was stabbed by a person unknown to him. He has blood stains on his shirt on the right side of his abdomen. At the scene the patient is responsive to commands and states that he has pain in the right side of his abdomen. He reports that the knife looked like a large kitchen knife.

When arriving in the emergency department, the patient's **A**irway and **B**reathing are normal he is phonating well and his chest is clear. Assessment of his **C**irculation finds him to be initially hypotensive: his heart rate is 98 beats per minute, blood pressure is 80/40 mm Hg. Respiratory rate is 18. He moves all extremities purposefully, and there are no discernible **D**isabilities; full **E**xposure permits assessment of a single stab wound with mild oozing in the right upper quadrant, 2 cm below the costal margin.

What Are the Initial Steps in the Workup of Penetrating Abdominal Wounds?

Patients with penetrating abdominal wounds should be assessed and treated according to the ABCs of the advanced trauma life support guidelines (see Chapter 32) as demonstrated previously.

Patients who are hypotensive on presentation should have two large-bore IVs placed and should receive either uncrossmatched packed red blood cells (PRBC) if immediately available or receive a bolus of normal saline or lactated Ringer's. If the patient remains hypotensive, the team should be prepared to massively transfuse with component therapy of PRBCs, fresh frozen plasma (FFP), and platelets in a 1:1:1 ratio.

Patients whose hemodynamics do not respond to fluid resuscitation should be taken to the operating room (OR) immediately for exploration.

If the patient is hemodynamically stable and the trajectory suggests that the liver may be the only abdominal organ injured, it is reasonable to obtain a CT of the chest, abdomen, and pelvis with IV contrast to evaluate the injury. If a bleeding liver laceration is presumed to be the only intraabdominal injury, the patient may be taken to the interventional radiology suite for intraarterial embolization. If additional injuries are suspected or the patient is hemodynamically unstable, operative exploration should be undertaken.

Patients who remain hypotensive despite volume resuscitation or who have obvious peritonitis should be taken emergently to the OR for exploration. Additionally, exploration is mandatory in the face of omental or visceral evisceration. When peritoneal penetration of a stab wound is equivocal, it can be assessed with a local wound exploration to determine whether the fascia is intact. At times when it is unclear whether peritoneal penetration has taken place, as in the case of an obese patient, laparoscopy may be a useful and minimally invasive method to determine whether the peritoneum is intact and to explore for intraabdominal injury. Figure 37.1 summarizes these steps in a flowsheet format.

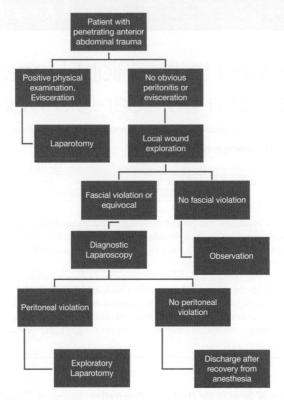

Fig. 37.1 Flow chart for the management of penetrating abdominal trauma.

CLINICAL PEARL (STEPS 1/2/3)

Successful embolization of bleeding from a liver laceration requires knowledge of the hepatic arterial system. The celiac trunk extends approximately 1.0 cm from the aorta and then divides into three major branches—left gastric, splenic, and common hepatic arteries. The proper hepatic artery enters the porta hepatis and then splits into the left and right hepatic arteries that supply the liver.

Despite being given 2 L of lactated Ringer's and 1 unit of packed red blood cells (PRBCs), the patient's blood pressure remains 80/40 mm Hg, so a decision is made to take the patient to the OR for an exploratory laparotomy given the concern for intraabdominal injury and bleeding (peritonitis and hypotension). Additional uncrossmatched PRBCs are transfused en route to the OR and a cooler with PRBCs, FFP, and platelets is requested from the blood bank.

What Are the Considerations in Performing a Trauma Laparotomy?

In the setting of an emergent laparotomy, the patient should be placed in a supine position with arms abducted at 90 degrees. In addition to adequate intravenous access, there should be uncross-matched PRBCs, FFP, and platelets in a 1:1:1 ratio immediately available as there will not be a completed type and screen due to the emergent nature of the procedure. The torso, neck, abdomen, and upper half of lower extremities should be included in the sterile prep.

The trauma laparotomy incision extends from the xiphoid process to the symphysis pubis. Subcostal extension, which involves extending the incision below the ribs, can be used at times to improve access to the liver on the right and provide better access to retrohepatic venous injuries.

Upon entry into the abdomen, all four quadrants (above and below the liver in the right upper quadrant, in the left upper quadrant by the spleen, and in the pelvis) are packed with laparotomy pads to provide compression. The packs are then removed in the order of the least to the most likely quadrant injured. The goal is to identify and stop any major sources of bleeding. Once active hemorrhage has been temporized, the operative team can undertake a more complete survey of the abdominal organs.

CLINICAL PEARL (STEPS 1/2/3)

Though good communication between the operating team and the anesthesia team is always essential, it is of paramount importance in the situation of an unstable, hypotensive patient. Patients may have significant hypotension on initiation of anesthesia and/or on opening of the abdominal cavity. Once the abdomen is opened and packed and ongoing blood loss is minimized, the operative team may need to pause to allow for further resuscitation by the anesthesia team.

The patient undergoes induction of general anesthesia without hemodynamic compromise. A laparotomy incision is made, and a large amount of intraabdominal blood is seen. Packs are placed in all four quadrants, including packs above and below the liver, and on survey of the abdomen, the right upper quadrant packs are removed last. There is a 3-cm liver laceration noted, from which active bleeding is able to be stopped temporarily with manual compression. Also noted was a 1.5-cm tangential injury to the right hepatic flexure of the colon. Minimal stool contamination was noted. The colon was repaired primarily with a two-layer primary closure. The liver laceration required three deep sutures for closure. Abdominal lavage was performed, and the abdomen was closed primarily.

CLINICAL PEARL (STEPS 2/3)

Two terms worthwhile knowing well when reading the trauma literature are the **lethal triad** of **coagulopathy, hypothermia, and acidosis** and the concept of a **damage control laparotomy**. In a patient with ongoing bleeding and ongoing transfusion requirement, there is a danger of developing coagulopathy, hypothermia, and acidosis. This triad of derangements has a very significant risk of mortality. Accordingly, it is now recognized that in such a desperate situation, it is often prudent to perform a "damage control laparotomy," the goal of which is rapid control of bleeding and control of any gastrointestinal contamination with early termination of the procedure and temporary abdominal closure. This technique has been shown to have improved survival outcomes. The timing of the return to the OR should be determined by physiologic reserve, complexity of the injuries, available resources, and the experience of the surgical team.

Are There Cases in Which a Penetrating Abdominal Wound Can Be Managed Nonoperatively?
Nonoperative management of an abdominal stab wound in a stable patient requires that other abdominal injuries—including bowel injuries—must be excluded. Based on clinical and CT corroboration of the absence of significant injury, one may elect to monitor a patient carefully with continued repeat abdominal examinations by skilled providers, using frequent vital signs and serial labs. Consistency in staff and individuals performing the abdominal examination is ideal. Multiple examiners may confound the reliability of accurate assessments in detecting intraabdominal injury.

In general, 24 hours of ICU monitoring should be a sufficient period for such evaluation. Any alterations in the patient's clinical status require a full reassessment with a high suspicion for intraabdominal pathology.

What Are the Potential Complications of Hepatic Trauma?

Clinicians should be aware of several complications that can develop after liver trauma. The most common complication is bile leak and can occur in as many as 20% of patients managed operatively. Hepatic necrosis occurs commonly after hepatic injury and is most likely to occur in patients undergoing angioembolization. Hepatic abscesses can develop in devascularized areas of hepatic parenchyma.

A rare complication of hepatic trauma is arteriobiliary or portobiliary fistula that results in hemobilia. Hemobilia can result in clot and obstruction of the biliary tree. Brisk bleeds can present similarly to classic GI bleed with the addition of jaundice and upper abdominal pain. Hemobilia can often be treated with selective angioembolization. More severe cases may require operative intervention with ligation of the feeding vessel or anatomic liver resection.

From the operating room, the patient is taken to the intensive care unit where the focus is on postoperative resuscitation with correction of the metabolic derangements was resuscitated with additional blood products, including FFP and platelets, and hemodynamics improved. The patient was observed for 2 days in the intensive care unit and for 2 days on the step-down unit and was ultimately discharged to home in stable condition.

BEYOND THE PEARLS

- The location of penetrating abdominal wounds dictates the intraabdominal organs that are most at risk for injury.
- Nonoperative management of penetrating abdominal wounds is possible, but care must be taken to standardize serial examinations and to quickly act upon any alterations to the patient's clinical status.
- Exploratory laparotomy is indicated in patients with penetrating abdominal wounds who have peritonitis or hemodynamic instability.
- The goals of damage control abdominal surgery include identifying and addressing life-threatening abdominal injuries and temporarily closing the abdomen with plans to return to the OR after resuscitation and correction of metabolic derangements.

Suggested Readings

Ahmed N, Vernick JJ: Management of liver trauma in adults, *J Emerg Trauma Shock* 4(1) Jan–Mar:114–119, 2011.

Inaba K, Okeye OT, Rosenheck T, et al: Prospective evaluation of the role of CT in assessment of abdominal stab wounds, *JAMA Surg* 148(9):810–816, 2013.

Kevric J, O'Reilly GM, Gocentas RA, et al: Management of hemodynamically stable patients with Q14 penetrating abdominal stab injuries: review of practice at an Australian major trauma centre, *Eur J Trauma Emerg Surg* 42(6) Dec:671-675, 2015.

Centers for Disease Control and Prevention, Sasser SM, Hunt RC, Faul M, et al: Guidelines for field triage of injured patients: recommendations of National Expert Panel on Field Triage, 2011. *MMWR Recomm Rep* 61(RR-1):1–20, 2012.

Snyder WH, Weigelt JA, Watkins WL, et al: The surgical management of duodenal trauma: precepts based on a review of 247 cases, *Arch Surg* 115:422–429, 1980.

Zafar SN, Rushing A, Haut ER, et al: Outcome of selective non-operative management of penetrating abdominal injuries from North American National Trauma Database, *Br J Surg* 99(Suppl 1):115–164, 2012.

CHAPTER 38

Blow to the Abdomen in a 19-Year-Old Male Football Player

James Pendleton ■ Joshua A. Marks

A 19-year-old, otherwise healthy athletic male was playing football when he was tackled and suffered a direct blow to the left side of his abdomen. He immediately reported feeling as though "the wind got knocked out" of him and was bent over, unable to stand up straight as a result of the abdominal pain. 911 was called, and he was transported to a nearby hospital by emergency medical services (EMS). In the emergency department, his heart rate is 114 bpm; his systolic blood pressure 96mm Hg; his respiratory rate 22; and his pulse oximeter 94% on room air.

How Should a Patient With Blunt Abdominal Trauma Be Triaged and Evaluated?
As with any patient presenting with a traumatic injury, assessment should take place according to the ABCs (see Chapter 32) following the model of the primary and secondary surveys: it is important in order to systematically identify injuries that are potentially life threatening. This approach compels clinicians not to be distracted by injuries that are easily appreciated and then to identify other occult injuries, which may not be obvious. The head-to-toe examination of the secondary survey is the time to focus special attention on anatomic locations and organ systems most at risk for injury based on patient complaints and the mechanism of injury. The most common mechanism of blunt abdominal trauma is the motor vehicle collision. Other common causes include falls and injuries due to vocational or recreational activities. On physical examination in patients with blunt abdominal trauma the examiner should look for signs that may herald significant intraabdominal injury: seat belt or steering wheel signs (ecchymosis caused by high-velocity impact); flank and periumbilical ecchymosis (Grey Turner and Cullen signs, respectively) that can signify pancreatic and/or retroperitoneal injury; and significant abdominal distension and peritoneal signs such as guarding and rebound tenderness, which are associated with hemoperitoneum and/or rupture of an intraabdominal viscus. Physical findings associated with abdominal injury resulting from blunt trauma may be subtle and require a high index of suspicion based on the mechanism of injury. Additionally, assessment of the abdomen in unstable patients can be undertaken quickly at the bedside using the focused assessment with sonography in trauma (FAST) (Fig. 38.1A).

What Is the Relevant Anatomy for Assessing Patients With Blunt Abdominal Injuries?
The abdominal injury pattern of blunt trauma is much different from that of penetrating wounds (see Chapter 37). Blunt vehicular trauma results from rapid acceleration or deceleration, where visceral damage may occur from a direct blow, shear forces, or a closed-loop phenomenon. Solid abdominal organs—liver, spleen, and kidney—are the structures most likely to be damaged after

blunt trauma. The relative incidence of hollow visceral perforation and lumbar spinal injuries is low, but increases with incorrect seat belt usage.

The abdomen can be split into regions—the peritoneal cavity, retroperitoneal space, and pelvis—all of which have important organs at risk for injury. The upper abdomen is that portion of the peritoneal cavity covered by the bony thorax and includes the diaphragm, liver, spleen, stomach, and transverse colon. Fractures of the lower ribs should increase suspicion for hepatic or splenic injury. The lower abdomen contains the small bowel and remaining portion of the intraabdominal colon. The retroperitoneal space contains the aorta, vena cava, pancreas, kidneys, ureters, and portions of the colon and duodenum. The pelvis contains the rectum, bladder, iliac vessels, and, in women, the internal genitalia. Organs that have points of fixation to the bony skeleton or other organs are at highest risk for deceleration injury as they can pull away from their tether points rapidly. The organs most commonly affected by blunt abdominal injuries are spleen, liver, small bowel, kidneys, bladder, rectum, diaphragm, and pancreas.

The injured football player is triaged to the trauma bay by the EMS providers based on his prehospital vital signs, mechanism of injury, and degree of pain. His airway is patent. He has bilateral breath sounds. Two large-bore peripheral IVs are established, and he receives a bolus of isotonic crystalloid solution for his relative hypotension. No external bleeding is observed. His Glasgow Coma Score is 15, and he is moving all extremities. He has some bruising along his left upper flank, and he is tender to palpation of the left upper quadrant of his abdomen. His abdomen is soft, and there is no rebound or guarding. The digital rectal examination shows no gross blood. A chest radiograph shows no pneumothorax or hemothorax but reveals two lateral left rib fractures. His pelvis radiograph reveals no abnormality. A FAST shows free fluid in the left and right upper quadrants of the abdomen but none in his pericardial space or pelvis (see Fig. 38.1B). Subsequent vital signs show that his systolic blood pressure has dropped to 70 mm Hg.

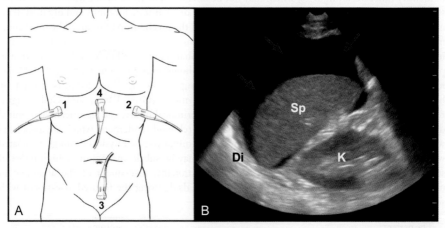

Fig. 38.1 (A) The four views for the original focused assessment with sonography in trauma (FAST) scan: 1) right upper quadrant also known as perihepatic space or Morison's pouch; 2) left upper quadrant or perisplenic space; 3) suprapubic view or pelvic space; and 4) subxiphoid view or pericardium. (B) An ultrasound of the perisplenic space demonstrating the spleen *(Sp)*, the left kidney *(K)*, the diaphragm *(Di)*, and free fluid (anechoic, *red arrows*) indicative of hemoperitoneum. (From Richards JR, McGahan JP: Focused assessment with sonography in trauma (FAST) in 2017: what radiologists can learn, *Radiology* 283(1):30–48, 2017. https://doi.org/10.1148/radiol.2017160107.)

What Are the Next Steps in Workup and Management for Blunt Trauma Patients?

Trauma patients must be assessed for their hemodynamic status to determine whether there is concern for hemorrhage and the development of shock. For patients who are hemodynamically stable, imaging such as a computed tomography (CT) scan of the abdomen and pelvis can be undertaken to further define the extent of injury. Intravenous contrast should be used unless contraindicated because it may reveal disruption of vascular structures or organ parenchyma (identified by the extravasation of contrast) and direct appropriate therapy.

For patients who are not hemodynamically stable on arrival or who become hemodynamically unstable bleeding into the abdominal cavity must be considered. The goal of the trauma team is to restore circulating volume and control hemorrhage. Until the hemorrhage is controlled, permissive hypotension should be pursued; that is, the blood pressure should be adequate to perfuse the brain, the patient need not be rendered "normotensive." Raising the blood pressure to normal runs the risk of disrupting clot formation and causing additional unnecessary blood loss. With this in mind, patients should be resuscitated using blood products, most commonly as component therapy—packed red blood cells, fresh frozen plasma, and pooled platelets. Most hospitals have a massive transfusion protocol that, once activated, delivers blood products in predefined ratios to permit a balanced resuscitation. Unstable patients, especially those in whom there is a positive FAST examination, should be taken emergently to the operating room for exploration.

What is the Operation of Choice for Blunt Abdominal Trauma?

Typically, an exploratory midline laparotomy for trauma is the operation of choice. Like in penetrating abdominal trauma (see Chapter 37), trauma laparotomy is indicated in patients with hemodynamic instability and peritonitis. In blunt trauma, injury prediction may be less obvious than in penetrating trauma because the location of the injury is often more diffuse, but solid organs are often the source. A full description of the trauma laparotomy can be found in Chapter 37, but in summary:

- Make a midline laparotomy incision from xiphoid to pubis (Fig. 38.2).
- Pack all four abdominal quadrants with laparotomy pads.
- Assess each quadrant for the site of bleeding from least to most likely to be the source.
- Address hemorrhage and gastrointestinal contamination.
- Temporarily (damage control) or permanently close the abdomen.
- Throughout, work closely with anesthesia to optimize hemodynamics.

CLINICAL PEARL (STEPS 2/3)

The unstable trauma patient belongs in the operating room. A negative laparotomy or nontherapeutic laparotomy may be acceptable in the trauma population.

The patient is taken emergently to the operating room for exploratory laparotomy given his progressive instability. The massive transfusion protocol was initiated, and transfusion is ongoing. Hemoperitoneum was encountered upon laparotomy. The abdomen is packed with laparotomy sponges, and the bleeding appeared to be coming from the left upper quadrant. After inspection of all other quadrants without identification of injury, exploration of the left upper quadrant reveals bleeding from a shattered spleen.

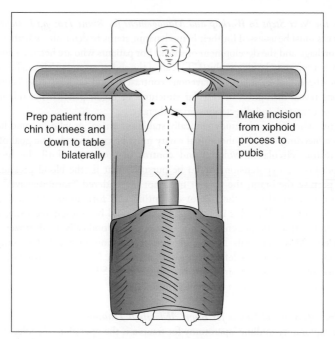

Prep patient from
chin to knees and
down to table
bilaterally

Make incision
from xiphoid
process to
pubis

Fig. 38.2   The trauma laparotomy is indicated in patients with hemodynamic instability, peritonitis, and penetrating abdominal wounds. To perform a trauma laparotomy, the patient should be positioned supine, a Foley catheter should be placed, and the patient should be prepped from chin to knees. This maximizes access for the surgeon to achieve his primary goal of hemorrhage control.

How Are Splenic Injuries Classified and Managed?

Splenic injuries can occur from either blunt or penetrating abdominal trauma, though blunt injuries are more common. Hematomas and lacerations are the most common splenic injuries and comprise the grading system for splenic injuries (Table 38.1). Regardless of the grade of injury, patients with unstable hemodynamics and a positive FAST require operative exploration—noting that injury to other organs may be the cause of the hemodynamic changes in patients with low-grade splenic injury. Stable patients typically undergo CT imaging whereby splenic injuries can be fully characterized. Management ranges from observation alone to splenic embolizationby by interventional radiology to operative exploration. Patients who have contrast extravasation on initial imaging are more likely to fail conservative management with observation. For patients who do fail observation (development of peritonitis or hemodynamic instability or progressive anemia), splenic artery embolization in interventional radiology may be an option to control bleeding and prevent the morbidity associated with operative exploration. Patients with more severe injuries may not be safe for observation or embolization and proceed to operative exploration, though most of these patients have significant hemorrhage and their significant hemodynamic compromise will dictate the need to proceed to the operating room. See Chapter 27 for a discussion of splenectomy.

TABLE 38.1 ■ American Association for the Surgery of Trauma Grading System for Splenic Injuries

Grade	Type of Injury[a]	Injury Description
I	Hematoma	Subcapsular, nonexpanding, < 10% surface area
	Laceration	Capsular tear, nonbleeding, < 1 cm parenchymal depth
II	Hematoma	Subcapsular, nonexpanding, 10%–50% surface area; intraparenchymal, nonexpanding < 5 cm diameter
	Laceration	Capsular tear, active bleeding; 1–3 cm parenchymal depth which does not involve a trabecular vessel
III	Hematoma	Subcapsular, > 50% surface area or expanding; ruptured subcapsular hematoma with active bleeding; intraparenchymal hematoma > 5 cm or expanding
	Laceration	> 3 cm parenchymal depth or involving trabecular vessels
IV	Hematoma	Ruptured intraparenchymal hematoma with active bleeding
	Laceration	Laceration involving segmental or hilar vessels producing major devascularization (> 25% of spleen)
V	Laceration	Completely shattered spleen
	Vascular	Hilar vascular injury that devascularized spleen

[a]The most common injuries are lacerations or hematomas and may include involvement of the splenic vasculature.
Courtesy of the American Association for the Surgery of Trauma, Chicago, IL.

CLINICAL PEARL (STEPS 1/2/3)

Patients undergoing splenectomy require vaccination against encapsulated organisms (*Streptococcus* pneumonia, *Haemophilus influenzae* type B, and *Neisseria meningitidis*) due to risk of postsplenectomy sepsis. Although vaccinations optimally take place preoperatively, in the traumatic setting they are typically given postoperatively before discharge from the hospital.

The patient undergoes a splenectomy, his vital signs remain stable, and no other injuries are identified on complete reexploration of the abdomen. He is taken to the surgery step-down in stable condition and is discharged home 4 days later in stable condition after receiving a series of postsplenectomy vaccines.

BEYOND THE PEARLS

- Blunt abdominal trauma has the potential to cause significant intraabdominal injuries.
- The spleen and liver are the most commonly injured organs in blunt abdominal trauma.
- Peritonitis and hemodynamic instability with a positive FAST are indications for trauma laparotomy in patients with blunt abdominal trauma.
- Hemodynamically unstable patients who have undergone blunt abdominal trauma should be given blood as the cause of their instability is most likely due to hemorrhagic shock.
- Splenic injury can be managed with observation alone, splenic artery embolization, or operative exploration with splenectomy, depending on the grade of the injury and the patient's clinical status.
- Splenectomy is more common than splenorrhaphy in patients with traumatic splenic injury.

Suggested Readings

ATLS Subcommittee (2013). American College of Surgeons' Committee on Trauma, International ATLS Working Group: Advanced trauma life support (ATLS®), the ninth edition. *J Trauma Acute Care Surg*, *74*(5), 1363–1366. https://doi.org/10.1097/TA.0b013e31828b82f5.

Cirocchi, R., Montedori, A., Farinella, E., et al. (2013). Damage control surgery for abdominal trauma. *Cochrane Database Syst Rev Mar. 28*(3). CD007438. https://doi.org/10.1002/14651858.CD007438.pub3.

Hirshberg, A., & Walden, R. (1997). Damage control for abdominal trauma. *Surg Clin North Am*, *77*(4), 813–820.

Jacobs, L., Burns, K., Luk, S., & Hull, S. (2010). Advanced trauma operative management course: Participant survey. *World J Surg*, *34*(1), 164–168. https://doi.org/10.1007/s00268-009-0276-z.

McCoy, C. E., Chakravarthy, B., & Lotfipour, S. (2013). Guidelines for field triage of injured patients: In conjunction with the Morbidity and Mortality Weekly Report published by the Center for Disease Control and Prevention. *West J Emerg Med*, *14*(1), 69–76. https://doi.org/10.5811/westjem.2013.1.15981.

Richards, J. R., & McGahan, J. P. (2017). Focused assessment with sonography in trauma (FAST) in 2017: What radiologists can learn. *Radiology*, *283*(1), 30–48. https://doi.org/10.1148/radiol.2017160107.

CHAPTER 39

Fall From Height Involving a 64-Year-Old Female

Colin Doyle ■ Susan Steinemann

A 64-year-old female is brought into the emergency department (ED) by ambulance after falling off a 10-foot ladder when picking mangos. She had no loss of consciousness and states she landed on her left side. On primary survey her heart rate is 120 bpm, her blood pressure is 90/40mm Hg, and her oxygen saturation is 94% on room air. She is pale and confused.

What Are the Important Considerations in Triage and Workup of a Patient Who Has Sustained a Fall?

As is the case for any trauma patients, a comprehensive primary survey should be performed with a focus on airway, breathing, and circulation (see Chapter 32). Triage in patients who have sustained falls should include protection of the spine until injuries have been conclusively ruled out. Injuries to the bony skeleton are common after falls, especially in the elderly, so a full musculoskeletal examination is important during the secondary survey. The secondary survey should also incorporate an examination of the pelvis, checking for stability to rotational and translational (AP and lateral) compression. Additionally, blunt injuries to the thorax and abdomen should be on the differential of potential injuries for patients who have sustained a fall (see Chapters 36 and 38). Stable patients can undergo adjunctive diagnostic tests such as chest, abdominal, and long bone radiographs, in order to fully assess the pattern of injury. An anterior-posterior pelvic x-ray should be performed to further assess any suspected fractures before leaving the ED.

As the examination proceeds, there are no abnormalities of the long bones of the extremities, but the trauma team notes that the patient's pelvis is mobile on lateral compression. On further examination, there is substantial ecchymosis and swelling of the perineum.

What Is the Clinical Significance of Pelvic Fractures in the Acute Trauma Patient?

Pelvic fractures by themselves can be lethal injuries due to their potential to cause hemorrhagic shock. Patients can present with hypotension and tachycardia, suggesting a significant blood loss and hemorrhagic shock; patients with hemodynamic instability secondary to a pelvic fracture have a mortality of 40%. More than 80% of patients who present with hypotension and pelvic fractures will not respond to initial fluid resuscitation. The venous and arterial networks in the pelvis can produce massive bleeding if disrupted, and, if the pelvic ring is not intact, there is decreased pressure to tamponade bleeding from these vessels. The majority of bleeding in patients with pelvic fractures comes from the bone itself or the presacral and paravesical venous plexuses, but arterial bleeding may also be present and require specific intervention. Although venous bleeding is more common, patients with arterial bleeding have the highest risk of mortality. Pelvic fractures also have a significant effect on a patient's quality of life. Fewer than half of patients admitted for pelvic fractures are discharged to home, and a significant number report frequent ongoing health concerns.

BASIC SCIENCE PEARL (STEP 1)

The internal iliac artery, a branch of the common iliac artery, is the major artery of the pelvis and gives rise to the majority of branches serving the pelvis. The structures are paired (Fig. 39.1). The gonadal arteries are branches directly from the aorta; the ovarian arteries remain intraabdominal in females, and the testicular arteries traverse the inguinal canal in males en route to the scrotum, so neither enters the bony pelvis.

CLINICAL PEARL (STEPS 2/3)

The diagnosis of sacral fractures is more difficult and can be delayed in up to 30% of patients.

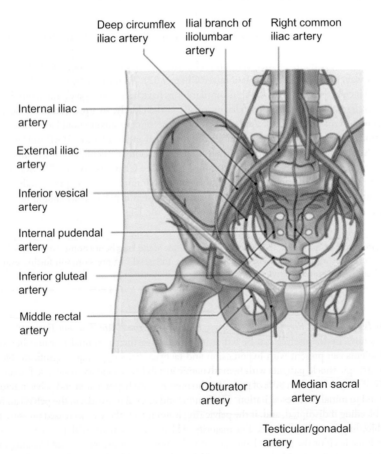

Fig. 39.1 Arterial anatomy of the pelvis. (From Moses: *Atlas of clinical gross anatomy*, ed 2, Philadelphia. 2013, Saunders, pp 446–459.)

How Are Pelvic Fractures Classified?

The Young-Burgess system classifies pelvic fractures into four patterns based on the translational and rotational vectors of force that caused the injury. They include anterior-posterior compression (APC), lateral compression (LC), vertical shear (VS), and combined injuries that are shown in Fig. 39.2. VS injuries are the result of massive axial loading, associated with high-speed automobile or motorcycle collisions, falls from height, or crush injuries. The VS pattern involves a complete disruption of both the pubic symphysis and the SI joint, with or without associated pubic rami, sacral, or iliac fractures. The fracture pattern is both rotationally and vertically unstable.

CLINICAL PEARL (STEPS 2/3)

An "open book" fracture pattern refers to disruption of the pubic symphysis with an external rotation deformity, similar to opening a book. This is an alternative term for more severe APC injuries.

What Other Injuries Are Associated With Pelvic Fractures?

The bony pelvis is in proximity to several organs that are at risk of injury from blunt force or laceration by bone fragments. These include the rectum, the vagina, the bladder, and the urethra. Digital vaginal and rectal examinations should be performed. Any signs of injury (blood, palpable bone fragments) should be further evaluated with rigid proctosigmoidoscopy and/or pelvic examination. A computed tomography (CT) cystogram is the preferred method of detecting a bladder injury. The bladder is instilled with 300 to 400 mL of contrast via a Foley catheter and CT imaging performed. Gross hematuria is almost universally present with bladder injury. Urethral injury may be suspected with the finding of blood at the urethral meatus. A retrograde urethrogram should be performed to evaluate suspected urethral injury.

How Are Pelvic Fractures Managed?

A patient's hemodynamic status dictates management after a pelvic fracture has been diagnosed. If a patient is hemodynamically stable on presentation, then a CT angiography of the pelvis may be performed followed by angioembolization if bleeding vessels are identified. It is important to note that angioembolization can cause gluteal claudication and pelvic necrosis due to reduction of pelvic blood flow and kidney injury due to the contrast used during angiography.

In patients with altered hemodynamics, control of hemorrhage, restoration of normal hemodynamics, and prompt diagnosis of other injuries are central to patient management. The treatment of these injuries requires a multidisciplinary approach with cooperation between the

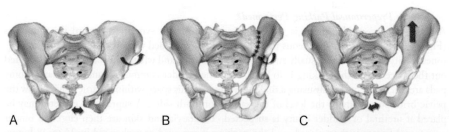

Fig. 39.2 Types of pelvic fractures: (A) anterior-posterior compression (APC) fracture; (B) lateral compression (LC) fracture; (C) vertical shear (VS) fracture. (From Molière S, Dosch JC, Bierry G: Pelvic, acetabular, and hip fractures: what the surgeon should expect from the radiologist, *Diagn Interv Imaging* 97(7–8):709–723, 2016.)

trauma/general surgeon, orthopedic surgeon, and interventional radiologist. Prompt administration of blood and blood products in a balanced fashion can help avoid coagulopathy. A focused assessment with sonography for trauma (FAST) examination or diagnostic peritoneal aspiration (DPA) are a critical aspect of the trauma assessment, especially in an unstable patient to assess for hemoperitoneum.

In open-book fractures the pelvis requires temporary stabilization, providing increasing force to tamponade the bleeding in the pelvis by wrapping a sheet (or commercial pelvic binder) tightly around the patient's pelvis at the level of the greater trochanters. This should be performed in the ED as soon as an open-book fracture is identified in an unstable patient. However, LC injuries are a relative contraindication to pelvic wrapping as it can worsen the deformity. Prolonged periods of tight immobilization can lead to abdominal or extremity compartment syndrome or soft tissue ischemia; pelvic wrapping, therefore, is only a temporary therapy.

If the patient is unstable, it is also critical to exclude an intraabdominal bleeding source. If there is evidence of hemoperitoneum the patient is brought to the operating room (OR) for laparotomy, and the pelvis can be addressed simultaneously with a preperitoneal pelvic packing procedure that can be performed with or without external fixation. Pelvic packing reduces the potential space that must be filled in order to cause tamponade and stop venous and bony bleeding. External fixation of the pelvis closes the volume of the pelvis and stabilizes the fractures. If the patient remains unstable after pelvic packing, pelvic angiography and embolization of arterial bleeding may be performed in interventional radiology. Once the patient is hemodynamically stable, definitive pelvic fixation (open reduction, internal fixation) may be performed.

The patient does not have blood at the urethral meatus on examination. A FAST examination reveals no intraabdominal fluid, but she remains hemodynamically unstable with a blood pressure of 94/56 mm Hg after the administration of two units of uncrossmatched packed red blood cells. Because there is concern for an LC fracture, the pelvis is not wrapped, and the orthopedic surgery team is called to come evaluate the patient. She is taken emergently to the operating room for preperitoneal packing with external fixation.

CLINICAL PEARL (STEPS 2/3)

Patients who have significant bleeding and require temporizing measures may have a resuscitative endovascular balloon occlusion of the aorta (REBOA) catheter placed via either femoral artery before proceeding to interventional radiology or the operating room for further treatment. The REBOA catheter has an occlusive balloon that is inflated just above the aortic bifurcation, serving to decrease arterial pelvic bleeding and helping maintain myocardial and cerebral perfusion.

How Is Preperitoneal Packing Performed?

A 6- to 8-cm vertical incision is made starting at the pubic symphysis toward the umbilicus (Fig. 39.3). The skin, subcutaneous tissue, and fascia are divided without entering into the peritoneal cavity. Hematoma is usually encountered at this time and will usually have already dissected out the space where the packing is to be placed. The bladder is retracted, and three laparotomy pads are inserted sequentially using a ringed forceps into this space within the true pelvis below the pelvic brim posteriorly to the level of the sacrum on both sides. A suprapubic catheter may be placed if urethral or bladder injury is suspected. The fascia and skin are then closed, a binder or external fixator is then placed, and the packing is removed or exchanged in 24 to 48 hours. If the patient requires a laparotomy, then a separate incision is made apart from the suprapubic incision.

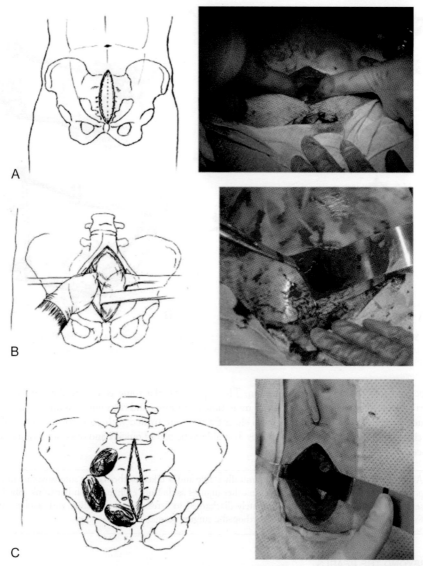

Fig. 39.3 Incision, exposure, and placement of laparotomy sponges to perform preperitoneal packing. (Redrawn from Burlew, CC, et al: Preperitoneal pelvic packing/external fixation with secondary angioembolization: optimal care for life-threatening hemorrhage from unstable pelvic fractures, *J Am Coll Surg* 212(4):628–635, 2011; discussion pp 635–637.)

How Is Pelvic External Fixation Performed?

Anterior fixation through the iliac wings or supraacetabular region is performed for open-book fractures with intact posterior ligaments (Fig. 39.4). Unstable LC fractures may also be treated via anterior fixation, but the force vector of the fixation serves to open the pathologically internally rotated pelvis. Pins placed via the iliac crest route do not require fluoroscopy and therefore may be more

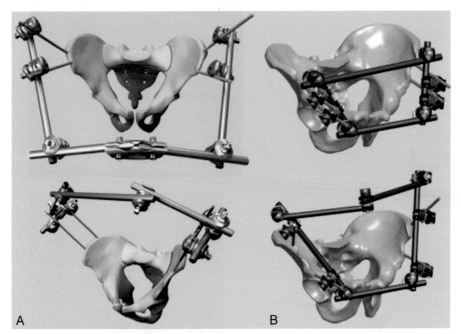

Fig. 39.4 Anterior fixation of the pelvis using iliac crest pins (A) and supraacetabular pins (B). (From Taylor DM, Tebby JM, Foster PA, Harwood PJ: Temporary skeletal stabilization in major trauma, *Orthopaedics and Trauma* 29(6):359–373, 2015.)

expedient in a damage control situation. The supraacetabular route is a more durable, stronger repair, but it requires fluoroscopy and is more time consuming and risks injury to the sciatic nerve, gluteal vessels, or the hip joint. Vertical shear fractures are treated with posterior fixation using a C-clamp applied to the dorsal iliac bones. It is able to be placed quickly and does not require fluoroscopy.

After fixation, the patient is hemodynamically stable and is taken to the trauma intensive care unit postoperatively. She is found to have no other injuries aside from ecchymosis on her trunk. She is seen by physical therapy and is ultimately discharged to a rehabilitation facility with a plan for follow-up with both the trauma and orthopedic surgery teams.

BEYOND THE PEARLS

- Mechanisms of blunt trauma, such as falls, have the potential to cause significant injury requiring operative intervention.
- The pelvis has a rich vascular network and has the ability to accumulate large amounts of blood after pelvic fracture.
- Pelvic binding with a bed sheet or commercial pelvic binder is an important step in triage for patients with open book pelvic fractures.
- Bleeding from pelvic fractures may be managed nonoperatively, with angioembolization or with surgical exploration (including packing and fixation), depending on the severity of the injury and the patient's hemodynamics.
- Pelvic fractures are associated with high rates of morbidity and mortality, requiring expert triage and management.

Suggested Readings

Biffl, W. L., Smith, W. R., Moore, E. E., Gonzalez, R. J., Morgan, S. J., Hennessey, T., et al. (2001). Evolution of a multidisciplinary clinical pathway for the management of unstable patients with pelvic fractures. *Ann Surg, 233*(6), 843–850.

Burlew, C. C., Moore, E. E., Smith, W. R., Johnson, J. L., Biffl, W. L., Barnett, C. C., et al. (2011). Preperitoneal pelvic packing/external fixation with secondary angioembolization: Optimal care for life-threatening hemorrhage from unstable pelvic fractures. *J Am Coll Surg, 212*(4), 628–635.

Saito, N., Matsumoto, H., Yagi, T., Hara, Y., Hayashida, K., Motomura, T., et al. (2015). Evaluation of the safety and feasibility of resuscitative endovascular balloon occlusion of the aorta. *J Trauma Acute Care Surg, 78*(5), 897–903.

Stahel, P. F., Mauffrey, C., Smith, W. R., McKean, J., Hao, J., Burlew, C. C., et al. (2013). External fixation for acute pelvic ring injuries: Decision making and technical options. *J Trauma Acute Care Surg, 75*(5), 882–887.

Tran, T. L., Brasel, K. J., Karmy-Jones, R., Rowell, S., Schreiber, M. A., Shatz, D. V., et al. (2016). Western Trauma Association critical decisions in trauma: Management of pelvic fracture with hemodynamic instability—2016 updates. *J Trauma Acute Care Surg, 81*(6), 1171–1174.

Thoracic and Cardiac Surgery

CHAPTER 40

Anterior Mediastinal Mass in a 61-Year-Old Male

Dustin J. Manchester ▪ Michael J. Walker

A 61-year-old male presents to his primary care physician with a 3-month history of cough. He has a past medical history significant for hypertension that is well controlled with medication. There are normal cardiac and respiratory sounds on auscultation of the chest, though the patient coughs each time he is prompted to take a deep inspiration. He is sent for chest radiograph, which shows a mediastinal density (Fig. 40.1A), prompting further workup. A computed tomography (CT) scan shows a 4-cm, well-circumscribed, round mass of the anterior mediastinum (see Fig. 40.1B).

What Is the Differential Diagnosis for a Mediastinal Mass?

Mediastinal masses are uncommon thoracic findings, accounting for 3% of all thoracic tumors. They are predominantly defined by their anatomic location: anterior, middle, and posterior mediastinum (see Fig. 40.1). Anatomic knowledge of their location assists in establishing a differential diagnosis and potential treatment options. Peak incidence of all mediastinal masses is in the fifth decade of life, but this varies by location. In adults, anterior mediastinal masses are most common (54%–68%), followed by middle (18%–20%) and posterior masses (15%–25%). In the pediatric population, posterior mediastinal masses are most common (50%), followed by anterior (35%) and middle masses (12%–15%). Anterior mediastinal masses are commonly referred to as the "4 T's", as thymic neoplasms, teratomas, "terrible" lymphomas, and thyroid masses account for 95% of all anterior mediastinal tumors. Table 40.1 outlines the differential diagnosis for mediastinal masses by location.

BASIC SCIENCE PEARL (STEP 1)

The mediastinum is anatomically divided into three compartments: anterior, middle, and posterior (Fig. 40.2). The anterior mediastinum is bordered by the posterior surface of the sternum, anterior surface of the great vessels/pericardium, innominate vessels, and diaphragm. The middle mediastinum includes all of the great vessels, pericardium, heart, descending thoracic aorta, esophagus, and related structures anterior to the vertebral column. The posterior mediastinum begins at the anterior vertebral body and extends posteriorly, containing the intercostal neurovascular bundle, sympathetic trunk, and portions of the azygos vein.

How Do Mediastinal Masses Typically Present?

The majority of mediastinal masses are asymptomatic and are often detected on routine imaging performed for some other indication. As these masses grow and compress surrounding structures, they may begin to cause symptoms such as cough, chest pain, and/or dyspnea; less than half ever become symptomatic. Physical examination findings are limited but may include facial swelling/plethora from superior vena cava compression. Similarly, large anterior mediastinal masses can cause airway compression manifesting as stridor on auscultation. One should also screen for ocular muscle weakness (diplopia, blurred vision), as these may be early symptoms of myasthenia gravis, which is

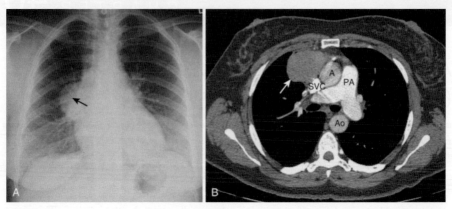

Fig. 40.1 Imaging of mediastinal masses. (A) CXR showing a mediastinal mass *(black arrow)*. (B) CT chest showing a well-circumscribed, anterior, soft tissue mass *(white arrow)*. Note its intimate relationship with the great vessels (A = ascending aorta; Ao = descending thoracic aorta; SVC = superior vena cava; PA = pulmonary artery). (From Herring W: *Learning radiology: recognizing the basics*, 2016, pp 97–113. Philadelphia, PA: Elsevier.)

TABLE 40.1 ■ **Differential Diagnosis for Mediastinal Masses by Location**

Mediastinal Compartment	Masses/Cysts
Anterior	Thymic mass (thymoma, thymic carcinoma)
	Lymphoma ("terrible" lymphoma)
	Germ cell tumor (teratoma, seminomatous, nonseminomatous tumor)
	Thymic hyperplasia/retained thymus
	Thymic cyst
	Thymolipoma
	Thyroid mass (thyroid goiter, thyroid adenoma, ectopic thyroid)
	Parathyroid adenoma
Middle	Bronchogenic cyst
	Pericardial cyst
	Enteric cyst
	Lymphoma
	Lymphangioma
	Fibroma
Posterior	Neurogenic tumor (schwannoma, neurofibroma, ganglioneuroma, neuroblastoma)
	Esophageal/enteric cyst
	Lymphoma

associated with thymoma. Posterior mediastinal masses, specifically neurogenic tumors, can be associated with pain and neurologic symptoms such as Horner's syndrome (manifesting as ptosis, anhidrosis, miosis) from sympathetic chain involvement. Hoarseness from recurrent laryngeal nerve involvement and diaphragm paralysis from phrenic nerve involvement can also be seen.

What Is the Workup for Patients With a Mediastinal Mass?

Albeit rare, mediastinal masses are most frequently detected incidentally on chest radiograph (CXR) (see Fig. 40.1A). Computed tomography (CT) of the chest with intravenous contrast is the imaging modality of choice to diagnose a mediastinal mass (see Fig. 40.1B). CT is particularly helpful in defining the characteristics of a mediastinal mass and its relationship to surrounding

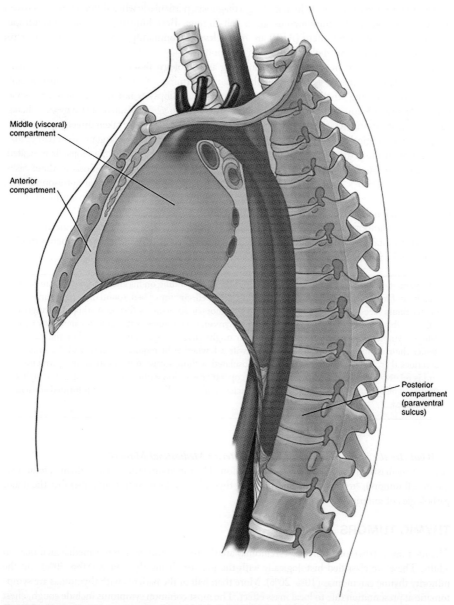

Middle (visceral) compartment

Anterior compartment

Posterior compartment (paraventral sulcus)

Fig. 40.2 Mediastinal compartments. (From Liu W, et al: Mediastinal divisions and compartments, *Thorac Surg Clin* 21(2):183–190, 2011.)

structures. Magnetic resonance imaging (MRI) may be helpful in defining posterior neurogenic tumors and their specific nerve involvement. MRI with and without gadolinium can also help separate solid tumors from cysts, as solid tumor will show enhancement. Positron emission tomography (PET) scan can be useful when evaluating for metastatic disease.

Serum tumor markers may help in making a diagnosis, particularly when differentiating between nonseminomatous and seminomatous germ cell tumors. Beta human chorionic gonadotropin (β-HCG) and alpha-fetoprotein (AFP) are more elevated commonly in nonseminomatous germ cell tumors and may have slight elevation in seminomas.

With advancements in cross-sectional imaging and serology, tissue biopsy is not always mandatory to establish a diagnosis. Additionally, when performing a tissue biopsy, one must be concerned about "seeding" the biopsy tract with tumor cells. Biopsy is not recommended for small masses (less than 5 cm) with distinctive features on CT, such as encapsulation (thymoma), heterogenous calcifications (teratoma), or cystic structures. These patients are taken directly to the operating room for surgical resection before establishing a tissue diagnosis. For larger masses (larger than 5 cm), those without distinctive features, or those suspicious for lymphoma, a biopsy is indicated. CT-guided core-needle biopsy is the standard of care for establishing a diagnosis in these cases. Additional modalities such as endobronchial ultrasound or endoesophageal ultrasound with fine-needle aspiration may be used to establish a diagnosis when anatomically convenient. Fine-needle aspiration alone may be insufficient to establish a diagnosis for processes in which tumor architecture is important (lymphoma, thymoma). In these cases, CT-guided core-needle biopsy is needed to establish a diagnosis. If all else proves insufficient or nondiagnostic, then a surgical biopsy may be indicated.

The patient is called by his physician and is told about the finding on his chest radiograph, and that he advises further workup. A CT scan shows a 4-cm, well-circumscribed, round mass of the anterior mediastinum (see Fig. 40.1B). He is referred to a thoracic surgeon for further workup; the surgeon tells him that the mass most likely represents a thymoma. The surgeon also inquires about any neurologic symptoms, especially weakness, which might suggest myasthenia gravis, but the patient denies these symptoms. The patient and his wife ask whether he requires surgery, and the surgeon describes that, because the mass is well encapsulated without invasion into surrounding structures and is relatively small size, he recommends an operative excision without biopsy or further imaging studies. The patient is scheduled for robotic excision of his mediastinal mass after informed consent is obtained.

What Are the Special Considerations for Anterior Mediastinal Masses?
Anterior mediastinal masses are the most common. The mnemonic the "4 Ts"—thymic, teratomas (germ cell tumors), "terrible" (lymphoma), and thyroid—can be used to help remember the major pathologies of anterior mediastinal masses.

THYMIC TUMORS

Thymic tumors (thymoma, thymic carcinoma) are the most common anterior mediastinal mass in adults. These are classified histologically with the majority being thymomas (80%–90%) and the minority thymic carcinomas (10%–20%). More than half of the patients with thymomas are symptomatic at presentation due to local mass effect. The most common symptoms include cough, chest pain, or dyspnea. Patients with thymomas must also be screened for associated paraneoplastic syndromes such as myasthenia gravis, hypogammaglobulinemia, or pure red cell aplasia. Importantly, 50% of patients with thymomas have myasthenia gravis, but only 15% to 20% of myasthenics will have a thymoma. Cross-sectional imaging characteristics include a well-defined, soft tissue mass, confined only to the anterior mediastinum. The mainstay of treatment for thymic tumors is complete surgical resection, though chemotherapy and radiation may be included for patients with advanced disease.

The thymus is a bilobed gland located in the anterior superior mediastinum in which T cells mature. Embryologically, the thymus develops from the third pharyngeal pouch (thymus epithelial cells) and migrating hematopoietic stem cells (lymphoid cells). T cells undergo positive selection within the thymus, which determines their capability of recognizing self major histocompatibility complex (MHC).

Patients with myasthenia gravis provide unique challenges when being evaluated for surgical thymectomy. Indications for surgery include myasthenics refractory to medical management (anticholinesterase inhibitors, immunosuppression, plasmapheresis, intravenous immunoglobulins (IVIG), etc.). Perioperative care must be individualized, and those with severe disease and/or respiratory depression may require preoperative plasmapheresis or IVIG. Anesthesia should be delivered by inhaled anesthetics alone, avoiding neuromuscular blocking agents altogether. Great care should be taken to protect the airway and hemodynamics on anesthesia induction, as large anterior masses can cause airway and great vessel compression. Postoperatively, these patients should be closely monitored and may require urgent reintubation and plasmapheresis or IVIG for respiratory distress.

TERATOMAS (PRIMARY MEDIASINAL GERM CELL TUMORS)

Overall, germ cell tumors (teratomas, seminomatous germ cell tumors, nonseminomatous germ cell tumors) account for 10% to 15% of anterior mediastinal masses. Teratomas, which contain tissue from all three germ cell layers, are the most common type of germ cell tumor found in the mediastinum. They have equal male–female prevalence and are more common in the pediatric population. Diagnosis is usually made via CT imaging demonstrating a heterogenous mass containing a mixture of soft tissue, fluid, and calcifications. Serum AFP, β-HCG, and LDH are typically normal. These masses are neither chemosensitive nor radiosensitive. The mainstay of treatment is complete surgical resection, after which recurrence is extremely rare.

Seminomatous germ cell tumors are predominantly diagnosed in 30- to 40-year-old males. Although slower growing than nonseminomatous germ cell tumors, 60% to 70% are metastatic at the time of presentation. CT imaging typically shows a large, lobulated, homogenous, soft tissue mass. Diagnosis is confirmed by biopsy, and serology shows normal β-HCG and LDH levels. AFP may be either normal or slightly elevated in seminomatous germ cell tumors. Physical examination of these patients must include a thorough testicular examination and possible testicular ultrasound. Systemic chemotherapy is the treatment of choice. After treatment, these patients should get routine surveillance cross-sectional imaging to evaluate for recurrence or residual disease.

Nonseminomatous germ cell tumors are also predominantly found in 30- to 40-year-old males. These are more rapid-growing tumors and lead to compressive symptoms such as dyspnea, chest pain, or SVC syndrome/plethora. CT imaging typically shows a heterogenous, complex, anterior mediastinal mass, and serology shows markedly elevated AFP, β-HCG and LDH. Together, these findings alone can often establish a diagnosis. The treatment for nonseminomatous germ cell tumors is systemic chemotherapy; however, survival is significantly worse than seminomatous tumors with only 50% 5-year survival. The use of adjuvant radiation after chemotherapy is still being evaluated and may improve survival.

All patients with treated primary mediastinal germ cell tumors should undergo surveillance cross-sectional imaging. Recurrence is rare but prompts further treatment. Mature teratomas almost never recur if completely resected. Immature teratomas can recur and require repeat resection. Seminomatous germ cell tumors are extremely chemosensitive, and a residual mediastinal mass may persist after treatment that is commonly benign. Mass enlargement on surveillance imaging should prompt an additional course of systemic chemotherapy or even radiation. Conversely, patients with nonseminomatous germ cell tumors found to have residual mediastinal disease after chemotherapy should go on to have complete surgical resection. This residual disease can often harbor a teratoma and resection improves survival.

"TERRIBLE" LYMPHOMA

Mediastinal lymphoma is rare disease process, accounting for only 5% to 10% of anterior mediastinal masses. These patients often exhibit constitutional symptoms of night sweats, fevers, and weight loss. The workup for mediastinal lymphoma includes a CT scan and possibly a PET scan to evaluate for distant disease. A tissue biopsy is necessary to establish a diagnosis and is most commonly performed by CT-guided core-needle biopsy. Once the diagnosis is established, treatment is systemic chemotherapy.

THYROID MASS

Thyroid masses (goiters) can be found in the anterior mediastinum. Enlarged, mediastinal, multinodular goiters can cause symptoms due to airway, esophageal, and/or great vessel compression. See Chapter 22 for more information about the treatment of thyroid disease.

What Are Operative Approaches for the Treatment of Mediastinal Masses?
Surgical approaches to the mediastinum are varied and include: cervical mediastinoscopy, anterior mediastinoscopy (Chamberlain procedure), sternotomy, thoracotomy, video-assisted thoracoscopy (VATS), and robotic-assisted thoracoscopy (RATS). Anterior mediastinal masses are easily accessed via minimally invasive surgical platforms. VATS and RATS both provide excellent visualization while minimizing patient morbidity. The key to a surgical thymectomy is careful identification and avoidance of bilateral phrenic nerves when resecting the rest of the thymus and surrounding fat in its entirety. Advanced imaging techniques such as near-infrared imaging and fluorescent dye can be used to help identify vascular structures and bilateral phrenic nerves if needed. Once extubated and stabilized, these patients recover quickly and can often go home the day after surgery.

The patient undergoes robotic excision of his anterior mediastinal mass without complication. He is extubated in the operating room and is discharged on the first postoperative day. At his 2-week follow-up appointment, the surgeon reviews the pathology of the mass that was a completely excised thymoma without evidence of malignancy. The patient and his wife are happy to hear that he will not require radiation or chemotherapy due to the low risk of recurrence but understand recommendations for surveillance with CT scan every 6 months.

- Anterior mediastinal masses are the most common mediastinal masses in adults and are classically known as the "4 T's": thymic mass, teratoma (germ cell tumor), "terrible" lymphoma, and thyroid mass.

- Ninety percent of thymic masses are thymomas.
- Thymomas are closely associated with myasthenia gravis.
- Indications for surgical thymectomy include CT evidence of a thymoma, compressive symptoms, medically refractory myasthenia gravis (with or without thymoma), and concerning features for thymic carcinoma.
- Outcome after thymectomy is based on pathologic stage.
- Video- or robot-assisted thoracoscopic surgery (VATS or RATS) are two important minimally invasive operative approaches to the mediastinum.

Suggested Readings

Detterbeck, F. C., & Parsons, A. M. (2004). Thymic tumors. *Ann Thoracic Surg, 77*, 1860–1869.

Detterbeck, F. C., & Parsons, A. M. (2008). Thymic tumors: A review of current diagnosis, classification and treatment. In G. A. Patterson, J. D. Cooper, J. Deslauriers, A. E. M. R. Lerut, J. D. Luketich, & T. W. Rice (Eds.), *Pearson's thoracic and esophageal surgery* (3rd ed., pp. 1589–1614). Philadelphia, PA: Churchill Livingstone.

Duwe, B. V., et al. (2005). Tumors of the mediastinum. *Chest, 128*(4), 2893–2909.

Thieben, M. J., et al. (2005). Pulmonary function tests and blood gases in worsening myasthenia gravis. *Muscle Nerve, 32*(5), 664–667.

Wood, D., & Bedzra, E. (2016). Mediastinal masses. In J. Cameron & A. Cameron (Eds.), *Current surgical therapy* (12th ed., pp. 871–877). Philadelphia: Elsevier Mosby.

CHAPTER 41

Solitary Pulmonary Nodule in a 65-Year-Old Female

Sourodeep Banarjee ■ Patrick Ross, Jr.

A 65-year-old woman with no significant past medical history comes to her physician with a complaint of a chronic nonproductive cough that recently has become productive of some blood-streaked sputum. She also reports overall malaise, reduced appetite, increased fatigability, and unintentional weight loss. She denies any fever, chills, or night sweats.

What Is the Differential Diagnosis for Cough Productive of Bloody Sputum?
Cough is a common complaint in both the outpatient and inpatient settings. It is a symptom that carries a lengthy differential diagnosis. Whether the cough is *productive* and the *quality* of the expectorated material both help shape the differential diagnosis. Whereas infectious, inflammatory, and neoplastic processes in the airways and lung parenchyma can lead to the production of bloody sputum, allergies, asthma, and simple upper respiratory infections are unlikely to lead to the production of bloody sputum. The patient's past medical history, social history, travel history, and occupational exposures are all relevant to the diagnosis.

Auscultation of the chest will detect alterations in breath sounds consistent with an infectious or obstructive process. Imaging should begin with a chest x-ray, but if abnormalities appear, a CT scan would be indicated for better anatomic definition of the abnormality.

BASIC SCIENCE PEARL (STEP 1)

Unlike most organs, the respiratory system has communication with systemic and pulmonary circulations. The pulmonary arteries bring deoxygenated blood to the lungs and branch into pulmonary capillaries, which participate in gas (oxygen and carbon dioxide) exchange at the alveoli. The bronchial arteries supply the lung parenchyma and airways with oxygenated blood.

On further questioning, the patient states that she has smoked 1 pack per day for 15 years. On physical examination the patient's lungs are normal to percussion and are clear to auscultation bilaterally with no wheezes, rales, or rhonchi. Chest radiography shows a solitary pulmonary nodule in the left lung (Fig. 41.1).

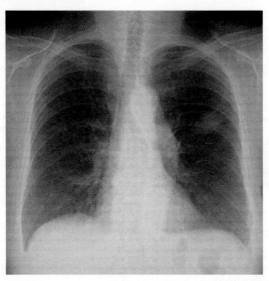

Fig. 41.1   Chest radiograph demonstrating a solitary pulmonary nodule in the left lung *(red arrow)*. (From: The lung. In Klatt EC: *Robbins and Cotran Atlas of Pathology*, ed 8, Philadephia, 2015, Saunders, pp 107–158).

What Is the Differential Diagnosis for a Solitary Pulmonary Nodule?

A solitary pulmonary nodule (SPN) is defined as a single, well-circumscribed lesion that measures less than 3.0 cm in diameter and is completely surrounded by pulmonary parenchyma. It is not associated with other pulmonary abnormalities such as atelectasis. Pulmonary lesions larger than 3.0 cm in diameter are defined as pulmonary *masses.*

The differential diagnoses for an SPN is lengthy (Table 41.1). Given its potential for malignancy, an SPN should be considered a cancer until proven otherwise. The diagnostic workup should be focused therefore on determining the likelihood of malignancy.

What Risk Factors Are Associated With Malignancy?

A history of smoking and older age increases the likelihood that an SPN is malignant. However, it is important to note that the absence of risk factors does not preclude malignancy. Smoking is the single most important risk factor, with a lifetime risk of 30% in smokers. The risk of lung cancer lessens after 5 years of abstinence, and it continues to decline progressively with time. As noted, the incidence of malignancy increases with increasing age. More than 50% of nodules in patients older than 60 years prove to be malignant compared with 3% in patients younger than 40 years. Other risk factors include exposure to environmental/workplace carcinogens (e.g., radon, asbestos, inhaled chemicals), the presence of chronic obstructive pulmonary disease, a history of prior lung cancer, or history of other malignancy.

How Are Imaging Modalities Used to Evaluate a Solitary Pulmonary Nodule?

Imaging modalities used to evaluate a solitary pulmonary nodule include chest radiography, chest computed tomography (CT), and fluorine-18-labeled fluorodeoxyglucose (FDG) positron emission tomography (PET) with CT (PET/CT). The majority of SPNs are found on chest radiographs (CXR) or as incidental findings on CT scan. The CXR is an excellent initial imaging study for patients with symptoms or for follow-up for patients with known pulmonary lesions. CXRs are inexpensive, readily available, quickly obtained, and can be read by both clinicians and radiologists. For patients with an SPN that is visible on CXR, all previous CXRs should be

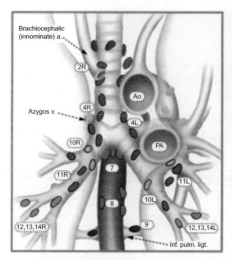

Superior Mediastinal Nodes

● 1 Highest Mediastinal

● 2 Upper Paratracheal

● 3 Pre-vascular and Retrotracheal

● 4 Lower Paratracheal
   (including Azygos Nodes)

N_2 = Single digit, ipsilateral
N_3 = Single digit, contralateral or supraclavicular

Aortic Nodes

● 5 Subaortic (A-P window)

● 6 Para-aortic (ascending
   aorta or phrenic)

Inferior Mediastinal Nodes

● 7 Subcarinal

● 8 Paraesophageal
   (below carina)

● 9 Pulmonary Ligament

N_1 Nodes

◐ 10 Hilar

● 11 Interlobar

◐ 12 Lobar

◐ 13 Segmental

◐ 14 Subsegmental

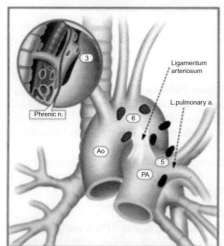

Fig. 41.2 Lymph node stations. (From Mountain CF, Dresler CM: Regional lymph node stations for lung cancer staging, *Chest* 111:1718–1723, 1997.)

reviewed. The presence of calcification or the absence of growth for more than 2 years is believed to be reliable indicators of benign disease. For patients with previous CXRs, an SPN that is unchanged for more than 2 years does not require further evaluation.

Spiral CT with intravenous (IV) contrast enhancement is the imaging modality of choice for SPNs and should be obtained on all newly diagnosed SPNs. The patient with a new finding of an SPN and a recent history of pneumonia may warrant tracking the lesion for 6 to 8 weeks to exclude an infectious etiology. Malignant pulmonary nodules may be ill-defined with irregular margins and spiculated borders. Air bronchograms and pseudocavitations are more common characteristics of malignant rather than benign lesions. Cavitation of a nodule may be indicative of a malignancy, but inflammatory and infectious disease may also present with this appearance.

TABLE 41.1 ■ **Differential Diagnosis for Solitary Pulmonary Nodule**

Differential Diagnosis	Example
Neoplastic	Malignant 1. Bronchogenic carcinoma (adenocarcinoma, squamous cell carcinoma, small cell carcinoma, large cell carcinoma) 2. Metastatic lesion 3. Extranodal lymphoma 4. Carcinoid tumor
	Benign 1. Hamartoma 2. Chondroma
Inflammatory	Rheumatoid nodule Sarcoidosis Granulomatosis with polyangiitis (Wegener's)
Infectious	Granuloma (necrotizing) Fungal
Congenital	Arteriovenous malformations Pulmonary cysts Bronchial atresia
Miscellaneous	Pulmonary amyloidosis Pulmonary hematoma Pulmonary infarct

PET with FDG is performed for proven or highly suspicious lesions. FDG is taken up by cells in glycolysis but is bound within these cells and cannot enter the normal glycolytic pathway. Increased activity is demonstrated in cells with high metabolic rates as is seen in tumors and areas of inflammation. PET scan is not only an excellent imaging study for tumor, but it can potentially change patient management by detecting unsuspected nodal spread and metastatic disease.

The patient undergoes a spiral CT scan with IV contrast that shows a solitary pulmonary nodule in the left upper lobe that is 1.5 cm in diameter. PET scan shows no metastasis and moderate uptake by the nodule.

CLINICAL PEARL (STEP 2/3)

For patients with an SPN that is visible on the CXR, all previous CXRs should be reviewed. For patients with previous CXRs, an SPN that is unchanged for more than 2 years does not require further diagnostic evaluation. CT can be useful in identifying nodules more likely to be benign and may obviate the need for further diagnostic evaluation. Low-risk nodules can be followed with a CT at 6-month intervals for a total of 2 years.

What Are Guidelines for Assessment of a Solitary Pulmonary Nodule?

The management of an SPN begins with evaluation of the patient's history and risk assessment followed by morphologic review of the SPN on CT scan. Important factors that suggest benign disease are the presence of characteristic calcification, the presence of fat within the SPN, the size, and the stability over time. CT evaluation is the imaging of choice, but in selected cases in which the nodule is indeterminate, PET may aid diagnosis. As the majority of SPNs smaller than 4 mm are benign, follow-up with CT at 6-month intervals for 2 years is appropriate. The management of SPNs involves both clinical and imaging assessment, including risk assessment and morphology of the nodule.

Obtaining an accurate diagnosis using the fewest possible resources, judiciously using biopsy procedures, and performing surgical resection when indicated should be considered best principles of management.

BASIC SCIENCE PEARL (STEP 1/2/3)

The hilum is the mediastinal connection for the lung. Evaluation of lymph nodes and assessing involvement of critical mediastinal structures enables determining timing of resection and of resectability.

What Are the Options for Pulmonary Tissue Biopsy?

Minimally invasive options for tissue biopsy include bronchoscopy, navigational bronchoscopy, CT-guided transthoracic needle-guided biopsy (TTNB), and endobronchial ultrasound (EBUS). It should be noted that a nonmalignant diagnosis on such a biopsy attempt could represent a false-negative result due to the possibility of sampling benign tissue surrounding the neoplasm. If the lesion is not accessible via these more minimally invasive methods or if there is high suspicion that the biopsy obtained may be a false negative, surgery may be required to establish the diagnosis.

Why Is Mediastinal Evaluation Important?

In a patient with lung cancer the purpose is to locate and biopsy mediastinal lymph nodes. Nodal status will determine the stage of the malignancy and its appropriate treatment. Mediastinoscopy is a procedure by which a rigid endoscope is passed anterior to the trachea to visualize the contents of the mediastinum. In many centers, EBUS has replaced mediastinoscopy as the staging procedure of choice.

The patient undergoes bronchoscopy and mediastinoscopy.

Bronchoscopy reveals an endobronchial lesion in the bronchus to the left upper lobe that corresponds to the lesion on chest x-ray. Under the same anesthetic, mediastinoscopy is performed. Two days later the endobronchial biopsy is reported to be "small fragment, but consistent with squamous cell carcinoma" and all mediastinal nodes were negative, consistent with a stage 1 malignancy.

What Are the Indications for Surgical Resection of a Pulmonary Mass?

Assessing cardiopulmonary reserve is essential before pulmonary resection. Many patients with pulmonary masses also have diminished pulmonary function at baseline due to a history of smoking or other exposures. It is important to use pulmonary function testing and information about the planned volume of lung tissue to be resected in order to predict the patient's postoperative pulmonary function.

CLINICAL PEARL (STEP 2/3)

It is of fundamental importance to be aware of the difference between small cell lung cancer (SCLC) and nonsmall cell lung cancer (NSCLC).
- Nonsmall cell lung cancer is divided into four main types: squamous cell carcinoma (25%), adenocarcinoma (40%), large cell carcinoma (10%), and adenosquamous (3%). These tumors are of bronchial origin; typically, squamous cells tumors are centrally located and adenocarcinomas are peripherally located. Mutational profiling further delineates the subsets of adenocarcinoma and guides therapy.
- Small cell lung cancers (SCLC) are rapidly growing and aggressive malignancies of bronchial origin that rarely present as an SPN. SCLC accounts for approximately 15% of lung cancer and has a median survival of 18 months. It is predominantly found centrally, associated early in its course, with diffuse mediastinal lymphadenopathy. Frequently, there is distant metastatic disease at the time of presentation. Surgery has a limited role in SCLC. Chemotherapy and/or radiation are definitive therapy.

Given the Variety of Diagnoses for a Solitary Pulmonary Nodule, What Should Be the Logic of Our Approach to Treatment?

Solitary Pulmonary Nodule Assessed to Be Malignant

An SPN that is new and does not have benign-appearing calcifications should be considered malignant until proven otherwise. If a diagnosis cannot be confirmed utilizing the nonoperative techniques, surgical resection can be the ideal approach, as it is both diagnostic and therapeutic.

Solitary Pulmonary Nodule Thought Likely to Be Metastatic

If, based on a patient's history, it is believed that the SPN may not be NSCLC, but rather metastatic disease, then wedge resection is an accepted initial surgical approach. The specimen should be sent for frozen section, so that completion lobectomy can be performed in the same setting should the nodule prove to be NSCLC and should lobectomy be indicated.

Solitary Pulmonary Nodule Proven to Be Nonsmall Cell Lung Cancer

For the surgical candidate with an SPN proven to be NSCLC, lobectomy and systematic mediastinal lymph node dissection is considered the standard of care for complete oncologic resection and staging.

For the patient who is a marginal surgical candidate and whose pulmonary or cardiac status precludes lobectomy, wedge resection or segmentectomy with lymphadenectomy is acceptable treatment. Such patients require close postoperative surveillance due to increased rates of recurrence.

Solitary Pulmonary Nodule Representing Small Cell Lung Cancer

Patients with SCLC found at the time of operation will be referred for definitive radiation and chemotherapy.

What Are the Types of Lung Resection Surgery?
The type of lung cancer surgery that is ideal for a patient depends on many factors including the location, size, whether the tumor has spread to nearby structures, the patient's medical comorbidities, and the status of pulmonary function at baseline. The three major methods of lung cancer surgery are: (1) via a thoracotomy; (2) by video-assisted thoracoscopic surgery (VATS); or (3) by robotic-assisted thoracoscopic surgery (RATS). Minimally invasive approaches (thoracoscopic or robotic) utilize ports inserted in the rib interspaces to access the pleural cavity. The majority of pulmonary resections are not performed minimally invasively.

A **wedge resection** removes a portion of the lung that contains the tumor as well as some surrounding tissue. It is usually performed for very small lung tumors such as early-stage nonsmall cell lung cancers (NSCLC) and those located in the periphery of the lungs. Sometimes a wedge resection is also performed as a means of lung biopsy. Patients who cannot tolerate having an entire lobe removed benefit from a sublobar resection so that as much lung tissue as possible can be preserved.

A **lobectomy** is the removal of an entire anatomic lobe of the lung and is the most common surgical procedure performed to treat lung cancer. Recurrence is less and survival is better after lobectomy than with sublobar resection.

A **pneumonectomy** is the removal of an entire lung.

Operation: Lobectomy

1. Intubate with a double lumen endotracheal tube and ventilate using the contralateral lung.
2. **Access the chest.**
   - Open lobectomy.
     - Posterolateral or anterolateral thoracotomy incision usually in the fifth interspace.
     - Retraction device is placed to fully expose the operative field.
   - Minimally invasive lobectomy
     - Insert trochars for camera and instruments in the appropriate intercostal spaces.
3. For both open and minimally invasive resections:
   - Remove the appropriate lobe by ligating its contributing pulmonary arteries, pulmonary veins, and lobar bronchi.
   - Complete resection may include parietal pleura, chest wall, or pericardium. Lymphadenectomy of hilar and mediastinal lymph nodes is essential.

What Are the Potential Complications of Lung Resection?

Complications that can occur immediately after pulmonary resection include air leak, atelectasis, pneumonia/mucous plugging, hemorrhage, tachyarrhythmias including atrial fibrillation, pulmonary embolus, phrenic nerve injury, and middle lobe torsion.

The patient is scheduled for a VATS lobectomy. The left upper lobe is resected, and systematic lymph node dissection is performed. Frozen section of the specimens reveals the nodule to be squamous cell carcinoma with no metastasis to the lymph nodes. One chest tube is placed, and the incisions for the ports are closed. The postoperative course is uneventful, and the chest tube is removed without difficulty. The patient is discharged on the third postoperative day. She is scheduled to see her surgeon and a medical oncologist in 2 weeks.

BEYOND THE PEARLS

- A solitary pulmonary nodule (SPN) is defined as a single, well-circumscribed lesion completely surrounded by pulmonary parenchyma that measures less than 3 cm in diameter.
- A history of smoking and older age increase the likelihood that an SPN is malignant.
- Spiral CT with IV contrast is the imaging modality of choice for an SPN.
- A new SPN that does not have benign-appearing calcifications should be considered malignant until proven otherwise.
- Surgical resection is indicated for nodules at high risk of malignancy.
- The type of lung cancer surgery that is ideal for a particular patient depends on many factors, including location and size of the tumor, extent of nodal spread, as well as the patient's medical comorbidities.

Suggested Readings

Gould MK, Donington J, Lynch WR, et al: Evaluation of individuals with pulmonary nodules: When is it lung cancer? Diagnosis and management of lung cancer, 3rd ed: American College of Chest Physicians evidence-based clinical practice guidelines, *Chest* 143(5 Suppl):e93S–e120S, 2013. https://doi.org/10.1378/chest.12-2351.

Khan, A. N., Al-Jahdali, H. H., Irion, K. L., Arabi, M., & Koteyar, S. S. (2011). Solitary pulmonary nodule: A diagnostic algorithm in the light of current imaging technique. *Avicenna J Med, 1*(2), 39–51. https://doi.org/10.4103/2231-0770.90915.

Roviaro, G., Varoli, F., Rebuffat, C., Vergani, C., D'Hoore, A., Scalambra, S. M., et al. (1993). Major pulmonary resections: Pneumonectomies and lobectomies. *Ann Thorac Surg*, *56*(3), 779–783.

Tan, B. B., Flaherty, K. R., Kazerooni, E. A., & Iannettoni, M. D. (2003). The solitary pulmonary nodule. *Chest*, *123*(1 Suppl), 89S–96S.

Ziarnik, E., & Grogan, E. L. (2015). Post-lobectomy early complications. *Thorac Surg Clin*, *25*(3), 355–364. https://doi.org/10.1016/j.thorsurg.2015.04.003.

CHAPTER 42

Shortness of Breath in a 78-Year-Old Female

Vishal Shah ■ Konstadinos Plestis ■ Scott Goldman

A 78-year-old female with a history of hypertension, hyperlipidemia, and hypothyroidism presents to the emergency department with increasing shortness of breath over the past several months, especially when doing household chores and running errands. She has a history of coronary artery disease (CAD), peripheral vascular disease, and chronic renal failure. This morning she woke up feeling breathless and was brought by a neighbor to be evaluated.

What Is the Differential Diagnosis for Shortness of Breath?

One of the most common complaints with which patients present to either an outpatient evaluation or the emergency department is of dyspnea, or shortness of breath. Although most frequently the etiology of a patient's dyspnea is cardiopulmonary, pathology in almost any organ system can lead to presentation with a complaint of dyspnea (Table 42.1). Therefore a comprehensive history and physical examination is required to help elucidate the true cause of the patient's complaint. One of the major ways that dyspnea is categorized is whether the dyspnea is acute or chronic, the latter being defined as present for 4 weeks or more. Although not comprehensive, Table 42.1 outlines the major acute and chronic etiologies of dyspnea. It should also be noted that etiologies of acute dyspnea are capable of presenting as chronic dyspnea, and vice versa. Additionally, because the majority of the etiologies of dyspnea are nonsurgical, differentiating between etiologies of dyspnea that do require surgical management is extremely important.

What Are the Important Aspects of History and Physical Examination to Evaluate a Patient With Shortness of Breath?

As always, a thorough history and physical examination are important in the assessment of patients with shortness of breath. Certainly, assessing the chronicity of the patient's symptoms helps differentiate acute from chronic dyspnea and therefore helps tailor the differential diagnosis. Associated symptoms and medical history will often narrow the focus to one or two organ systems. If there is concern for an acute, life-threatening cause of dyspnea such as myocardial or cerebral ischemia or tension pneumothorax, indicated assessment and treatment (electrocardiogram and troponins, tissue plasminogen activator, and needle thoracostomy, respectively) should not be delayed.

As the most common causes of dyspnea are cardiopulmonary in nature, examination of the cardiovascular and pulmonary systems is of great importance. Auscultation to assess the rate, rhythm, and the presence of murmurs can reveal underlying cardiac pathology such as arrhythmias or structural cardiac problems such as valvular or septal pathology. Auscultating and percussing bilateral lung fields can detect areas of consolidation, rhonchi, and wheezes suggestive of primary pulmonary pathology.

TABLE 42.1 ■ Causes of Acute and Chronic Dyspnea by Organ System

System	Acute	Chronic
Neurologic	Stroke Neuromuscular disease	Amyotrophic lateral sclerosis
HEENT	Foreign body Trauma Angioedema Vocal cord dysfunction	Laryngeal tumor Goiter
Cardiac	Myocardial infarction Arrhythmia Pericardial tamponade	Congestive heart failure Valvular heart disease
Pulmonary	COPD exacerbation Asthma attack Airway obstruction (mucus, foreign body, etc.) Trauma Pneumonia Empyema Pneumothorax Pleural effusion Acute respiratory failure	Lung cancer Chronic bronchitis/emphysema Interstitial lung disease Cystic fibrosis Pulmonary hypertension
Gastrointestinal	Abdominal distension Diaphragmatic hernia/rupture	
Renal	Acute renal failure	Chronic renal failure
Immune	Anaphylaxis Sepsis	
Other	Toxin ingestion	Metabolic diseases

On physical examination, the patient's heart rate is 88 bpm and regular, her blood pressure is 140/72 mm Hg, her respiratory rate is 28 breaths per minute, pulse oximetry is 90% on room air, and she is afebrile. Auscultation reveals a harsh crescendo-decrescendo systolic murmur best heard in the right second intercostal space. The murmur radiates to both carotid arteries, and palpation of the carotids bilaterally reveals a delayed upstroke. She has 2+ pitting edema in her lower extremities bilaterally. Lung examination reveals coarse crackles bilaterally. The remainder of the physical examination is unremarkable. Chest radiograph demonstrates moderate left ventricular enlargement with bilateral small effusions. Based on the physical examination, the physician tells the patient that she most likely is suffering from aortic stenosis.

What Are the Cardinal Symptoms of Aortic Stenosis?

The classic triad of symptoms in patients with aortic stenosis (AS) includes chest pain, heart failure, and syncope, and patients typically present experiencing at least one of these symptoms. Angina occurs in two-thirds of patients and results from an imbalance in myocardial oxygen supply and an increased demand secondary to increased left ventricular mass. Left ventricular failure occurs as the ventricle hypertrophies to compensate for increased afterload. In turn, elevated left ventricular filling pressures are transmitted to the left atrium and pulmonary capillary bed, resulting in clinical symptoms of LV failure and pulmonary edema. Patients then experience progressive dyspnea. Finally, syncope, which can result when standing from sitting or other exertion, occurs when arterial blood pressure decreases as a result of systemic vasodilation in the face of fixed cardiac output resulting in inadequate cerebral perfusion.

Patients with aortic stenosis may remain asymptomatic for 10 to 20 years; however, patients who develop symptoms can rapidly deteriorate, leading to increased mortality. The time from onset of symptoms to death in patients without surgical treatment presenting with angina, syncope, and heart failure is 5 years, 3 years, and 2 years, respectively.

What Are the Causes of Aortic Stenosis?

Degenerative AS is the most common cause of AS, especially in the elderly population over age 65. It is characterized by immobilization of the aortic valve cusps by deposits of calcium. Bicuspid aortic valve is the most common cause of stenosis in patients younger than 65 years of age. It is an inherited form of heart disease in which two of the leaflets of the aortic valve fuse during development, resulting in a two-leaflet valve (bicuspid valve) instead of a normal three-leaflet valve (tricuspid). The resulting turbulent flow in a bicuspid valve leads to leaflet fibrosis and subsequent stenosis. Rheumatic fever, although previously prevalent, is now a rare cause of AS in which antistreptococcal antibodies cross-react with host-tissue epitopes, which results in prolonged inflammation and collagen deposition, resulting in a stenotic valve.

BASIC SCIENCE PEARL (STEP 1)

The atrioventricular valves separate the atria and ventricles from one another on both sides of the heart (Fig. 42.1). The tricuspid valve typically has three leaflets whereas the mitral valve has two. The semilunar valves (pulmonic and aortic) both typically have three leaflets. A congenital bicuspid aortic valve confers increased risk for developing AS.

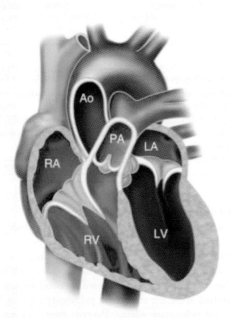

Fig. 42.1 Cardiac valvular anatomy. Atrioventricular valves: the tricuspid valve separates the right atrium (RA) and right ventricle (RV) and the mitral valve separates the left atrium (LA) and left ventricle (LV). Semilunar valves: the pulmonic valve separates the RV and pulmonary artery (PA) and the aortic valve separates the LV from the aorta. (Redrawn from Otto CM: The adult with congenital heart disease. In *Textbook of Clinical Echocardiography*, Philadelphia, 2018, Elsevier, pp 479–506.)

What Are the Physical Examination Findings in Patients With Aortic Stenosis?

The physical examination findings in patients with AS result from turbulent and decreased flow of blood through the aortic valve. A carotid arterial pulse that is weak and rises slowly (pulsus tardus et parvus) reflects the obstruction of blood entering the peripheral arterial circulation. A harsh crescendo-decrescendo systolic ejection murmur, heard best at the right second intercostal space, is classically associated with AS. The murmur can radiate to both carotid arteries. Some patients may have a fourth heart sound (S4) and a palpable systolic thrill at the sternal notch or second intercostal space secondary to increased left atrial contraction into a stiff left ventricle.

What Is the Appropriate Diagnostic Workup for Patients With Aortic Stenosis?

Patients who present with symptomatic AS diagnosed on physical examination should be admitted to the hospital for further workup. Intravenous diuretics are started immediately and cardiac markers such as troponin levels should be assessed to rule out myocardial infarction (MI). An electrocardiogram (ECG) is also routinely performed to evaluate for concomitant conditions such as atrial fibrillation or ST-elevation MI. The ECG typically reveals normal sinus rhythm with left ventricular hypertrophy and left axis deviation.

A two-dimensional transthoracic echocardiogram (TTE) is the primary test for evaluation of AS. The echocardiogram evaluates valvular structure and function, left ventricular size, aortic valve

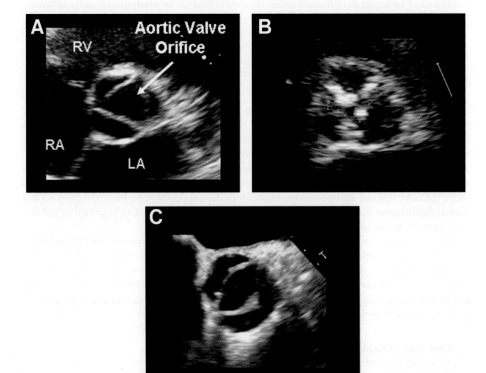

Fig. 42.2 Echocardiography of the aortic valve. Normal valve (A) with labeled left atrium (LA), right atrium (RA), and right ventricle (RV). Stenotic valve with markedly decreased vale area (B). Bicuspid aortic valve without stenosis (C). (From Pandian NG, Ramamurthi A, Applebaum S: Role of echocardiography in aortic stenosis, *Prog Cardiovasc Dis* Jul–Aug;57(1):47–54, 2014.)

area, and left ventricular outflow tract (Fig. 42.2). TTE in AS usually reveals concentric left ventricular hypertrophy with a mildly diminished ejection fraction suggestive of severe aortic stenosis. Diminished valve area and increased velocity of blood across the valve are also indicators of stenosis.

Cardiac catheterization should be utilized when there is a discrepancy between clinical evaluation and echocardiogram, because the use of intravascular contrast is able to better assess flow dynamics across the aortic valve. Cardiac catheterization may also diagnosis concomitant coronary artery disease and patients who may need coronary artery bypass grafting in addition to aortic valve replacement.

BASIC SCIENCE PEARL (STEPS 1/2/3)

Ejection fraction (EF) is reported from echocardiogram as an estimation of the percentage of blood pumped from the left ventricle during systole. Quantitatively, EF can be calculated by the formula:

$$Ejection\ fraction = \frac{(End\ systolic\ volume - End\ diastolic\ volume)}{End\ systolic\ volume} \times 100$$

An EF of 55% or greater is considered normal.

The patient undergoes an electrocardiogram and chest radiograph on which she is found to have no abnormalities. A transthoracic echocardiogram is performed that reveals a tricuspid aortic valve with severe aortic stenosis. Due to her risk factors and a strong family history of coronary artery disease, she undergoes cardiac catheterization that reveals no coronary artery disease but confirms the diagnosis of significant aortic stenosis.

What Are the Treatment Options for Patients With Aortic Stenosis?
Sole medical management is not appropriate for symptomatic patients. The mainstay of treatment for symptomatic aortic stenosis is aortic valve replacement, though there are several other, less invasive options for patients who have prohibitively high surgical risk.

Percutaneous aortic balloon dilation (percutaneous aortic balloon valvotomy) is a procedure in which one or more balloons are placed across the stenotic aortic valve and inflated in an attempt to widen the valve area and disrupt calcium and collagen deposits in the valve leaflets. Restenosis and clinical deterioration occur in most cases within a half-year. This procedure is limited to patients with short-life expectancy with a prohibitive surgical risk.

More commonly, a choice is made between surgical aortic valve replacement (SAVR) and transcatheter aortic valve replacement (TAVR). A multidisciplinary heart valve team should provide the decision making as to which option is indicated in the appropriate patient. The decision making takes into consideration a patient's life expectancy, frailty, comorbidities, specific anatomy, values, and preferences, and a risk score is calculated. A high surgical risk score may preclude an open surgical approach and favor TAVR.

What Types of Replacement Aortic Valves Are Available?
There are two types of valves: mechanical and biologic.

Mechanical valves are bileaflet and made from pyrolytic carbon. The primary advantage of mechanical valves is life-long durability and avoiding another aortic valve replacement later in one's life. Mechanical valves have excellent blood flow performance, which may benefit a patient's quality of life and ability for exercise. The main drawback, however, is the requirement of life-long anticoagulation with its accompanying risk of bleeding. A mechanical prosthesis is suggested for surgical aortic valve replacement for patients less than 60 to 65 years of age who do not have a contraindication to anticoagulation, although this is controversial.

Biologic or tissue valves are harvested from porcine or bovine heart valves. The primary advantage of tissue valves is that they do not require life-long anticoagulation therapy. However, these valves last only 15 to 20 years, and younger patients with biologic valve replacements may require another operation later in life. A biologic valve is suggested for patients more than 70 years old and for those with life expectancy lower than the expected durability of the bioprosthesis.

What Is a Transcatheter Aortic Valve Replacement?

Transcatheter aortic valve replacement (TAVR) is a minimally invasive procedure that utilizes a catheter to thread a new valve over an existing native aortic valve. There are three major catheter-based techniques for replacing the aortic valve: the most common transfemoral access; direct aortic access (via either ministernotomy or right anterior thoracotomy); and direct transapical access through the apex of the left ventricle.

Preoperative planning includes computed tomography angiography (CTA) to assess aortic annulus geometry and peripheral access and a multidisciplinary approach involving cardiac surgeons, interventional cardiologists, and cardiologists.

Procedural considerations include antibiotic prophylaxis, a temporary pacing lead in patients who may develop heart block postoperatively, intravenous access, intraoperative transesophageal echocardiography, and fluoroscopy and a heart-lung machine in the case emergent cardiopulmonary bypass is required.

Postprocedural care includes telemetry monitoring to diagnosis heart block or arrhythmias and dual pacemaker implantation in patients with heart block. Possible complications include: vascular injury (including injury at the arterial access site or ventricular perforation); incorrect valve deployment (including malpositioning, coronary obstruction, or annular rupture); poor valve function (including paravalvular leak); organ injury (including stroke or MI); and arrhythmic complications (including high degree heart block and atrial fibrillation).

CLINICAL PEARL (STEPS 2/3)

When performing a SAVR or TAVR, native calcium deposits, which are a main contributing factor to aortic stenosis, can dislodge and travel to the brain, causing stroke.

After a discussion of her options with her cardiologist and the cardiothoracic surgeon and given her significant comorbidities and age, the patient successfully undergoes a TAVR procedure. She does not experience any arrhythmia or postprocedure complications. She is discharged from the hospital the next day. She is seen by her cardiologist 1 week later and reports improvement of her symptoms and independent resumption of many of her activities of daily living.

BEYOND THE PEARLS

- The most common cause of aortic stenosis, especially in patients over 65, is calcification of the aortic valve.
- The presence of symptoms in the setting of aortic stenosis is a poor prognostic indicator.
- The decision for SAVR vs TAVR requires a multidisciplinary team consisting of cardiac surgeons, interventional cardiologists, general cardiologists, and echocardiologists.
- TAVR is an increasingly popular approach in high-risk patients needing aortic valve replacement.

Suggested Readings

Lieberman, E. B., et al. (1995). Balloon aortic valvuloplasty in adults: failure of procedure to improve long-term survival, *J Am Coll Cardiol* Nov 15;26(6):1522–1528.

Nishimura, R. A., et al. (2017). 2014 AHA/ACC guideline for the management of patients with valvular heart disease: A report of the American College of Cardiology/American Heart Association Task Force on Practice Guidelines. *J Am Coll Cardiol, 70*(2), 252–289.

Turina, J., et al. (1987). Spontaneous course of aortic valve disease. *Eur Heart J, 8*(5), 471–483.

Vandvik, P. O., et al. (2016). Transcatheter or surgical aortic valve replacement for patients with severe, symptomatic, aortic stenosis at low to intermediate surgical risk: A clinical practice guideline. *BMJ (Clinical Research Ed), 354*, i5085.

CHAPTER 43

Unstable Angina in a 67-Year-Old Male

Christopher E. Greenleaf ■ Erin Kenning

A 67-year-old male with a past medical history significant for diabetes and hypertension presents to the emergency department with a complaint of chest pain. The pain is intermittent and seems to worsen with walking. He has had some pain in his chest for about 6 months—it has always been with exertion—but he has recently been experiencing the pain when at rest. Upon further questioning, he admits to not taking his medications for diabetes and hypertension consistently.

What Is the Differential Diagnosis for Chest Pain?

There are acute, subacute, and chronic pathologies that can produce chest pain. Pathology of any organ within the thorax and mediastinum can cause chest pain, and it is important to distinguish between them (Table 43.1). Acute problems usually require urgent intervention, whether it is medical or surgical. Acute surgical problems include pneumothorax, massive pulmonary embolism with hemodynamic compromise, myocardial ischemia requiring surgical revascularization, esophageal perforation, and type A aortic dissections.

What Are the Primary Physical Examination Techniques to Evaluate Chest Pain?

Most etiologies of chest pain can be diagnosed with a thorough history and physical examination. It is imperative to have a differential diagnosis in mind after obtaining the patient's history so that a focused physical examination can be performed. Cardiac auscultation should identify new murmurs and abnormal rhythms. Physical examination of other organ systems revealing carotid bruits and peripheral vascular disease suggests cardiac disease. Jugular venous distension and extremity edema could indicate right heart failure due to increased preload. Aortic dissection could lead to differential blood pressures in the four extremities. The patient's respiratory effort and pulmonary auscultation may reveal decreased breath sounds or crackles.

The physical examination reveals obesity, a normal cardiopulmonary examination, no carotid bruits, and palpable but diminished dorsalis pedis and posterior tibial pulses in the both legs. An electrocardiogram shows a normal sinus rhythm without ST changes, and a chest radiograph shows no cardiopulmonary abnormality. On laboratory analyses, the serum troponin T is 0.1 ng/mL (normal < 0.01 ng/mL). The patient's chest pain resolves with one 0.4 mg sublingual nitroglycerin tablet. The patient is diagnosed with a non-ST elevation myocardial infarction. He is evaluated by a cardiologist and is taken to the catheterization laboratory where coronary angiography shows 80% to 90% proximal and midstenoses in the left anterior descending (LAD) artery, the left circumflex (LCX) artery, and the right coronary artery (RCA), or so-called three-vessel coronary disease.

TABLE 43.1 ■ Differential Diagnosis of Chest Pain

	Pathology	Clinical Findings
Lung	Pneumothorax	Unilateral decreased breath sounds
	Pulmonary embolism	Elevated D-dimer, dyspnea, swollen leg
Cardiac	Myocardial ischemia	ECG changes, exertional chest pain
	Pericarditis	Cardiac rub, distended neck veins
Esophagus	Esophageal perforation	Excessive vomiting, chest trauma
Thoracic aorta	Aortic dissection	Tearing pain, radiating to the back

BASIC SCIENCE PEARL (STEPS 1/2/3)

Anatomists define coronary dominance by whichever coronary artery has the sinoatrial node artery as a branch. By this definition, 55% of hearts are right dominant. Clinicians define coronary dominance by the posterior descending artery because this supplies the artery to the atrioventricular node. By this definition, 85% to 90% of hearts are right dominant.

CLINICAL PEARL (STEPS 2/3)

The World Health Organization defines the diagnosis of myocardial infarction on the presence of at least two of three features including ischemia-type chest discomfort, changes on electrocardiography, and a rise in serum cardiac markers.

What Are the Mechanical Complications of Myocardial Infarction?

Due to tissue death after a myocardial infarction, several structures are at risk for disruption. Postinfarction ventricular free wall rupture, ventricular septal defect, and acute mitral insufficiency constitute surgical emergencies because they are life-threatening. With the advent of quicker revascularizations, these complications have decreased over time.

A newly infarcted ventricular wall can be weakened by necrosis. Because of the higher pressures generated by the left ventricle, it is typically the left ventricle that ruptures in this situation. This usually happens within the first week after myocardial infarction, and there is a very high early mortality with this complication. If the rupture does not cause tamponade and death because it happens more gradually, then the patient will have a hematoma on the ventricular free wall. This is treated with either resection and plication with pledgeted sutures or with patching with polytetrafluoroethylene.

A pansystolic murmur after myocardial infarction is concerning for ischemic ventricular septal defect. Increased ventricular afterload over right ventricular afterload promotes a left-to-right shunt that increases the volume workload of the heart. There are typically signs of right ventricular failure with liver congestion, peripheral edema, and elevated jugular venous distension. If there is a pulmonary artery catheter in place, there will be an oxygen step-up between the right atrium and the pulmonary artery due to oxygenated blood returning from the left to the right ventricle. The diagnosis is made by echocardiography. Repair involves debridement of the necrotic tissue and patch repair of the defect through the ventricle.

Rupture of a papillary muscle after myocardial infarction can lead to acute mitral insufficiency. The posteromedial papillary muscle is usually the one involved because it usually has a single blood supply from the posterior descending artery. The usual patient with acute mitral insufficiency has single-vessel right coronary thrombosis without collaterals. This occurs within a week of the infarction. Treatment is usually mitral valve replacement or repair with or without coronary revascularization.

After Initial Stabilization, What Are the Treatment Options for Patients With a Myocardial Infarction?

Depending on patient factors, presentation, and extent of disease, the treatment options include percutaneous coronary intervention (PCI) or coronary artery bypass grafting (CABG). Although less invasive, PCI (which includes stent placement) has a higher rate of restenosis than the more invasive CABG. Many studies have been performed to determine which populations of patients (comorbidities, pattern of disease, residual heart function) do best with which intervention. The SYNTAX score is one system that allows physicians to gather data about the patient and their disease and help determine the optimal treatment.

With regard to CABG, there are multiple randomized trials showing that surgery has a survival advantage over medical therapy in patients with left main stenosis, three-vessel disease, two-vessel disease with proximal left anterior descending disease, coronary artery disease with depressed ventricular function, coronary artery disease with concomitant valvular pathology that needs to be addressed, and failed coronary angioplasty.

What Workup Should Be Completed Before a Coronary Artery Bypass Graft Surgery?

Patients with coronary atherosclerosis typically have multiple other comorbidities, so medical suitability for surgery is important for nonemergent surgery. Optimization of diabetes and blood pressure is crucial. All patients should have a chest radiograph preoperatively to assess for pulmonary disease. Significant aortic calcification noted on chest radiograph should prompt chest computed tomography. Evidence of peripheral arterial disease should prompt evaluation of the lower extremity arteries with ankle-brachial indices and pulse volume recordings. Because the preferred conduits for bypass graft are native vessels (i.e., internal mammary artery and saphenous vein), they should be assessed for suitability. The vast majority of conduits used in the United States are saphenous veins, and these should be assessed by physical examination with or without ultrasound depending on if there are any findings of lower extremity venous insufficiency. Similarly, most patients undergoing coronary artery bypass grafting should be evaluated for carotid artery disease with ultrasound. Concomitant valvular pathology is present in about one-third of patients requiring coronary artery bypass grafting, so all patients should undergo echocardiography to assess valvular and ventricular function. Other workup should be prompted by the history and physical examination, including evaluation for pulmonary, renal, hepatic, infectious, and bleeding disorders.

The patient is scheduled for coronary artery bypass grafting. Workup revealed no valvular pathology, normal ventricular function, short-segment superficial femoral artery stenosis, and no carotid artery disease. At the time of surgery the aorta was soft and without atherosclerosis, and the distal coronary arteries beyond the blockages were adequate targets for distal anastomosis. A reversed saphenous vein graft was anastomosed to the distal right coronary artery and one to an obtuse marginal branch of the left circumflex artery. The proximal saphenous vein grafts were anastomosed to the ascending aorta. The left internal mammary artery was anastomosed to the left anterior descending artery in an *in situ* fashion. The patient weaned from cardiopulmonary bypass without issue.

CLINICAL PEARL

Risk factors associated with poor outcome after coronary artery bypass grafting have included decreased ejection fraction, older age, emergency surgery, preoperative shock, female sex, diabetes, and previous cardiac surgery, among others. The Society of Thoracic Surgeons has maintained a database of adult cardiac surgical procedures since 1989. Powerful statistical methods have allowed a risk calculator for most coronary and valvular procedures in adult cardiac surgery. The calculator can be found at www.sts.org and will give the risk of major morbidity and mortality within 30 days of operation.

On-pump Coronary Artery Bypass Grafting (Fig. 43.1)

1. Perform a median sternotomy.
2. Dissect and prepare the bypass vessel being used (left internal mammary artery or saphenous vein).
3. Cannulate the ascending aorta and right atrium and initiate cardiopulmonary bypass.
4. Cross-clamp the ascending aorta.
5. Administer potassium-containing antegrade, with or without retrograde cardioplegia.
6. Perform distal and proximal coronary anastomoses.
7. Remove the aortic cross-clamp.
8. Wean from cardiopulmonary bypass.
9. Place chest tubes.
10. Close the chest in layers.

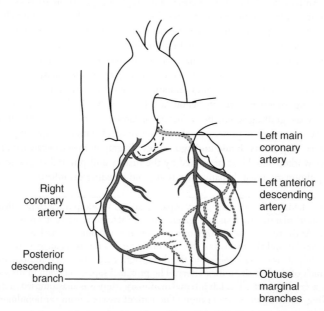

Fig. 43.1 Coronary arteries and their major branches. (From Hsia T-Y, Peck EA, Conte JV: Coronary artery disease. In Conte JV, Baumgartner, WA, Dorman T, Owens SG, editors: *The Johns Hopkins Manual of Cardiac Surgical Care*, Philadelphia, 2008, Elsevier, Fig. 3.1.)

CLINICAL PEARL

The goal of coronary artery bypass grafting is to revascularize all vessels with greater than 60% stenosis and that are greater than 1 mm in diameter. There are multiple options for conduits to use during coronary artery bypass grafting. The left internal mammary artery to the left anterior descending artery anastomosis is the single most important portion of the coronary artery bypass in determining long-term outcome and has been the strongest association with survival improvement postoperatively (Tables 43.2 and 43.3).

The patient is transferred to the cardiac intensive care unit after chest closure. The patient is extubated within 6 hours of the conclusion of the operation. Postoperatively, he is started on aspirin, a statin, and a beta blocker. His blood glucoses are well controlled with diet. His chest tubes are removed, and he ambulates without difficulty. He is discharged from the hospital on the sixth postoperative day.

What Are the Potential Immediate and Delayed Complications of Coronary Artery Bypass Grafting?

Bleeding and infection are risks with any invasive procedure. The blood's interaction with the artificial surface of the cardiopulmonary bypass machine leads to coagulopathy that continues postoperatively, so surveillance of postoperative bleeding and transfusion of blood products as needed is an important part of postoperative care. In addition to bleeding, the risk for developing blood clots, including deep venous thrombosis and pulmonary embolism, is high in nonmobile, critically ill patients. There is typically a decrease in the cardiac output precipitated by the inflammatory cascade from the bypass machine that occurs approximately 6 to 18 hours postoperatively. Failure to extubate can occur in patients with underlying pulmonary disease; prolonged ventilation is defined as being mechanically ventilated after 24 hours. Delirium and neurocognitive decline are possible, especially with the use of narcotics, and are more likely in the elderly population. Arrhythmias, especially atrial fibrillation, are common after any cardiothoracic surgery. Most can be treated pharmacologically, but some may require procedural treatment with ablation or pacemaker insertion. Other risks related to a patient's medical comorbities are also important to acknowledge. The delayed complications of graft stenosis and the need for subsequent procedure should be discussed with the patient preoperatively.

Two weeks later the patient presents for his postoperative visit. His sternotomy wound is healing well. He has been walking daily with his wife and states that he has no episodes of chest pain despite increasing his walking distance daily. He has had no adverse reaction to the new medications. He is schedule for follow-up with his primary care physician and his cardiologist.

BEYOND THE PEARLS

- Cardiovascular disease is the leading cause of death in the United States.
- For patients with complex coronary disease or impaired ventricular function, surgical therapy provides improved symptomatic relief and survival.
- The risk profile of the "typical" coronary bypass grafting patient has increased over time, but the outcomes with surgery have improved with better surgical techniques and perioperative care.
- Surgical emergencies after myocardial infarction include ventricular free wall rupture, ventricular septal defect, and acute mitral regurgitation.
- Atrial fibrillation is a common complication after any cardiothoracic surgery.

TABLE 43.2 ■ American College of Cardiology/American Heart Association Guidelines for Coronary Artery Bypass Graft Surgery: Indications

Disease	Stage
Asymptomatic or mild angina	*Class I* Significant left main coronary artery stenosis Left main equivalent: Significant (> 70%) stenosis of proximal LAD and proximal left circumflex artery Three-vessel disease (survival benefit is greater in patients with abnormal left ventricular [LV] function [e.g., with an EF < 0.50]) *Class IIa* Proximal LAD stenosis with 1- or 2-vessel disease *Class IIb* One- or two-vessel disease not involving the proximal LAD
Stable angina	*Class I* Significant left main coronary artery stenosis Left main equivalent: Significant (> 70%) stenosis of proximal LAD and proximal left circumflex artery Three-vessel disease (survival benefit is greater when LVEF is < 0.50). Two-vessel disease with significant proximal LAD stenosis and either EF < 0.50 or demonstrable ischemia on noninvasive testing One- or two-vessel coronary artery disease without significant proximal LAD stenosis but with a large area of viable myocardium and high-risk criteria on noninvasive testing Disabling angina despite maximal medical therapy, when surgery can be performed with acceptable risk; if angina is not typical, objective evidence of ischemia should be obtained *Class IIa* Proximal LAD stenosis with one-vessel disease One- or two-vessel coronary artery disease without significant proximal LAD stenosis but with a moderate area of viable myocardium and demonstrable ischemia on noninvasive testing *Class III* One- or two-vessel disease not involving significant proximal LAD stenosis in patients who have mild symptoms that are unlikely due to myocardial ischemia or have not received an adequate trial of medical therapy and (1) have only a small area of viable myocardium or (2) have no demonstrable ischemia on noninvasive testing Borderline coronary stenoses (50%–60% diameter in locations other than the left main coronary artery) and no demonstrable ischemia on noninvasive testing Insignificant (< 50% diameter) coronary stenosis
Unstable angina or non–Q-wave MI	*Class I* Significant left main coronary artery stenosis Left main equivalent: Significant (> 70%) stenosis of proximal LAD and proximal left circumflex artery Ongoing ischemia not responsive to maximal nonsurgical therapy *Class IIa* Proximal LAD stenosis with 1- or 2-vessel disease *Class IIb* One- or two-vessel disease not involving the proximal LAD
S-T–segment elevation (Q wave) MI	*Class I* None *Class IIa* Ongoing ischemia or infarction not responsive to maximal nonsurgical therapy *Class IIb* Progressive LV pump failure with coronary stenosis compromising viable myocardium outside the initial infarct area Primary reperfusion in the early hours (< 6–12 hours) of an evolving S-T–segment elevation MI *Class III* Primary reperfusion late (> 12 hours) in evolving S-T–segment elevation MI without ongoing ischemia

TABLE 43.2 ■ American College of Cardiology/American Heart Association Guidelines for Coronary Artery Bypass Graft Surgery: Indications (Continued)

Disease	Stage
Poor LV function	*Class I* Significant left main coronary artery stenosis Left main equivalent: Significant (> 70%) stenosis of proximal LAD and proximal left circumflex artery Proximal LAD stenosis with 2- or 3-vessel disease *Class IIa* Poor LV function with significant viable, noncontracting, revascularizable myocardium without any of the aforementioned anatomic patterns *Class III* Poor LV function without evidence of intermittent ischemia and without evidence of significant revascularizable, viable myocardium
Life-threatening ventricular arrhythmias	*Class I* Left main coronary artery stenosis Three-vessel coronary disease *Class IIa* Bypassable 1- or 2-vessel disease causing life-threatening ventricular arrhythmias Proximal LAD disease with 1- or 2-vessel disease *Class III* Ventricular tachycardia with scar and no evidence of ischemia
After failed percutaneous transluminal coronary angioplasty	*Class I* Ongoing ischemia or threatened occlusion with significant myocardium at risk Hemodynamic compromise *Class IIa* Foreign body in crucial anatomic position Hemodynamic compromise in patients with impairment of coagulation system and without previous **sternotomy** *Class IIb* Hemodynamic compromise in patients with impairment of coagulation system and with previous sternotomy *Class III* Absence of ischemia Inability to revascularize owing to target anatomy or no-reflow state
Patients with previous CABG	*Class I* Disabling angina despite maximal noninvasive therapy (if angina is not typical, then objective evidence of ischemia should be obtained) *Class IIa* Bypassable distal vessel(s) with a large area of threatened myocardium on noninvasive studies *Class IIb* Ischemia in the non-LAD distribution with a patent internal mammary graft to the LAD supplying functioning myocardium and without an aggressive attempt at medical management or percutaneous revascularization

CABG, Coronary artery bypass grafting; *EF,* ejection fraction; *LAD,* left anterior descending; *LV,* left ventricular; *MI,* myocardial infarction.
Class I: Conditions for which there is evidence or general agreement that a given procedure or treatment is useful and effective.
Class II: Conditions for which there is conflicting evidence or a divergence of opinion about the usefulness or efficacy of a procedure.
Class IIa: Weight of evidence and opinion is in favor of usefulness and efficacy.
Class IIb: Usefulness and efficacy is less well established by evidence and opinion.
Class III: Conditions for which there is evidence or general agreement that the procedure or treatment is not useful or effective and in some cases may be harmful.
(From Hsia T-Y, Peck EA, Conte JV: Coronary artery disease. In Conte JV, Baumgartner, WA, Dorman T, Owens SG, editors: *The Johns Hopkins Manual of Cardiac Surgical Care*, Philadelphia, 2008, Elsevier, Table 3.1.)

TABLE 43.3 ■ **Coronary Artery Bypass Conduit Indications, Contraindications, and Graft Failure Rate**

	Indication	Contraindication	Failure Rate
Left internal mammary artery	Whenever feasible	Emergency surgery	3%–8% at 1 year
		Poor flow or injury	4%–12% at 5 years
		Subclavian artery stenosis or occlusion	7%–12% at 10 years
Right internal mammary artery	Young patient	Diabetes (relative)	
Free internal mammary artery graft	When internal mammary artery cannot be used as pedicled graft	Atherosclerotic or dissection	8%–25% intermediate term
Radial artery	Arterial conduit	Positive Allen test	15% at 3 months; further 7% during next 6 months
		Incomplete palmer arch Prior carpal tunnel operation Prior radial arterial cannulation (relative)	
Gastroepiploic artery	Additional arterial conduit	Prior gastric resection	4% at 2 months
		Atherosclerosis of celiac axis Emergency surgery Large heart Severe LV dysfunction	8% between 2 and 5 years
Inferior epigastric artery	Lack of other conduits	Paramedian abdominal incision	21% at 5 years
	Prior use of internal mammary	Atherosclerosis Previous groin incision (relative)	
Greater saphenous vein	Best venous conduit	Too small (< 2 mm)	10%–15% in first month
			2%–3% per year between 1 and 5 years 5% per year after 5 years 50% in 10 years + 25% with stenosis

(From Hsia T-Y, Peck EA, Conte JV: Coronary artery disease. In Conte JV, Baumgartner, WA, Dorman T, Owens SG, editors: *The Johns Hopkins Manual of Cardiac Surgical Care*, Philadelphia, 2008, Elsevier, Table 3.2.)

Suggested Reading

Hannan, E. L., et al. (2008). Drug-eluting stents vs coronary artery bypass grafting in multivessel coronary disease. *N Engl J Med*, *358*, 331–341.

Hillis, L. D., et al. (2011). ACCF/AHA guideline for coronary artery bypass graft surgery: A report of the American College of Cardiology Foundation/American Heart Association Task Force on Practice Guidelines. *Circulation*, *124*(23), e652–e735.

Serruys, P. W., et al. (2009). Percutaneous coronary intervention versus coronary artery bypass grafting for severe coronary artery disease. *N Engl J Med*, *360*, 961–972.

Veterans Administration Coronary Artery Bypass Surgery Cooperative Study Group (1984). Eleven-year survival in the Veterans Administration randomized trial of coronary bypass surgery for stable angina. *N Engl J Med*, *311*(21), 1333–1339.

Critical Care

CHAPTER 44

Lethargy After Bowel Resection in a 55-Year-Old Male

Yan Zhong ■ Hui Yi Shan

A 55-year-old male high school teacher with a 10-year history of ulcerative colitis has plans to have an elective total proctocolectomy and J-pouch performed when the school year finishes in 3 months. Unfortunately, he presented to the emergency department four days ago with hypotension, fever, leukocytosis and significant colonic distension. A diagnosis of toxic megacolon was made by clinical and radiographic features (Figure 44.1) and he underwent emergency total abdominal colectomy and end ileostomy. As presented by his surgeon, the revised plan for his definitive treatment will be for elective rectal mucosectomy and J-pouch reconstruction on an elective basis sometime next year.

What is Toxic Megacolon?

Toxic megacolon is a serious, nonobstructive dilation of the colon caused as a complication of inflammatory bowel disease or infectious colitis (e.g. *Clostridium difficile* colitis). While there are many pathophysiologic mechanisms that lead to toxic megacolon, diffuse mucosal inflammation can cause both systemic and local inflammatory reactions. Specifically, inflammatory mediators are thought to induce synthesis of nitric oxide, an inhibitor of smooth muscle tone, and lead to colonic dilation. Patients typically present with abdominal pain and distension, and often have

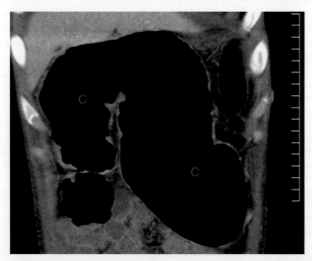

Fig. 44.1 Computed tomography (CT) scan demonstrating severe dilation of the colon (C) with thinning of its walls (red arrows) consistent with toxic megacolon.

349

systemic signs and symptoms of sepsis. Diagnosis is made using physical examination and radiographic evidence of colonic distension. Treatment includes supportive care (hydration, and antibiotics), anti-inflammatory agents for inflammatory bowel disease (e.g. glucocorticoids, infliximab, cyclosporine), and, if there is a failure to respond or if the patient is unstable, a colectomy and end ileostomy. The goal of surgery in patients with toxic megacolon is to remove the offending bowel (which eliminates the source of inflammation and prevents perforation of a severely dilated colon) and create an ostomy since primary anastomosis in this setting would be inappropriate due to the high risk of anastomotic leak.

In a subtotal colectomy, the rectum is left as a rectal stump and is used at the point of anastomosis at the time of ileostomy reversal. While the rectum is typically spared in infectious colitis, the rectal mucosa is usually affected in ulcerative colitis. A mucosectomy (removal of the rectal mucosa only) may be performed at the time of ileostomy reversal in order to decrease the possibility of a relapse of ulcerative colitis in the rectum and to eliminate the future risk of rectal carcinoma based on a history of longstanding ulcerative colitis.

The patient did well in the initial postoperative period achieving hemodynamic stability and symptomatic improvement. He has peri-incisional pain as well as high nasogastric tube (NGT) outputs through post-operative day 3. His NGT is removed on the fourth post-operative day, and his ileostomy began to work on post-operative day 3, though the volume of ileostomy output was very high. On morning rounds on postoperative day 5, he is found to be more lethargic and is difficult to arouse.

What Are the Common Causes of Lethargy in Postoperative Patients?

The common causes of lethargy that should be considered within the first post-operative week are: (1) oral or intravenous **pain medications**, (2) **infections**, and (3) **electrolyte abnormalities**. Narcotic pain medications are often necessary after surgery, though the use of nonopioids, such as ketorolac and acetaminophen, is important when indicated in order to decrease the effect on mental status and gastrointestinal transit issues of opioids, especially in patients at the extremes of age. Postoperative infections, especially pulmonary, urinary, and wound infections, are also somewhat common: and, in addition to common symptoms of each, lethargy can be the first identifiable symptom, especially in the elderly. Due to gastrointestinal losses, fluid shifts, and patients being kept nothing by mouth (NPO), postoperative patients are also at risk for electrolyte abnormalities.

Less likely is the development of an intracranial process (e.g., ischemic stroke or intracranial bleed), though a full assessment, including a neurologic examination, should be performed to identify any abnormalities.

On physical examination, blood pressure is 120/65 mm Hg, pulse rate is 90 bpm, respiration rate is 14/min, temperature is 101.5°F, and weight is 100 kg. The patient is somnolent but responsive and alert, and oriented to time, place, and person when aroused. A neurologic examination is nonfocal. On auscultation, the patient has coarse breath sounds at the bilateral lung bases. His abdomen is soft, nontender, and nondistended, and his laparotomy incision is clean, dry, and nonerythematous. An ileostomy bag is in place with 750 mL output (high), and he has made 1500 mL of clear yellow urine in the past 24 hours. The patient has no peripheral edema, and the remainder of the examination is unremarkable. The patient's last dose of intravenous hydromorphone was 12 hours ago. He was advanced to a clear liquid diet this morning, though he has not been drinking very much according to the nurse, and his intravenous fluids had been reduced to 80 cc/hr.

What Is the Workup for Postoperative Lethargy?

The first step in evaluation is to perform a thorough physical examination and to review the patient's medication list. The examination should include an evaluation of recent vital signs, including trends from the past 24 hours, and a review of a comprehensive record of intakes and outputs, including those from any lines, tubes, or ostomies. If a thorough bedside evaluation of the patient does not reveal clinical concerns that would prompt imaging or reversible causes of somnolence (such as overuse of narcotic medications), laboratory evaluation should be undertaken. The initial laboratory workup may include complete blood count, basic metabolic panel, and urinalysis to look for potential infections, occult bleeding, or electrolyte abnormalities.

A basic metabolic panel reveals: sodium 158 mEq/L, chloride 123 mEq/L, potassium 3.9 mEq/L, calcium 8.2 mEq/L, serum bicarbonate 22 mEq/L, blood urea nitrogen 20 mg/dL, and creatinine 0.8 mg/dL. Serum glucose is 102 mg/dL. Complete blood count and urinalysis are within normal limits except for a leukocytosis of 13,000/μL. The patient is diagnosed with hypernatremia.

What Is the Definition of Hypernatremia and What Is Its Clinical Presentation?

Hypernatremia is defined as a plasma sodium greater than 145 mEq/L. It implies a deficiency of total body water relative to total body sodium. Acute hypernatremia (developed less than 48 hours) may induce neurologic symptoms, such as lethargy, confusion, weakness, irritability, seizure, and coma, due to relatively fast loss of intracellular water (from the brain and other tissues) to the serum by osmosis (Fig. 44.2). Chronic hypernatremia (developed longer than 48 hours) may be relatively asymptomatic, as this water shift occurs more gradually.

What Are the Mechanisms That Can Lead to Hypernatremia?

Hypernatremia develops with increased total body sodium and/or decreased total body water. The main mechanisms resulting in decreased total body water are losses of body fluid. Table 44.1 summarizes the sodium content of common body fluids. The loss of hypoosmolar fluid (<140 mmol Na+/L) tends to exacerbate the development of hypernatremia because more water is lost in relation to sodium. Insensible losses via the skin, such as sweating with a fever, or via the respiratory tract, such as in those who are mechanically ventilated, may also contribute to the development of hypernatremia if water loss was not replaced.

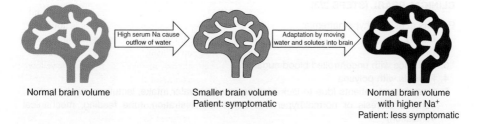

Fig. 44.2 Brain adaptation to hypernatremia. The high serum sodium causes outflow of water, resulting in brain shrinkage. Patients become lethargic and confused. The brain counteracts osmotic shrinkage by increasing the intracellular content of solutes, and water subsequently moves back into the brain cell. This adaptive mechanism prevents the brain cell from excessive shrinkage. Patients become less symptomatic at this time.

TABLE 44.1 ■ Types of Body Fluid Loss and Their Sodium Content

Type of Body Fluid Loss	Na Content
Gastric fluid (vomiting/nasogastric tube)	20–60 mmol Na$^+$/L
Biliary drainage	145 mmol Na$^+$/L
Pancreatic drain or fistula	125–138 mmol Na$^+$/L
Jejunal loss via stoma or fistula	140 mmol Na$^+$/L
Diarrhea or excess colostomy loss	30–140 mmol Na$^+$/L
High-volume ileal loss via new stoma, high stoma or fistula	100–140 mmol Na$^+$/L
Lower-volume ileal loss via established stoma or low fistula	50–100 mmol Na$^+$/L

Isoosmolar fluid 140 mmol Na$^+$/L; hypoosmolar fluid <140 mmol Na$^+$/L.

CLINICAL PEARL (STEP 1/2/3)

Na$^+$ cannot freely traverse cell membranes and is restricted to the extracellular fluid compartment. It is an "effective osmole": it has the ability to create osmotic pressure gradient across cell membrane and shift water from intracellular fluid compartment to the extracellular fluid compartment.

CLINICAL PEARL/BASIC SCIENCE PEARL (STEPS 2/3)

The neurologic symptoms associated with hypernatremia are mostly due to brain cell shrinkage. When serum Na+ increases, the brain cell volume decreases due to outflow of water (see Fig. 44.1). The brain counteracts osmotic shrinkage by increasing the intracellular content of solutes, and water subsequently moves back into the brain cell. This adaptive mechanism prevents the brain cell from excessive shrinkage. Severe neurologic symptoms usually develop when there is acute elevation of serum Na+ higher than 158 mEq/L. Values higher than 180 mEq/L are associated with high mortality, especially in adults.

In healthy individuals, salt intake and water loss seldom result in hypernatremia because the ensuing rise in plasma tonicity stimulates both the release of antidiuretic hormone (ADH) and thirst, thereby minimizing further water loss and increasing water intake. The decrease in water loss and increase in water intake lower the serum sodium concentration back to normal. Hypernatremia develops when the individual cannot respond to thirst, has no access to water, or has salt loading.

CLINICAL PEARL (STEPS 2/3)

Patients at risk for hypernatremia:
1. Elderly
2. Children
3. Diabetics with uncontrolled blood sugar
4. Patients with polyuria
5. Hospitalized patients (due to lack of adequate free water intake, lactulose administration, osmotic diuresis or normal/hypertonic saline administration, tube feeding, mechanical ventilation)

What Is the Approach to Assess a Patient With Hypernatremia?

After the laboratory diagnosis of hypernatremia has been established, further history and physical examination is needed in order to establish the specific cause(s), as this dictates the treatment. History should focus on an assessment of the patient's water intake, potential causes of water loss

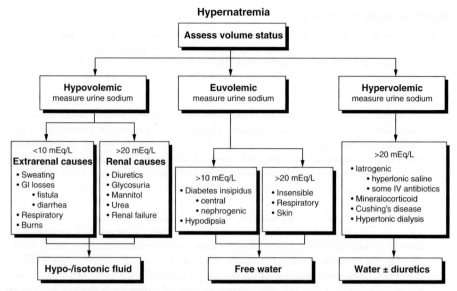

Fig. 44.3 Classification of hypernatremia based on volume status and treatment. (Redrawn from Cameron JL: Electrolyte disorders. In *Current surgical therapy*, ed 10, Philadelphia, 2011, Saunders, pp. 1412–1420.)

(polyuria, diarrhea, increased insensible loss, diuretics, lactulose), assessment for the possibility of salt loading (hypertonic saline, sodium bicarbonate, tube feeding, etc.), and whether patient is symptomatic from the hypernatremia.

Next, utilizing historical laboratory values, the determination needs to be made whether the hypernatremia is chronic or acute.

Finally, the patient's volume status should be assessed. Based on volume status, hypernatremia is classified into hypovolemic hypernatremia (water loss greater than Na^+ loss), hypervolemic hypernatremia (Na^+ gain greater than water gain), or euvolemic hypernatremia (pure water loss) (Fig. 44.3).

What Are the Treatments for Hypernatremia?
The treatment of hypernatremia is composed of five steps:

1. The correction of the underlying causes such as diarrhea, hyperglycemia, diuretic uses, hypokalemia, and hypercalcemia.
2. Estimation of volume status, which is extremely important. For hypovolemic hypernatremia, normal saline should be administered initially until hemodynamic stability is established. In this setting, restoration of the tissue perfusion is more urgent than correction of the serum sodium. Normal saline may actually lower the plasma sodium concentration because it is hypoosmolar relative to the hypernatremic patient. More diluted solutions can be used once tissue perfusion is adequate.
3. Calculation of water deficit.

$$water\ deficit = TBW \times \left[\frac{actual\ serum\,Na^+}{desired\ serum\,Na^+} - 1 \right]$$

Total body water (TBW): 0.5 × body weight in female; 0.6 × body weight in male

CLINICAL PEARL (STEPS 2/3)

The major complication of overly rapid correction of hypernatremia is cerebral edema. As the serum sodium concentration is rapidly lowered, the relative osmolarity inside the brain cell becomes higher, and this leads to water influx into the brain cell. It is generally agreed that the rate of correction of hypernatremia does not exceed 12 mEq/L in the first 24 hours.

The patient's insensible water losses and losses from other sources must also be considered (insensible loss: 0.5 L/day in floor patients, 1L/day in ICU patients, or patients with high-grade fever). Urine output, surgical drainage, ileostomy/colostomy output, and nasogastric tube suction, if large in volume, need to be replaced adequately. Because the majority of these fluids are hypoosmolar, significant losses will lead to hypernatremia (see Table 44.1).

4. Selection and route of fluid administration. If the patient can tolerate oral fluids, giving free water by mouth or nasogastric tube is preferred. Otherwise, the water deficit can be replaced intravenously. Several fluids are available, though they differ in osmolarity, and therefore the volume of the administered fluid that remains intravascularly (Table 44.2). A solution of 5% dextrose in water (D5W) is an ideal fluid for correcting hypernatremia. After being metabolized by the liver, the free water is equally distributed among all compartments of TBW; only 84 mL (one-twelfth of 1 L of D5W) stays intravascularly. On the other hand, after 1 L of 0.9% normal saline infusion, one-fourth (250 mL) stays intravascularly and can be used for volume repletion, but it is not ideal for the treatment of hypernatremia. Other solutions that may be used to treat hypernatremia include 0.45% or 0.225% saline.

5. Rate of correction. A reduction of 6 to 8 mEq/L per 24 hours in serum sodium concentration is appropriate for chronic hypernatremia that developed over a period longer than 48 hours. For acute hypernatremia that develops within 48 hours, the rate of correction can be 1 mEq/L/h. It is important to remember that free water deficit equation only provides an approximation of patient's water deficit. Serial measurements of the plasma sodium concentration every 4 to 6 hours are required to ascertain that the desired rate of correction is being achieved and to avoid overcorrection.

CLINICAL PEARL (STEPS 1/2/3)

Infusion of dextrose-containing fluid in treating hypernatremia may exacerbate hyperglycemia, particularly in diabetic patients. Uncontrolled blood glucose can cause osmotic diuresis. More free water is lost in the urine, thereby raising serum Na+. This could be avoided by giving free water orally or through a nasogastric tube.

TABLE 44.2 ■ Types of Intravenous Fluids (IVF) and Their Effect on Intravascular Space: Approximate Distribution of 250 mL of IVF in Body Compartments

Fluid	Intracellular (mL)	Interstitial (mL)	Intravascular (mL)
D5W	166	63	21
Normal saline (0.9%)	0	188	62
Ringer's lactate	0	188	62
Albumin (5%)	0	25	225
Albumin (25%)	0	−750	1000
Hetastarch (6%)	0	0	250
Packed red blood cells	0	0	250

CLINICAL PEARL (STEPS 1/2/3)

Direct intravenous infusion of water (not oral intake) can cause significant hemolysis. Five percent dextrose in water is essentially iso-osmolar at the time of infusion. Dextrose is quickly metabolized by the liver, which leaves the free water behind to dilute serum Na^+ without causing hemolysis.

On examination, the patient has no signs or symptoms of volume depletion/overload; he is euvolemic. The patient's surgical team calculates his free water deficit:
- His actual serum Na^+ is 158 mEq/L and a target serum sodium is set at 150 mEq/L (to be achieved in the next 24 hours).
- His body weight: 100 kg
- His water deficit $= 0.6 \times 100\,kg \times (158/150 - 1) = 3.2$ L
- The patient's insensible losses are estimated to be 1 L per day because he is febrile. After adding the insensible loss of 1 L, water deficit is about 4.2 L.

Because the patient is not tolerating liquids by mouth due to the recent bowel resection, he is started on intravenous 5% dextrose at 175 mL/hour (4.2 L/24hours = 0.175 L/h) initially. Basic metabolic panel is monitored every 6 hours. The intravenous rate of 5% dextrose is subsequently adjusted based on the serial serum Na^+ concentration. His serum sodium is corrected to 140 mEq/L over 72 hours and his mentation is back to baseline after serum sodium is corrected. Concurrently, his mental status improves. He is ultimately advanced to a regular diet, his serum sodium stabilizes off IV fluids, and he is discharged home without complication.

BEYOND THE PEARLS

- It is important to understand the difference between dehydration and volume depletion. Dehydration is defined as a reduction in TBW without proportional reduction in serum Na^+ and K, whereas volume depletion is defined as the loss of both serum Na^+ and TBW.
- Diabetes insipidus (DI) is an important cause of euvolemic hypernatremia if water intake does not match the patient's water loss via urine output.
- Hypercalcemia (serum Ca^{2+} > 11 mg/dL) and hypokalemia (serum K^+ < 3 mmol/L) may cause nephrogenic diabetes insipidus, leading to hypernatremia.
- Common drugs that may cause hypernatremia are cisplatin, aminoglycosides, Dilantin, ethanol, corticosteroids or vasopressin receptor inhibitors (vaptans), lithium, and vitamins A and D.
- D5W, 0.45% saline, or 0.225% saline can be utilized for correction of hypernatremia.
- A reduction of 6 to 8 mEq/L per 24 hours in serum sodium concentration is appropriate for chronic hypernatremia, whereas a reduction 1 mEq/L/h is appropriate for acute hypernatremia.

Suggested Readings

Brenner, B. M., & Clarkson, M. R. (2005). *Brenner & Rector's the kidney* (7th ed.). Philadephia: Elsevier Saunders.

Cameron, J. L. (2011). Electrolyte disorders. In *Current surgical therapy* (10th ed.). Philadelphia: Saunders, pp. 1412–1420.

National Institute for Health and Care Excellence (NICE). (December 10, 2013). *Intravenous fluid therapy in Q7 adults in hospital (CG174)*. https://www.nice.org.uk/guidance/cg174.

Preston, R. (2018). Hypernatremia. In *Acid-base, fluids, and electrolytes made ridiculously, simple*. Miami, FL: MedMaster Inc. pp. 57–62.

Reddi, A. S. (2014). *Fluid, electrolyte and acid-base disorders*. New York: Springer, pp. 133–144.

CHAPTER 45

Acidosis in an Intubated 45-Year-Old Male

Kelly Fan ■ Reza Ronaghi ■ Raj Dasgupta

A 45-year-old male with a past medical history of diabetes mellitus presents to the emergency department complaining of shortness of breath, fever, and productive cough for the past week. On initial assessment, the patient appears to be using accessory muscles of respiration, and his pulse oximetry reading is 82%. He is intubated for increased work of breathing and hypoxia and is transferred to the intensive care unit (ICU). Upon arrival, the ICU team orders a chest radiograph (Fig. 45.1) and laboratory evaluation, including an arterial blood gas (ABG), which are shown here.

White blood cells 34.1
Hemoglobin 10.4,
Platelets 242
Sodium 134
Bicarbonate 26
Creatinine 0.29
Albumin 3.0
Lactate 1.1
ABG: pH 7.15; P_{CO_2} 85; P_{O_2} 64; HCO_3^- 13.8
Ventilator Settings: Volume Control: volume: 450, rate: 18, F_{IO_2}: 100%, PEEP: 10

How Does One Interpret an Arterial Blood Gas?

When analyzing an arterial blood gas (ABG), similar to many complex tasks in medicine, it is important to follow an organized method every time.

1. Look at the pH and determine whether it is within normal range or represents an acidosis or alkalosis:
   a. Normal pH range: 7.35 to 7.45
   b. Acidosis less than 7.35
   c. Alkalosis greater than 7.45
2. If the pH is abnormal, determine whether it is a respiratory or metabolic process.
   a. Normal values and expected alterations
      i. A normal P_{CO_2} is 40, and any alteration indicates a respiratory process. CO_2 generates acidic ions, so an increase in P_{CO_2} results in a drop in the pH.
      ii. A normal bicarbonate is 24, and any alteration indicates a metabolic process. Bicarbonate (HCO_3^-) is a basic ion, so an increase in bicarbonate results in an increase in the pH.
   b. If the patient is acidotic, look for an increased P_{CO_2} (respiratory) or decreased bicarbonate (metabolic) primary cause for the acidosis.
   c. If the patient is alkalotic, look for a decreased P_{CO_2} (respiratory) or increased bicarbonate (metabolic) primary cause for the acidosis.

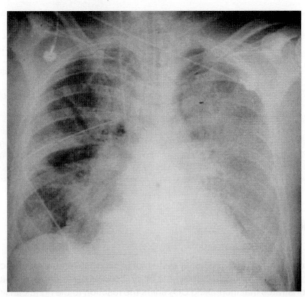

Fig. 45.1   Chest radiograph demonstrating diffuse bilateral opacities. (From Ware LB, Bastarache JA, Bernard GR: Acute respiratory distress syndrome. In Vincent J-L, Abraham E, Moore FA, et al., editors: *Textbook of critical care*, ed 4, Philadelphia, 2017, Elsevier, pp 413–424.)

Example: Respiratory acidosis—low pH with high P_{CO_2}
Respiratory alkalosis: high pH with low P_{CO_2}
Metabolic acidosis: low pH with low HCO_3^-
Metabolic alkalosis: high pH with high HCO_3^-

3. Determine whether there is compensation or a secondary process occurring.
   a. Compensation is a normal process utilized by the body in an attempt to correct an abnormal pH. Compensation is unable to bring the pH back to the normal range.
      i. The compensation for a metabolic process would be respiratory (increasing or decreasing the rate of pulmonary CO_2 exhalation). This can be accomplished rapidly. For example, the compensation for a metabolic alkalosis would be CO_2 retention by decreasing ventilation.
      ii. The compensation for a respiratory process would be metabolic (increasing or decreasing the rate of renal HCO_3^- secretion). This often takes time. For example, the compensation for a respiratory acidosis would be increasing HCO_3^- reabsorption in the kidneys.
      iii. There are several methods to determine whether the compensation observed is appropriate.
   b. A secondary process is an abnormal process affecting the pH and can possibly bring the pH back into the normal range (e.g., a respiratory alkalosis superimposed on a metabolic acidosis).
4. If there is a metabolic acidosis, determine whether there is an anion gap in order to inform the differential diagnosis of the cause:

$$\text{Anion gap} = Na^+ - (Cl^- + HCO_3^-); \text{ normal is 8 to 12}$$

5. After a thorough analyses of primary and secondary disturbances and whether there is compensation, determining the underlying cause(s) is important in order to treat and correct them. Table 45.1 lists the differential diagnosis for each type of disturbance.

TABLE 45.1 ■ Causes of Metabolic and Respiratory Acidosis and Alkalosis

Metabolic Acidosis	Nonanion gap: diarrhea and GI loss, RTA, acetazolamide, urethral diversion, hyperalimentation. Anion gap: methanol, uremia, DKA, paraldehyde, INH, lactic acidosis, ethylene glycol or ethanol and salicylate
Metabolic Alkalosis	GI loss (vomiting, loose HCL), loop and thiazide diuretics, renal loss of H^+ (increase aldosterone, increase cortisol, CHF, cirrhosis)
Respiratory Acidosis	Decreased airway drive, COPD, asthma, OSA/OHS, anything that causes decreased breathing drive, increased CO_2 production: sepsis, hypermetabolism
Respiratory Alkalosis	Hypoxia from lung disease, fever, pain, anxiety, panic attack (anything that would increase respiratory drive), anemia, increased ICP, PE, PTX, pneumonia, effusion, salicylates, progesterone, sepsis, pregnancy

BASIC SCIENCE PEARL

$$CO_2 + H_2O <\!-\!-> H_2CO_3 <\!-\!-> H^+ + HCO_3^-$$

This equation demonstrates the buffer system of bicarbonate and carbonic acid in the blood that allows for the balance of acid-base in the body. Le Chatelier's principle related to shifting equilibria demonstrates that increasing CO_2 shifts the reaction to the right, causing an increase in H^+ (acidosis), whereas increasing HCO_3^- shifts the reaction to the left, decreasing H^+ (alkalosis).

The patient's arterial blood gas is analyzed:

With a pH of 7.14, he is acidotic. His P_{CO_2} is 85 indicating that he is retaining carbon dioxide and has a primary respiratory acidosis. His bicarbonate is 26, within the normal range, indicating that this is an acute respiratory acidosis, as there has not been time for any major metabolic compensation.

Importantly, it is noted that the patient's P_{O_2} is only 64 despite being supported with 100% oxygen. Remember a P_{O_2} on 100% oxygen should normally be close to 500. This raises concern for a primary pulmonary disease, specifically acute respiratory failure.

Given that the patient was already intubated, he was placed on 100% oxygen with a positive end expiratory pressure (PEEP) of 5, and his respiratory rate was set at 22 breaths per minute and a tidal volume of 450 cc/breath.

What Are the Therapeutic Options Available for Correcting Acid-Base Disturbances?

In a nonventilated patient with respiratory acidosis, noninvasive ventilation (i.e., BIPAP or CPAP) can be used to improve ventilation and allow for reduction in the partial pressure of arterial carbon dioxide. Most patients will also receive the additional benefit of improved oxygenation. Those who fail noninvasive ventilation should undergo endotracheal intubation. The goal of intubation and noninvasive ventilation is to increase ventilation (either the respiratory rate, the tidal volume, or both) and to increase exhalation of CO_2 in an acidotic patient. Conversely, in an alkalotic patient, ventilation can be decreased, thus allowing for the retention of CO_2. The patient's oxygenation can be increased by increasing the oxygen content of inspired air or by increasing the positive end expiratory pressure (PEEP), which keeps alveoli open and available for gas exchange at the end of expiration. Monitoring serial ABGs allows the clinician to alter these settings in real time to correct respiratory derangements in acid-base status and oxygenation.

Sodium bicarbonate can be used in metabolic acidosis with a pH less than 7.1 to buffer the acidosis until the primary process is reversed; however its role in respiratory acidosis is limited. Bicarbonate does have some negative side effects, which include increased arterial and capillary P_{CO_2}, increased lactate generation, hypocalcemia, hypernatremia, and extracellular volume expansion. Referring to the acid-base equilibrium discussed earlier, the bicarbonate first must combine with hydrogen ion to form H_2CO_3, which dehydrates to CO_2 and H_2O. Finally, the CO_2 can be exhaled from the body. This elimination depends on adequate ventilation to be effective.

Hemodialysis can more quickly improve metabolic derangements in patients with chronic kidney disease than other available treatments, though its role is limited in the treatment of primary respiratory disorders.

Finally, patients with hypercarbia and poor ventilation despite intubation can undergo extracorporeal CO_2 removal. A large venous catheter is inserted, and an extracorporeal membrane diffusion device is utilized to remove CO_2 from the body. Patients with poor ventilation are likely to have problems with oxygenation as well, and this device can also oxygenate the blood simultaneously in a (better-known) process called extracorporeal membrane oxygenation (ECMO) (see later in this chapter for more details).

BASIC SCIENCE PEARL

In patient with acidosis and a low pH, the low pH will inhibit the enzyme phosphofructokinase that inhibits glycolysis and inhibits the production of lactate. Infusion of bicarbonate will temporarily increase the pH, remove the inhibition on the enzyme, and cause an increase in lactate production.

What Is the Differential Diagnosis for a Patient Who Presents in Respiratory Failure?

It is important to address the ABCs (airway, breathing, and circulation) in patients who present with a critical illness such as acute respiratory failure. Once stabilized, the underlying causes of the respiratory failure can be uncovered. The differential diagnosis for acute respiratory failure includes pneumonia, pulmonary edema, and acute respiratory distress syndrome (ARDS). Chest radiograph may reveal some findings, such as lobar consolidation in pneumonia, that may favor one diagnosis over another, but it is often difficult to determine the exact cause without adjunct diagnostic methods. Diffuse alveolar infiltrates (such as in this case) can be identified on many chest radiographs of patients in acute respiratory failure, and this can be caused by fluid from pulmonary edema, the inflammatory process related to an infection, or represent blood in diffuse alveolar hemorrhage.

What Are the Diagnostic Criteria for Acute Respiratory Distress Syndrome?

ARDS is a diffuse, inflammatory lung disease that occurs within 1 week of a known risk factor and leads to diffuse alveolar damage. Risk factors for development of ARDS are classified by either indirect (via increased vascular permeability) or direct (via pulmonary epithelial damage) modes of lung injury (Box 45.1). Management remains consistent regardless of the underlying risk factor. Although the definition and categorization of ARDS has evolved, the Berlin definition (Box 45.2), established in 2012, is the current standard. The severity of ARDS, as defined by the partial pressure of oxygen to fraction of inspired oxygen ratio (PaO_2/FiO_2), is assessed in intubated patients at a minimum positive end expiratory pressure (PEEP) of 5 cm of water.

BOX 45.1 ■ Risk Factors for Development of ARDS

Risk Factors Causing Increased Vascular Permeability

Septic shock
Pancreatitis
Major burn injury
Blood transfusions
Extrapulmonary trauma/hemorrhagic shock
Drug overdose
Cardiopulmonary bypass
Reperfusion/reexpansion pulmonary edema

Risk Factors Causing Direct Epithelial Injury

Pneumonia
Acute aspiration
Direct pulmonary trauma/lung contusion
Drowning
Inhalation injury

BOX 45.2 ■ Berlin Definition 2012 for ARDS

Timing	Onset within 1 week of a known risk factor
Radiographic findings	Bilateral opacities not explained by effusions, nodules, or atelectasis
Cardiac involvement	Respiratory pathology cannot be fully explained by cardiac causes; objective evaluation of cardiac function with echocardiography or pulmonary artery catheterization is recommended in patients without a known risk factor
Severity	PaO_2/FiO_2 at minimum PEEP of 5 cm of water
	201–300: Mild
	101–200: Moderate
	0–100: Severe

What Are Specific Ventilator Strategies Used in Patients With ARDS?

The focus of mechanical ventilation in ARDS patients is to prevent further volutrauma (regional overdistension of the lung), atelectrauma (repetitive opening and closing of lung units, amplifying strain and denaturing surfactant), and oxygen toxicity. Perhaps the most significant finding from the ARDS network study was that patients ventilated with lower tidal volumes (4 to 6 mL/kg) showed a significant mortality benefit and increased number of ventilator-free days compared with traditional tidal volume (12 mL/kg) ventilation.

Additional recommendations from the ARDS network investigation include optimizing plateau pressure (measure of lung compliance to lower than 30 cm of water, adjusting FiO_2 and PEEP to achieve an oxygen saturation of 88% to 95%, and adjusting respiratory rate to achieve a pH of 7.30 to 7.45. Permissive hypercapnia should be tolerated to maintain low tidal volume strategy and a respiratory rate lower than 35 breaths per minute. Implementation of these recommendations will increase the likelihood of remaining in the lung protective zone of the pressure volume curve. Risk of atelectrauma will be minimized with addition of PEEP, and risk of volutrauma will minimized with low tidal volume ventilation.

TABLE 45.2 ■ Therapies Beneficial in Management of ARDS Patients

Therapy	Benefit	Theoretical Risk
Conservative fluid management	Decreases pulmonary edema, more ventilator and ICU-free days	Electrolyte disorders and metabolic alkalosis
Corticosteroids	Moderate doses for a longer duration may decrease inflammation	Not useful in patients after 13 days of respiratory failure onset, as these patients likely already progressed to fibrotic stage
Pulmonary vasodilators	Improve oxygenation by increasing alveolar blood flow	Can worsen ventilation perfusion mismatch by perfusing dead space
Paralytics	Lower mortality, increase ventilator-free days, and decrease risk of pneumothorax	Prolonged use increases the risk of myopathy
Proning	Improves distribution of ventilation, trend toward decreased mortality in severe ARDS	Difficult for nurses to manage, often requires specialized hospital beds

In addition to lung-protective ventilation, the ARDS network investigators have described additional strategies to be beneficial in management of patients with ARDS (Table 45.2).

Perhaps the most aggressive tool that should be considered in patients with severe refractory ARDS after all measures have failed is the use of veno-venous extracorporeal membrane oxygenation (V-V ECMO). A large cannula is placed in a central vein. Blood is mechanically pumped from the vein through the extracorporeal circuit into an oxygenator. The oxygenator contains a blood-gas interface for oxygenation and carbon dioxide removal. The oxygenated blood is then returned to the central vein for systemic distribution. When on V-V ECMO, mechanical ventilator settings should be adjusted to minimize the risk of further lung injury. Anticoagulation is required in all patients on ECMO therapy. In patients with cardiogenic shock in addition to refractory respiratory failure, veno-arterial extracorporeal membrane oxygenation (V-A ECMO) in which blood is returned to the arterial circulation can be considered.

ECMO use has been expanding in the last decade, and more centers are acquiring this technology. Because of the expense involving ECMO usage, patient selection is critical. Optimal V-V or V-A ECMO candidates should include patients without significant comorbidities and with a reversible cause of the underlying cardiac or respiratory failure. ECMO can also be used as a bridge to heart or lung transplant. Irreversible brain injury, metastatic cancer, and conditions precluding the use of anticoagulation are contraindications.

A sputum analysis is performed, which demonstrates Gram-positive cocci on Gram stain. The patient is diagnosed with pneumonia complicated by acute respiratory distress syndrome given his bilateral pulmonary infiltrates and low PaO_2/FiO_2 ratio. Antibiotics are initiated in addition to lung-protective ventilation strategies. Despite these, his Po_2 on ABG remains lower than 85% over the next 24 hours. The decision is made to initiate ECMO. Over the course of the next week, the patient's oxygenation improves, daily chest radiographs reveal improvement in parenchymal consolidation, and he is able to be extubated. After transfer from the ICU to the step-down unit, the patient is discharged home on hospital day 16.

BEYOND THE PEARLS

- Acid-base disturbances can be characterized as respiratory or metabolic in nature. A secondary process may be superimposed on the primary process and normalize the pH. Compensatory mechanisms help bring the pH back toward normal but are unable to completely normalize the pH.
- Hypoxemia can be caused by problems with primary pulmonary diseases or other conditions (e.g., cardiovascular and neuromuscular) that affect the ability to oxygenate.
- Aberrations in a patient's acid-base status and oxygenation are most accurately monitored via serial arterial blood gases (ABGs).
- Acidosis, alkalosis, and hypoxemia can be addressed in an intubated patient by adjusting ventilator settings. Tidal volume and respiratory rate can be adjusted to increase or decrease P_{CO_2}, and the inhaled air's oxygen content (F_{iO_2}) and positive end expiratory pressure (PEEP) can be adjusted to increase or decrease P_{O_2}.
- Acute respiratory distress syndrome (ARDS) is a diffuse inflammatory lung disease with many underlying causes. Treatment options include those related to changes in ventilation as well as physical and systemic therapies aimed at improving ventilation.
- Extracorporeal membrane oxygenation (ECMO) can be used to maintain adequate gas exchange through membrane exchange in patients in whom maximal respiratory support is insufficient.

References

Acute Respiratory Distress Syndrome Network. (2000). Ventilation with lower tidal volumes as compared with traditional tidal volumes for acute lung injury and the acute respiratory distress syndrome. *N Engl J Med, 342* (18), 1301–1308.

Amato, M. B. P., et al. (2015). Driving pressure and survival in the acute respiratory distress syndrome. *N Engl J Med, 372*(8), 747–755.

Brodie, D., & Bacchetta, M. (2011). Extracorporeal membrane oxygenation for ARDS in adults. *N Engl J Med, 365*(20), 1905–1914.

Guerin, C., et al. (2013). Prone positioning in severe acute respiratory distress syndrome. *N Engl J Med, 368*(23), 2159–2168.

National Heart, Lung, and Blood Institute. (2006). Acute Respiratory Distress Syndrome Clinical Trials Network: Comparison of two fluid-management strategies in acute lung injury. *N Engl J Med, 354*(24), 2564–2575.

Papazian, L., et al. (2010). Neuromuscular blockers in early acute respiratory distress syndrome. *N Engl J Med, 363*(12), 1107–1116.

Peek, G. J., et al. (2009). Efficacy and economic assessment of conventional ventilatory support versus extracorporeal membrane oxygenation for severe adult respiratory failure (CESAR): A multicentre randomised controlled trial. *Lancet., 374*(9698), 1351–1363.

Thompson, B. T., et al. (2017). Acute respiratory distress syndrome. *N Engl J Med, 377*(6), 562–572.

CHAPTER 46

Chest Pain, Aortic Dissection and ATN in a 52-Year-Old Male

Annika Khine ■ Hui Yi Shan

A 52-year-old male with a past medical history of poorly controlled hypertension presents to the emergency department with an acute onset of chest pain radiating to the back and neck. The pain started shortly after eating dinner, and the intensity is 8 out of 10. He describes the pain as being tearing and substernal. The patient also reports associated lightheadedness and intermittent left arm numbness. There were no alleviating factors at home, but since his arrival to the hospital, IV morphine seems to help with the pain. Otherwise, patient denies shortness of breath, hemoptysis, nausea, or vomiting. He denies any recent illnesses. He is a social drinker and does not use tobacco or illicit drugs. He also does not take any medications at home.

What Is the Differential Diagnosis of Chest Pain?

There are several conditions to consider in a patient with an acute onset of chest pain. Myocardial infarction, unstable angina, aortic dissection, pulmonary embolism, and pneumothorax are potential life-threatening conditions that need an urgent evaluation and intervention. It is worth noting that pneumonia and pericarditis could also present with chest pain; however, the intensity of pain may not be as severe. Boerhaave syndrome, which is a spontaneous esophageal wall rupture that typically occurs after forceful emesis, could present with intense chest pain as well. Other potential gastrointestinal causes of chest pain include pancreatitis, peptic ulcer disease, and cholecystitis— patients may complain of "chest" pain that is actually located in the upper abdomen or abdominal pain that radiates to the chest.

What Are the Important Aspects of the History and Physical Examination in a Patient With Chest Pain?

It is important to discern as much detail from the history as possible about the severity, location and duration of the pain, as well as any other associated symptoms because one must rule out life-threatening etiologies of chest pain quickly. A history of cardiovascular disease (myocardial ischemia, peripheral vascular disease) and other associated medical comorbidities (hypertension, hyperlipidemia, diabetes) should raise suspicion for a cardiovascular etiology. Physical examination should be directed at the evaluation of the heart (rate, rhythm) and lungs (auscultation bilaterally). Although abnormalities may be detected on physical (e.g. hypertension, tachycardia, wheezing), most are nonspecific physical findings, and further workup is necessary to fully assess the patient.

Vital signs on admission include a temperature of 97.5 °F, heart rate of 90 bpm, blood pressure 198/115 mm Hg with O_2 saturation 99% on 2 L nasal cannula. On initial assessment, the patient appears diaphoretic and is in moderate distress. The physical examination is significant for sinus tachycardia, and no murmur is detected. Lungs are clear to auscultation except for mild inspiratory crackles at the left lower lung field. His abdomen is nontender and nondistended. There is no peripheral edema on examination. Cranial nerves are intact, and motor strength is 5 out of 5 in all four extremities. The rest of the neurologic examination is unremarkable.

Based on the Differential Diagnosis, What Laboratory Tests and Imaging Should Be Ordered Initially?

Basic laboratory analyses such as complete blood count (CBC) and basic metabolic panel (BMP) should be routinely ordered but may not reveal specific pathologies. However, cardiac markers (troponin), d-dimer, electrocardiogram (ECG), and chest radiograph are all important adjuncts to the initial assessment that can help reveal the underlying cause of the patient's symptoms. For both ECG and chest radiography, it is helpful to compare to historical studies if available, because the assessment of changes from baseline is often important. For example, new bundle branch blocks or the increase in the size of a pulmonary effusion can help inform the differential diagnosis.

On laboratory analysis the patient's troponin is mildly elevated at 0.12, and his ECG is notable for sinus tachycardia without ST segment changes. Chest radiograph reveals a small left-sided pleural effusion with a widened mediastinum (Fig. 46.1). After a discussion with the emergency physician about the concern for aortic pathology, the patient undergoes a CT angiogram and is found to have Type A aortic dissection. Cardiothoracic surgery is consulted; they recommend operative repair, and, after informed consent is obtained, the patient is taken to the operating room for sternotomy and open repair of his dissection.

CLINICAL PEARL (STEP 1/2)

Aortic dissection is typically caused by a circumferential or transverse tear of the intima (Fig. 46.2). The Stanford classification divides aortic dissections into two types. Stanford Type A involves the ascending aorta, regardless of the site of primary intimal tear. All other dissections are classified as Stanford Type B (Fig. 46.3).

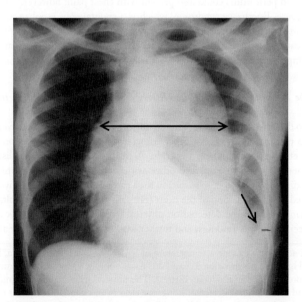

Fig. 46.1   Chest radiograph revealing an enlarged mediastinum *(double arrow)* and left pleural effusion *(single arrow)*. (From Herring W: Recognizing adult heart disease. In *Learning radiology*, ed 3, Philadelphia, 2016, Elsevier, pp 114–128.)

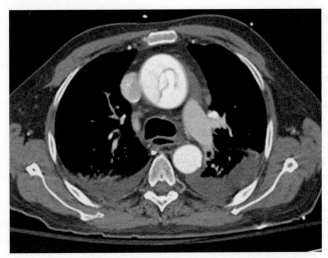

Fig. 46.2   Thin-slice CT image of a classic ascending dissection with aneurysmal dilation. (From Cameron AM, Cameron JL: *Current surgical therapy*, Philadelphia, 2011, Elsevier Saunders.)

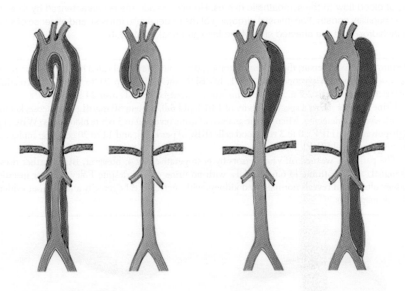

Stanford Type A   Stanford Type B

Fig. 46.3   Stanford classification of aortic dissection. (From Conrad M, Cambria R: Aortic dissection. In J. L. Cronenwett & K. W. Johnston (Eds.) *Rutherford's vascular surgery*, ed 4, Philadelphia, 2015, Elsevier, pp 2169–2188.)

CLINICAL PEARL (STEP 1/2/3)

Risk factors for aortic dissections include:
- Long-standing hypertension
- Genetic or developmental disorders such as Marfan syndrome, Loeys-Dietz syndrome, and Ehlers Danlos syndrome
- Bicuspid aortic valve
- Aortitis such as Takayasu's arteritis, giant cell arteritis
- Pregnancy (especially third trimester)
- Cocaine use (can be remote history)

What Are Common Complications of Aortic Dissection?

Aortic dissections and their repair both have high rates of morbidity. Based on the pathophysiology, dissections involving the aortic root can bleed into the pericardium and may lead to cardiac tamponade. Patients may also develop acute aortic insufficiency or regurgitation as a result of aortic dissection, which may be diagnosed by auscultating a new low-pitched early diastolic murmur. More globally, hypoperfusion of vital organs can occur when there is end-organ ischemia from aortic branch compromise or hypotension due to blood loss or low flow pre- or intraoperatively. Depending on the affected vessels, complications can include strokes, paralysis, mesenteric and bowel ischemia, extremity ischemia, and renal failure.

CLINICAL PEARL (STEP 1/2/3)

Horner syndrome could manifest when blood supply to the carotid artery is affected, resulting in loss of blood flow to the sympathetic nerves. Horner's syndrome is characterized by three features: pupillary constriction (miosis), drooping of the upper eyelid (ptosis), and absence of sweating (anhidrosis) on the affected side of the face and neck (Fig. 46.4).

Despite a successful repair, the patient's intraoperative course is complicated by hypotension requiring vasopressors. On postoperative day 1, his BUN increases from 21 to 35 mg/dL, creatinine increases from 0.98 to 2.2 mg/dL, and his urine output is 380 mL over 24 hours.

Urine analysis shows a specific gravity of 1.010, pH 6.0, protein 30 mg/dL; no glucose, ketones, or leukocytes are detected. Microscopic analysis of urine reveals 0 to 5 white blood cells (WBCs) per high-power field (HPF), 0 to 3 red blood cells (RBCs) per HPF, and 11 to 20 coarse granular casts per low-power field (LPF).

The patient is weaned off vasopressors by postoperative day 4; however, BUN further rises to 80 mg/dL and creatinine to 6.64 mg/dL, with no urine output despite Foley catheter insertion. Kidney ultrasound reveals normal-sized kidneys with increased echogenicity and without evidence of hydronephrosis.

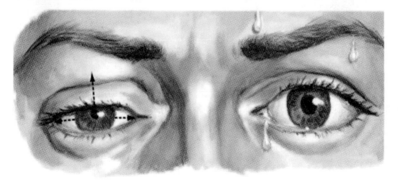

Fig. 46.4 Horner's syndrome is due to interruption of the sympathetic fibers outside of the brain, resulting in ipsilateral miosis, ptosis, and anhidrosis without abnormal ocular mobility. (From Hansen JT: *Netter's clinical anatomy*, ed 4, Philadelphia, 2014, Elsevier.)

What Is the Differential Diagnosis for the Cause of Postoperative Renal Failure?

Acute Kidney Injury (AKI) is characterized by rapid loss of kidney function over hours to days, resulting in accumulation of creatinine, urea, and other waste products and/or decreased urine output. It is associated with significant in-hospital morbidity and mortality. The most common cause of hospital-acquired AKI is acute tubular necrosis (ATN), which represents damage and destruction of the renal tubular epithelial cells, and is most commonly caused by ischemia or toxins.

For patients experiencing postoperative renal failure, Prerenal azotemia from reduced renal perfusion and acute tubular necrosis (ATN) from various nephrotoxic insults would be the top two differential diagnoses. The patient's medication list should be thoroughly reviewed, and any agents that have nephrotoxic properties should be avoided. Hypotension and the use of vasopressors are an important contributors to postoperative renal failure, as a significant decrease in renal blood flow can result in acute tubular necrosis. Additionally, contrast exposure CT scan and any intraoperative exposure during endovascular cases can lead to of kidney injury.

What Is the Significance of Coarse Granular Casts in Urine Sediment?

The presence of coarse granular casts, otherwise known as "muddy-brown casts" (Fig. 46.5), in urine sediment supports the diagnosis of acute tubular necrosis. These casts are a result of necrotic tubular cells sloughing into the tubular lumen and can cause tubular obstruction (Fig. 46.6 and 46.7). Associated anuria and rapid increase of BUN and creatinine support the diagnosis of ATN. Common causes of ATN are severe ischemia due to prolonged prerenal state and exposure to nephrotoxic agents.

CLINICAL PEARL (STEP 3)

Postoperative patients are especially at an increased risk for developing ATN due to preexisting intravascular volume depletion, anesthesia-induced hemodynamic changes, intraoperative blood loss, or fluid loss. Procedures that are commonly associated with high rates of acute kidney injury (AKI) are cardiopulmonary bypass, vascular procedures with aortic cross-clamping, and intraperitoneal procedures. Repetitive prerenal insults and combined injury from nephrotoxins may further increase risk of AKI and progression to ATN.

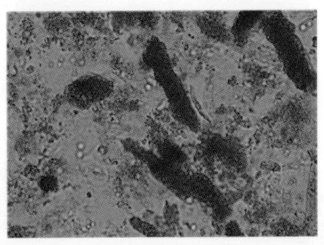

Fig. 46.5 Muddy-brown casts in acute tubular necrosis. (From Ferri FF: *Ferri's color atlas and text of clinical medicine*, Philadelphia, 2009, Elsevier Saunders.)

Tubular Factors in the Development of Acute Tubular Necrosis

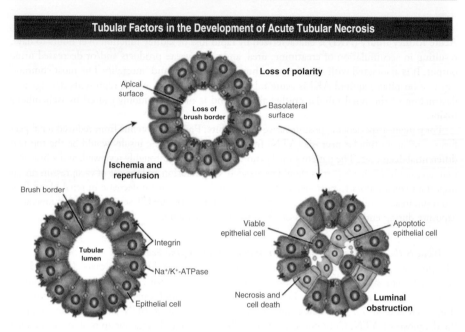

Fig. 46.6 Pathogenesis of ATN. Loss of cell polarity results in weakening of cell-to-cell and cell matrix adhesion, resulting in cast obstruction and eventual renal dysfunction. (From Johnson RJ, Feehally J, Flöge J, editors:. *Comprehensive clinical nephrology*, ed 5, Philadelphia, 2015, Elsevier Saunders, pp 802–817.)

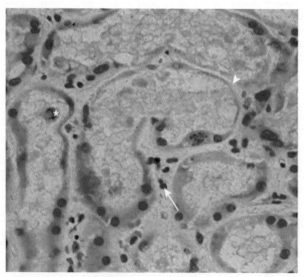

Fig. 46.7 Morphology of acute tubular necrosis in human biopsy specimen. There is a significant proximal tubular cell damage with intraluminal accumulation of apical membrane fragments and detached cells (*), as well as thinning of proximal cells to maintain monolayer tubule integrity *(arrow)*. (From Molitoris BA: Actin cytoskeleton in ischemic acute renal failure, *Kidney Intl* 66(2):871–883, 2004.)

TABLE 46.1 ■ **Comparison of Prerenal vs ATN Urinary Indices**

	Prerenal	ATN
Fractional sodium excretion (FeNa)	< 1%	> 1%*
Urine sodium	< 20 mmol/L	> 40 mmol/L
Urine specific gravity	> 1.018	1.010
Urine osmolality	> 500 mOsm/kg H_2O	300mOsm/kg H_2O

*Note that Fe_{Na} may be affected if diuretics are being used. Also, Fe_{Na} can be less than 1% in ATN associated with radiocontrast media.

BASIC SCIENCE/CLINICAL PEARL (STEP 1/2)

In acute tubular necrosis, the damaged tubules lose their ability to concentrate urine and reabsorb sodium. In contrast, in cases of prerenal injuries such as volume depletion, the tubular functions still remain intact. Therefore in addition to urine sediment, urinary indices are also useful diagnostic tools that can help differentiate prerenal azotemia from acute tubular necrosis (Table 46.1).

What Is the Natural Progression of Acute Tubular Necrosis?

There are typically three phases of acute tubular necrosis: oliguric phase, diuretic phase, and recovery phase.

The *oliguric phase*, defined by urine output less than 400 mL in 24 hrs, can even precede a rise in serum creatinine. This phase of ATN can last up to 7 days or more. However, some cases of ATN, especially ATN associated with aminoglycosides, can have nonoliguric ATN.

Nonoliguric ATN generally has a better prognosis.

The oliguric phase is followed by the *diuretic phase*, which is characterized by an increase in urine volume without providing much clearance of toxic metabolites. Although the diuretic phase often indicates a sign of clinical improvement, there is usually no significant improvement in either serum urea concentration or creatinine, as there is no significant filtration or reabsorption occurring.

The *recovery phase* follows the diuretic phase after tubular cells regenerate and regain their functionality. Depending on the extent of injury, however, there may be some residual impairment of renal function.

What Are the Clinical Consequences and Management of Acute Tubular Necrosis?

The most common complications of acute kidney injury as a result of ATN are volume overload (especially in the setting of oliguria or anuria) and electrolyte imbalances.

Despite the consequences of volume overload and electrolyte abnormalities, the management of acute tubular necrosis consists of mainly supportive measures. It is important to maintain strict sodium and fluid intake in order to maintain euvolemia. Hyperkalemia can be managed with loop diuretics (if nonoliguric) or with potassium-binding resins. With metabolic acidosis, sodium bicarbonate is generally given if serum bicarbonate is less than 15 mmol/L. Hyperphosphatemia can be managed by restricting dietary phosphate intake and by adding phosphate-binding agents.

Further nephrotoxic insults should be minimized or avoided, if possible. Medications will need to be dose adjusted based on patient's kidney function at the time.

CLINICAL PEARL (STEP 3)

There are two general types of nephrotoxic agents: endogenous and exogenous toxins.
    Examples of endogenous toxins are myoglobin from muscle breakdown, hemoglobin, and paraproteins (multiple myeloma). Exogenous toxins include commonly used antimicrobials such as aminoglycosides, vancomycin, amphotericin, acyclovir, and tenofovir. Certain chemotherapy classes, namely platinum-based cisplatin, can also cause nephrotoxic injury. Radiocontrast material is important to consider among the broad differentials of nephrotoxic agents as well.

When Is Dialysis Indicated in the Setting of Acute Kidney Injury?

Because dialysis is not without its consequences (e.g., infection from large-bore intravenous access for hemodialysis), it is important to initiate this therapy only if indicated. There are evidence-based indications for when dialysis is indicated:

1. Volume overload refractory to diuretics;
2. Severe intractable metabolic acidosis with pH less than 7.2;
3. Hyperkalemia with potassium levels higher than 6.5 mEq/L, refractory to medical treatment;
4. Symptomatic uremia (i.e, pericarditis, encephalopathy);
5. Platelet dysfunction, bleeding diathesis; or
6. Acute kidney injury in the setting of dialyzable drugs or toxins.

After placement of a dialysis catheter in the right internal jugular vein, the patient is initiated on intermittent renal replacement therapy on postoperative day 5 due to worsening azotemia and severe volume overload in the setting of anuria. After three sessions of renal replacement therapy, he begins to have urine output, and creatinine downtrends to 1.8 mg/dL. He is able to remain off dialysis for the remainder of the hospitalization. The dialysis catheter is removed on postoperative day 9, and he is transferred from the intensive care unit to the step-down unit. He works with physical therapy and is discharged to a rehabilitation facility on postoperative day 15. His creatinine is 2.4 mg/dL, his electrolytes are within the normal range, and he is making an appropriate amount of urine at the time of discharge.

BEYOND THE PEARLS: AORTIC DISSECTION

- Patients with acute aortic dissections should be started on intravenous opioids (morphine or hydromorphone), not only for pain control but also to attenuate catecholamine surge triggered by pain. Although management steps diverge based on the types of dissection, medical management with antiimpulse therapy can be applied as a means of bridging until surgical repair takes place.
- The 10-year survival rate of patients with aortic dissection posthospitalization ranges from 30% to 60% in studies. It is important to continue beta blockers in order to minimize aortic wall stress.
- Serial imaging with either thoracic magnetic resonance (MR) CTA is typically recommended before discharge, with follow-up imaging at 3, 6, and 12 months post discharge, and then annually thereafter. Imaging signs to monitor include: progressive increase in diameter, aneurysm formation, and hemorrhage at surgical anastomosis or graft sites.

BEYOND THE PEARLS: ACUTE TUBULAR NECROSIS

- Renal vascular supply in the setting of fluctuations in systemic blood pressures is an important factor in maintaining both renal blood flow (RBF) and renal function. This autoregulation is achieved by stretch receptors in the afferent arterioles in response to increased or decreased perfusion pressure. Renal autoregulation can withstand between systolic blood pressures of approximately 80 mm Hg to 160 mm Hg. Lower than or higher than these parameters, the autoregulation fails.

- Patients with long standing hypertension, diabetes, and chronic kidney disease, who have chronic severe elevation of blood pressure, can sustain acute kidney injury without evidence of overt hypotension. Relative hypotension compared with baseline blood pressure can lead to kidney injury and functional decline as a result of impairment in their renal vascular autoregulation.
- Fluid overload in critically ill patients with AKI is associated with increased morbidity and mortality and therefore, should be avoided.
- Although diuretics are typically used in managing positive fluid balance in the setting of AKI, they have not been shown to have mortality benefit or lead to earlier recovery of renal function.
- Intermittent hemodialysis is the conventional mode of renal replacement therapy in which volume and/or solutes are removed at a high flow rate typically over 3 to 4 hours. However, intradialytic hypotension is quite common. As such, continuous renal replacement therapy (CRRT) is an alternate modality that has a better hemodynamic tolerance in critically ill patients requiring vasopressors, and it has been shown to be more effective in fluid removal compared with intermittent hemodialysis.

Suggested Readings

Hueng, M. (2017). Acute kidney injury. In F. F. Ferri (Ed.), *Ferri's clinical advisor 2018* (pp. 37–41). Philadelphia: Elsevier.

Johnson, R. J., Feehally, J., & Flöge, J. (2015). *Comprehensive clinical nephrology.* Philadelphia: Elsevier Saunders.

Nienaber, C., Akin, I., Kische, S., & Rehders, T. (2014). Nonoperative medical management of acute aortic dissection. In J. C. Stanely, F. J. Veith, & T. W. Wakefield (Eds.), *Current therapy in vascular and endovascular surgery* (5th ed., pp. 361–365). Philadelphia: Elsevier.

Sharfuddin, A., Weisbord, S., Palevsky, P., & Molitoris, B. (2016). Acute kidney injury. In K. Skorecki, G. Chertow, P. Marsden, M. Taal, & A. Yu (Eds.), *Brenner and Rector's the kidney* (10th ed., pp. 958–1011). Philadelphia: Elsevier.

CHAPTER 47

Third-Degree Burns in a 22-Year-Old Female

Nathan L'Etoile ■ Jonah D. Klein ■ William B. Hughes

A 22-year-old-woman with a history of anxiety and depression presents to the emergency department with burns to her bilateral upper extremities. She is accompanied by her boyfriend. He explains that she was cooking dinner in the kitchen when a pot of boiling water fell off the stove onto her bilateral upper extremities. She is in moderate pain but refuses to let any person touch the affected area.

What Is the Clinical Evaluation and Assessment of a Burn Patient?

The initial evaluation of a burn patient is similar to that of a trauma patient: airway, breathing, and circulation. Assess the airway for any thermal injury or mucosal damage by inhaled smoke from combustion. Airway damage can lead to severe edema; therefore patients with perioral burns, hoarse voice, wheezing, singed nasal hairs, and stridor should raise concern for mucosal injuries, and intubation should be considered. If the burn injury has led to poor airway visualization, consideration is made for a surgical airway. After the airway has been deemed stable, assess breathing with equal chest rise and breathe sounds. If a mechanical airway device was inserted previously, ensure adequate oxygen exchange via end tidal CO_2 measurement. Now assess circulation and volume status by checking pulses, blood pressure, and insertion of large-bore intravenous lines. At this point, it is not uncommon to place a urinary catheter for close monitoring of urine output and volume status; additionally, an ECG may be performed to evaluate cardiac injury and/or arrhythmia.

After initial evaluation, a full head-to-toe examination is performed, with specific attention to burned body surface area. In assessing burned total surface area (TBSA), there is the Wallace rule of nines (Fig. 47.1). The head is 9%; each upper extremity is 9%; anterior and posterior torso are each 18%; and each lower extremity is 18%. The palms and genitals are each 1%, and the ratios are different with children and adults (see Fig. 47.1). The alternative is to use the patient's palm to be 1% TBSA when examining the burn wound. TBSA is important as it in part dictates the patient's resuscitation, treatment, grafting, and prognosis.

When evaluating a burn patient, special attention needs to be given to burns of the hands, feet, genitals, and joints. These patients need to be in a specialty burn facility experienced with the contractures, disfigurements, and grafting associated with these body regions. Additional special considerations need to be made in the setting of suspected abuse, both pediatric and adult. Although less than 5% of burn injuries are considered intentional, this patient's history may necessitate evaluation for abuse.

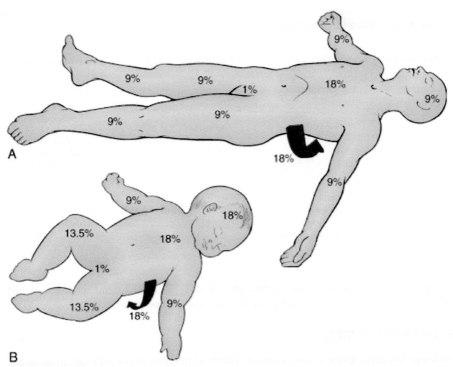

Fig. 47.1   Rule of nines for estimating burned surface area. (A) Adult. (B) Infant. (From Mosier MJ, Sheridan RL, Heimbach DM: Emergency care of the burned patient. In Auerbach PS, Cushing TA, editors: *Auerbach's wilderness medicine*, ed 7, Philadelphia, 2017, Elsevier, p 319.)

CLINICAL PEARL (STEPS 2/3)

Each evaluating clinician needs to consider abuse during the evaluation of both infant/children and adult/geriatric burn injuries. History should be obtained regarding the mechanism of injury, location of injury, and who was present at the time of the injury. Physical examination findings concerning for abuse include demarcated margins, flexor sparing, lack of splash marks, classic stocking-and-glove pattern, and any localized injury. All clinicians treating burn patients should be familiar with how to report suspected abuse at their institution.

The patient's airway, breathing, and circulation are stable and intravenous access has been obtained. Initial vital signs are temperature 99.8°F, heart rate 87 bpm, blood pressure 94/52, respiratory rate 20, and oxygen saturation 100% on room air. On physical examination the affected skin on her bilateral upper arms through fingertips appears mottled, pink-white, dry and blanching with a calculated burned TBSA of 18%. Additionally, her mucous membranes are dry. The patient's sister was also present at the time of the incident and verifies the accidental nature of the injury.

What Are the Classifications of Burns and How Are They Distinguished?

Thermal burn classification and the TBSA that is affected by a burn are the two most important factors in the mortality of burn patients. Burns are classified by the depth of tissue that is affected,

TABLE 47.1 ■ Classifications of Burns

Burn Classification	Layers Affected	Clinical Presentation	Typical Management
First Degree	Epidermis	Pain, erythema	Lotion, aloe
Second Degree	Epidermis and papillary dermis	Pain, erythema, blistering, blanches	Topical antimicrobial such as silver sulfadiazine; greasy gauze
• Superficial	Epidermis through to reticular dermis	Decreased sensation, mottled pink and white, dry, loss of hair follicles	
• Deep			Silver sulfadiazine; possible surgical excision and skin grafting
Third Degree	Epidermis, full thickness of the dermis, and possibly deeper tissues	Lack of pain, black or white, dry, exposed subcutaneous fat	Silver sulfadiazine, surgical excision and skin graft
Fourth Degree	Full skin thickness and involvement of muscle, bone, etc.	Similar to third degree	Excision and grafting (cannot graft on avascular structure)

and the management of burns varies by these classifications. Table 47.1 shows the layers affected, clinical presentation, and typical management regimen of each burn classification.

ELECTRICAL BURNS

Although thermal burns are far more common, electrical burns have important implications including the risk of cardiac arrhythmias and compartment syndrome with rhabdomyolysis, among other complications. Additionally, in comparison to thermal burns, infection by anaerobic bacteria is more common in electrical burns. These patients should be managed with an ECG and careful observation for vascular or renal compromise as well as neurologic symptoms. Lightning-associated burns can also cause serious cardiac arrhythmias or sudden death, and patients should be monitored on telemetry. Mechanical forces, for example if the patient is thrown by a shockwave, should be considered, and patients should have a complete physical examination for any possible associated trauma. These patients are also susceptible to intracranial hemorrhage in the basal ganglia and brainstem, and direct electrical damage to nerve cells can occur. Therefore observation for focal neurologic defects should be done to screen for possible complications.

CHEMICAL BURNS

Chemical burns also are less common, though many chemicals can cause severe burns. An important distinction should be made between the types of chemical burns. Acid burns, such as those caused by formic and hydrofluoric acid, are recognized by a hard eschar that prevents deep extravasation by the chemical. Therefore acid burns are generally less severe than alkaline burns. They should be treated with copious irrigation to remove the offending substance. Formic acid burn victims should be carefully monitored for electrolyte abnormalities, including metabolic acidosis, and are often treated with mannitol diuresis. Hydrofluoric acid burn victims should be treated with irrigation and calcium gluconate gel, which neutralizes the acid. These patients should also be admitted for cardiac monitoring. On the other hand, alkali burns are generally more severe than acid burns for the reason described previously, as well as causing protein denaturation. They must be copiously irrigated and possibly debrided in the operating room. Importantly, neutralization with weak acids is contraindicated due to the thermal injury that can result from the exothermic reaction.

What Other Pathologies Can Appear Similar to Burns?

Staph scalded skin syndrome. Staph scalded skin syndrome (SSSS) is pathology caused by epidermolytic toxins released by *S. aureus* that typically affects infants and young children. The result is a desquamating rash that is painful to touch and affects all layers of the epidermis. This is treated with IV antibiotics and moist dressings to control the infection, and generally surgical management is not warranted.

STEVEN-JOHNSON SYNDROME

Steven-Johnson syndrome (SJS) and the more severe toxic epidermal necrolysis are dangerous idiopathic drug reactions that involve less than 10% or greater than 30% of the body surface area, respectively. Both conditions are life-threatening. Patients present with mucosal erosions followed by confluent lesions with a positive Nikolsky sign on examination. These conditions can affect the mucosal surfaces as well. Many drugs on first exposure have been implicated, including sulfonamides, penicillins, phenytoin, carbamazepine, quinolones, steroids, and NSAIDs. The treatment for this condition is immediate discontinuation of the offending drug. Aside from any surgical management, the treatment for these patients is similar to that of burn patients, including thermoregulation, fluid and electrolyte resuscitation, and skin coverings.

FROSTBITE

Frostbite is a type of thermal damage that is characterized by ischemia and reperfusion injuries. The surgical management of frostbite is with delayed debridement after demarcation. More serious or progressed frostbite may require appendage or limb amputation.

What Is the Pathophysiology Behind Burn Wounds?

The tissue associated with a burn injury may progress to necrosis (associated with protein denaturation), ischemia, or inflammation. The inflamed and ischemic areas are the primary source of cytokine release. This cytokine release increases capillary permeability, enabling recruitment of cell adhesion molecules and platelets for remodeling. This physiologic phase is present for about 72 hours and is also associated with fluid shifts, electrolyte abnormalities, and organ hypoperfusion, requiring appropriate unique fluid resuscitation and supportive care. After the first 72 hours, there is a catabolic and inflammatory phase that is associated with a hyperdynamic physiology. This is the time when the wound can be complicated by infection, eschar formation, and more intense pain.

BASIC SCIENCE PEARL (STEP 1)

The most abundant proteins in the skin are collagen, keratin, and elastin. Collagen is secreted by fibroblasts, and type I is the most abundant type in normal skin. During wound healing, type III collagen (which has less tensile strength) is secreted by fibroblasts initially and, during the course of remodeling, is replaced by type I collagen.

How Are Burn Patients Appropriately Resuscitated?

Due to the previously discussed inflammatory response and capillary leak, there is a taxing effect on the cardiovascular and renal systems, and there is a high morbidity associated with burn sepsis. Appropriate resuscitation is absolutely key for the management of a burn patient. A few principles, including the estimation of appropriate volume, the type of fluid resuscitation, and evaluation of the efficacy of fluid management, are essential to understand.

PARKLAND AND CONSENSUS FORMULAE

Once venous access has been obtained (unburned skin is preferred, but burned skin is acceptable with no other option), the Parkland formula can be used to estimate the amount of replacement fluid required in the first 24 hours after a burn. The formula is:

$$24\,\text{hour fluid volume} = 4\text{mL} \times \text{weight in kilograms} \times \%\text{ TBSA burned}$$

Once the volume is calculated, half the volume should be given in the first 8 hours after the burn. Both hypernatremia and hyperkalemia are possible electrolyte abnormalities due to third spacing and acute renal failure, thus fluid resuscitation should be tailored to correct these electrolyte abnormalities. There is continuous change on the fluid used for resuscitation, but a general consensus is lactate ringers in the first 24 hours followed by colloid and/or crystalloid. The most critical aspect of resuscitation is hour-by-hour assessment of end organ perfusion, including vital signs, urine output (0.5–2 cc/kg/hr depending on age), mental status, and base deficit.

The consensus formula is:

$$24\,\text{hour fluid volume} = 2 \text{ to } 4\text{mL} \times \text{weight in kilograms} \times \%\text{ TBSA burned}$$

Two mL is used for adults; 3 mL is used for children; and 4 mL is used in electrical burns.

As with the Parkland formula, half of this volume is given in the first 8 hours after the burn and the balance is infused over the next 24 hours.

After evaluation the patient is given the respective amount of resuscitative fluids over the first 24 hours. Her urine output has remained greater than 0.5 cc/kg/hr, and she remained hemodynamically stable over the next 48 hours. She has been given medication for pain but now complains of increasing pain in her bilateral upper extremities. On repeat examination, her forearms appear tight, and there is now thick circumferential leathery eschar formation.

What Is the Nonsurgical Treatment for Burns?

Supportive care Ensuring adequate pain control is paramount in burn patients. Additionally, the body temperature should remain as physiologic as possible, especially in patients with large burn surface areas. The wound area should be cleansed with an aseptic solution. After debridement, additional antimicrobial ointments such as silver sulfadiazine or antibiotic ointment can be applied. Supportive care includes electrolyte repletion and continued monitoring and maintenance of a euvolemic state.

NUTRITION

Burn injuries can induce a hypermetabolic state requiring adequate nutritional support. Enteral feeding support should be initiated in burns greater than 20% of TBSA. An average of 2.5 g/kg/day of protein are adequate for the majority of burn patients. To calculate the caloric needs of patients, the Curreri formula, which is most accurate for patients with less than 40% TBSA affected. The formula for an adult is represented by:

$$\text{Enteral Nutrition} = 25\,\text{kcal/kg/day} + 40\,\text{kcal/\%TBSA affected/day}$$

CLINICAL PEARL (STEPS 2/3)

Topical treatment of superficial burns is something that all clinicians from surgeons to family practitioners need to be aware of as it is often an outpatient treatment. The goal of topical treatment is to serve as an antimicrobial barrier and to create an environment for reepithelization. Silver sulfadiazine has antimicrobial activity against gram-positive and gram-negative organisms, including pseudomonas. Its common side effect is transient neutropenia when used in large surface area wounds, and it should be avoided in patients allergic to sulfa drugs. Other antimicrobials agents include antibiotic ointments.

What Is the Surgical Treatment for Burns?

Escharotomy An escharotomy is performed using several tangential incisions and removal of necrotic tissue until bleeding tissue is encountered. This is indicated after a partially or fully circumferential burn forms an eschar, leading to pain, firmness of the compartment, or any other signs of neurovascular compromise. This procedure can be performed at the bedside or the operating room, often with minimal analgesia. Using electrocautery, the eschar is incised down to the subcutaneous fat in order to release the nonexpandable inelastic tissue. If the symptoms present before the escharotomy have not been relieved, the patient will require formal operative fasciotomy.

SURGICAL EXCISION

Surgical excision of burn wounds must occur after fluid and electrolyte resuscitation and when the patient is hemodynamically stable. Surgical management should be initiated within the first few days of the injury. Early debridement and excision can help with the prevention of burn wound–associated sepsis. Initial debridement of the wound can take place after cleansing and involves sharp excision of nonviable skin and blisters. Superficial wounds often do not require debridement or excision. Larger wounds may require serial debridement. If wound healing after resuscitation and debridement appears unlikely to occur, then excision may be indicated. Two techniques for excision of the graft include fascial excision and tangential excision. Fascial excision is achieved by removing the damaged and necrotic tissue, subcutaneous tissue, and preservation of fascia. This gives an excellent plane that is well vascularized for acceptance of a graft. This procedure has less blood loss but poorer cosmesis. Tangential excision is preferred over fascial excision as it removes only affected tissue while leaving more viable tissue. Serial tangential cuts of the affected area are performed until bleeding tissue is encountered. This is achieved by using a calibrated guarded knife. Disadvantages include increased blood loss and a level of uncertainty as to whether sufficient amounts of viable tissue are present to support a graft. To decrease blood loss during tangential excision, a proximal tourniquet is often placed before excision.

WOUND CLOSURE AND SKIN GRAFTING

Split thickness autologous skin grafts (STSGs) are the preferred technique. The donor site can be the thigh, buttock, or back and is harvested via a powered or handheld dermatome. Split-thickness grafts have a greater risk of contracture, whereas full-thickness grafts have a longer healing time at the donor site due to deeper dermal excision. STGSs are often meshed, enabling larger surface area coverage and deceased risk of seroma, although they are less cosmetic. Sheet grafts (unmeshed STSGs) are the graft of choice for the face, neck, and other exposed areas of skin. They are more cosmetically desirable and have a faster healing rate compared to meshed grafts. Revascularization of the skin grafts is based on the serial processes of plasmatic imbibition, inosculation, and neovascularization. Allograft, instead of autograft, can be used as a bridge graft in hemodynamically unstable patients. After graft placement, the burn wounds are covered with a moist pressure dressing or negative pressure wound therapy device. Definitive grafting of wounds to the hands, face, and genitals is deferred after the first week of injury. Graft failure is a dangerous and a possibly costly complication of surgically incised burns. It is primarily prevented with hemostasis at the time of grafting to prevent excessive blood loss and to ensure adequate nutrient supply to the graft.

CLINICAL PEARL (STEPS 2/3)

There are different kinds of grafts that can be used for closure, most commonly split-thickness skin grafts (STSGs) and full-thickness skin grafts (FTSGs). STSG does not include the full dermis, whereas FTSG includes the entire dermis (Fig. 47.2). These are both examples of autografts. STSGs have a better survival as the thinness of 0.12 to 0.15 mm enables better imbibition and revascularization. They can be meshed and cover a larger surface area but are more prone to contracture. FTSGs have less contracture and are indicated for coverage of smaller surface areas and closer to joints such as the palms and soles.

An escharotomy is performed. After 7 days of admission, the patient begins to complain of some tenderness around the burn site on her left forearm. On physical examination, there is erythema and induration on the eschar and surrounding area. The wound site is cultured via punch biopsy and results are consistent with bacterial cellulitis. The wound is not satisfactorily healing and must be excised and grafted.

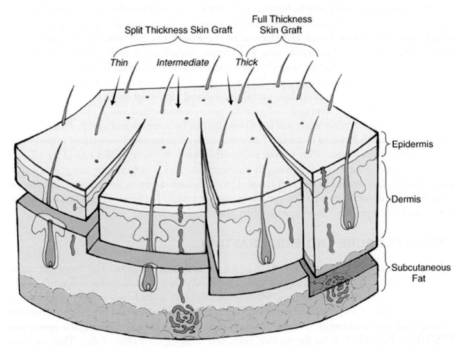

Fig. 47.2 Relationship of skin graft type to thickness of skin. (Jewett BS: Skin and composite grafts. In Baker SR, editor: *Local flaps in facial reconstruction*, Philadelphia, 2014, Elsevier, Chapter 15.)

What Complications Can Be Seen in Burn Patients and How Are They Managed?

Wound infection Infections are of great concern in a burn patient, and these patients should be closely monitored for signs and symptoms of an infection. Wound infection is a common complication and can be heralded by erythema, edema, and increased pain around the wound site as well as systemic symptoms of an infection. The larger the surface area of burn, the higher the risk of infection. The most common organism isolated in a burn wounds is *Pseudomonas aeruginosa;* however, *Staphylococcus aureus* is also a pathogen of concern. Later colonization by fungi, especially *Candida albicans,* is also a possible complication. Treatment of a burn patient with topical silver sulfadiazine or antibiotic ointment is paramount in decreasing the risk of colonization and infection. Sepsis is a feared complication of burns due to the presence of a possible wound infection and the immunosuppressive effects of burns. Herpes simplex virus (HSV) or cytomegalovirus (CMV) can often reactivate in burn patients due to a suppressed immune system.

RESPIRATORY COMPLICATIONS

Patients with inhalation injury, especially those requiring intubation, are at increased risk for pneumonia. Patients may develop pneumonia due to hyperventilation and atelectasis due to eschar formation on the chest wall, or they may develop ventilator-associated pneumonia (VAP), which is defined as pneumonia occurring more than 48 hours after intubation. Also, ciliary clearance mechanisms can be lost with inhalation injuries. Workup for these patients includes sputum culture or bronchoalveolar lavage. Before culture results, empiric antibiotics should be given. Additionally, aggressive pulmonary toilet is critical.

COMPARTMENT SYNDROME

If a full-thickness, circumferential burn occurs, the eschar can act like a tourniquet, increasing the pressure in a fascial compartment. This can lead to compartment syndrome. Thoracic compartment syndrome may present with hypotension, increased airway pressures, and hypoventilation. Additionally, abdominal compartment syndrome may present with decreased urine output, hypotension, and increased ventilator airway pressures. This complication often requires urgent escharotomy and/or surgical decompression of the compartment. Rhabdomyolysis and myoglobinuria are further complications of compartment syndrome that can lead to renal failure.

OTHER MEDICAL COMPLICATIONS

Thrombosis and embolization are both concerns due to restriction of movement either because of burn location or immobilization in promotion of healing. Studies have shown that for these patients, prophylactic heparin is safe and should be administered. Renal failure, as described previously, is common due to a decreased plasma volume as well as the release of toxic metabolites after a burn. Curling ulcers are a type of gastric erosion after a burn injury. These are caused by hypovolemia and an increased cortisol levels via pituitary stimulation. These ulcers, also called stress ulcers, are often prevented with enteral feeding and proton pump inhibitors.

After 2 weeks in the hospital and additional skin grafts to slowly healing areas, the patient is discharged with instructions on daily dressing changes. She is instructed to dress the meshed skin graft sites with greasy gauze and pressure dressings. Appropriate follow-up has been arranged.

BEYOND THE PEARLS

- Initial evaluation of the burn patient involves assessment of the airway, breathing, and circulation. Signs of impending airway compromise include singed hairs, perioral burns and hoarseness, and intubation must be considered in these patients.
- An estimation of the TBSA burned is important in guiding initial fluid management, although continuous assessment of end-organ perfusion is key, including urine output and mental status.
- Burn wounds must be continuously evaluated for need for debridement of nonviable tissue, eschar development and compartment syndrome requiring escharotomy, and the development of wound infection.
- Autograft coverage is the preferred method of wound closure, with utilization of STSG or FTSG. Temporary allograft closure can be performed in patients that are unstable, or with wounds in specialized body regions.

Suggested Readings

Church, D., et al. (2006). Burn wound infections. *Clin Microbiol Rev, 19*(2), 403–434.

Cooper, M. A., Andrews, C. J., & Holle, R. L. (2006). Lightning injury. In P. S. Auerbach & T. A. Cushing (Eds.), *Auerbach's wilderness medicine*. CV Mosby. Chapter 3.

Forjuoh, S. N. (1998). The mechanisms, intensity of treatment, and outcomes of hospitalized burns: Issues for prevention. *J Burn Care Rehabil, 19*(5), 456–460.

Friedstat J, Endorf FW, Gibran NS: Burns. In *Schwartz's Principles of Surgery*, ed 10.

Jeschke, M. G., & Herndon, D. N. (2017). Burns. In C. Townsend et al. (Eds.), *Sabiston textbook of surgery: The biological basis of modern surgical practice* (20th ed., pp. 505–531). Philadelphia: Elsevier Saunders.

Kao, Y., et al. (2018). Fluid resuscitation in patients with severe burns: A meta-analysis of randomized controlled trials. *Acad Emerg Med, 25*(3), 320–329.

Mishra, A. K., Yadav, P., & Mishra, A. (2016). A systemic review on staphylococcal scalded skin syndrome (SSSS): A rare and critical disease of neonates. *Open Microbiol J, 10*, 150–159.

Monstrey, S., et al. (2008). Assessment of burn depth and burn wound healing potential. *Burns, 34*, 761–769.

Murphy, J. V., Banwell, P. E., Roberts, A. H., & McGrouther, D. A. (2000). Frostbite: Pathogenesis and treatment. *J Trauma, 48*, 171–178.

Sheridan, R. (2014). Practical management of the burn patient. In J. L. Cameron & A. M. Cameron (Eds.), *Current surgical therapy* (pp. 1131–1138). Philadelphia: Elsevier Saunders.

CHAPTER 48

Necrotizing Soft Tissue Infection in a 57-Year-Old Male

Amanda Teichman ■ Dane Scantling ■ Michael S. Weingarten

A 57-year-old male presents to the emergency department with a complaint of increasing pain and redness of his left medial thigh. He remembers having a bug bite in the area about 5 days prior and scratching the area vigorously. Since that time, the thigh has become gradually more red, swollen, and tender to palpation. On the morning of presentation to the hospital, he complains of subjective fever and chills but denies any drainage from the area. The patient states the pain is currently 10/10 and constant. He has a past medical history of diabetes, hypertension, obesity, and asthma. He denies the use of alcohol or illicit drugs and has a 17-pack-year history of smoking. He has never had surgery and has no significant past family history. He works as a cashier at a grocery store, and over the last day the pain in his thigh has made it increasingly difficult to stand at work. He denies history of any other skin lesions and reports that his diabetes is poorly controlled.

What Clinical Findings Are Important in a Patient Who Presents With a Painful Skin Lesion or Extremity?

There are many potential etiologies for a patient who presents with a red, painful skin lesion or extremity from infectious to inflammatory to vascular. Diabetic patients are at especially high risk for developing any number of skin and soft tissue diseases, including necrotizing infections at the severe end of the spectrum. Necrotizing soft tissue infections (NSTIs) are rapidly progressive, resulting in widespread soft tissue necrosis and systemic illness. Physical examination findings are inconsistent but may include crepitus, bullae, pain out of proportion to examination, and hemodynamic instability. An early sign of NSTI is anesthesia of the overlying skin, though it may appear to be normal. Pain out of proportion is one of the most common examination findings and is found in 72% of cases. Laboratory findings may demonstrate an elevated white blood cell count (WBC), elevated blood glucose, hyponatremia, elevated creatinine, and potentially a lactic acidosis.

The Laboratory Risk Indicator of Necrotizing Fasciitis (LRINEC) was developed as a predictive tool to help guide the diagnosis of NSTI (Table 48.1). Patients with a LRINEC score of 6 or higher have been shown to have a greater likelihood of NSTI diagnosed. But if there is a high index of suspicion, a lower score should not preclude operative intervention, as NSTIs are primarily clinical diagnoses.

What Are Some Other Skin and Soft Tissue Infections to Keep in Mind?

NSTIs (including necrotizing fasciitis and myositis; see later in this chapter) comprise some of the worst skin/soft tissue infections; however, other entities may present in a similar fashion and need to be differentiated.

For example, pyomyositis, an infection isolated to the muscle, typically results from hematogenous bacterial spread. It manifests with fever, anorexia, muscle pain, and swelling and is

TABLE 48.1 ■ The Laboratory Risk Indicator of Necrotizing Fasciitis

LRINEC Variable	Value	Score
CRP[a]	< 150	0
	> 150	4
WBC	< 15	0
	15–25	1
	> 25	2
Hemoglobin	> 13.5	0
	11–13.5	1
	< 11	2
Sodium	> 135	0
	< 135	2
Creatinine	≤ 1.6	0
	> 1.6	2
Glucose	≤ 180	0
	> 180	1
Points	Risk Category	NSTI Probability
≤ 5	Low	< 50%
6–7	Intermediate	> 75%
≥ 7	High	> 75%

[a]C reactive protein

often managed effectively with antibiotics alone or, rarely, surgical drainage if it is associated with an abscess.

Gas gangrene, or Clostridial myonecrosis, is a rapidly progressive, necrotizing soft tissue infection caused by Clostridial species. Risk factors include penetrating trauma or crush injury with disruption of blood flow. The anaerobic environment promotes proliferation of the toxins that cause tissue damage. Clinical manifestations of this disease are similar to those of other NSTI's; however, gas is often the distinguishing finding on clinical examination and radiographic imaging. Note, however, that gas may also be seen on radiography in those patients with NSTIs.

Lastly, cellulitis is an infection involving the skin and subcutaneous tissue but rarely results in severe systemic effects. Occasionally, there is an underlying abscess or osteomyelitis, and fever, tachycardia, or leukocytosis may be observed. Cellulitis is characterized by edema, erythema, heat, and induration. It is often caused by Gram-positive organisms and is often managed successfully with antibiotics alone. Patients who appear to have cellulitis but have evidence of severe systemic toxicity should be evaluated for a potentially more severe underlying process, such as NSTI.

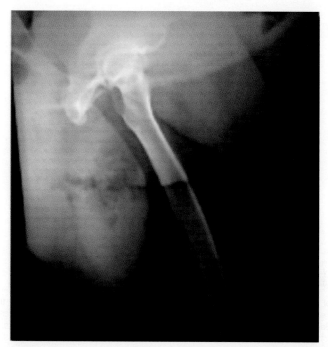

Fig. 48.1   Radiograph of the femur demonstrating a large amount of gas in the surrounding soft tissue.

On physical examination, the patient is febrile to 102.3°F, with a pulse rate of 108/min and blood pressure of 135/74 mm Hg. His left medial thigh is erythematous, exquisitely tender, and indurated. There is no appreciable crepitus or drainage. The entire thigh is tender, even beyond the borders of erythema. Laboratory values are significant for a white blood cell count of 21,600/mm^3, glucose of 255 mg/dL, and hemoglobin A1C of 10.9%. A radiograph of the femur demonstrates a large amount of gas in the surrounding soft tissue (Fig. 48.1).

What Are the Next Steps in Management in a Patient for Whom There Is Concern for a Necrotizing Soft Tissue Infection?

The suspicion for the diagnosis of a NSTI should be raised on the initial clinical examination, and all steps in diagnosis and management should work to rule in or out a necrotizing infection. Plain radiographs of an extremity may be sufficient to demonstrate subcutaneous air (a hallmark of NSTIs; see later in this chapter); however, if there is doubt in the clinical assessment and if the radiograph is inconclusive (in the pelvis, it can be difficult to evaluate with plain radiograph), a computed tomography (CT) scan (Fig. 48.2) or magnetic resonance image (MRI) (Fig. 48.3) may aid in the diagnosis. If there is a high index of suspicion, imaging is not mandatory in the workup of NSTI. When a diagnosis of NSTI is suspected based on clinical evaluation and/or imaging, the next step in management includes initiation of broad-spectrum antibiotics and emergent operative debridement of the necrotic tissue. An algorithm for management of NSTIs is shown in Fig. 48.4.

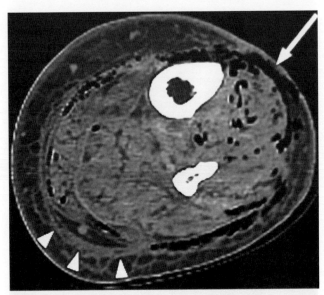

Fig. 48.2 Axial CT image of the left lower extremity of a patient with necrotizing soft tissue infection, demonstrating edema in the soft tissues *(arrowheads)* and air tracking along the fascial planes *(arrow)*. From Chaudhry A, Baker K, Gould E, et al. Necrotizing fasciitis and it's mimics: what radiologists need to know. AJR 2015;204:133; with permission.

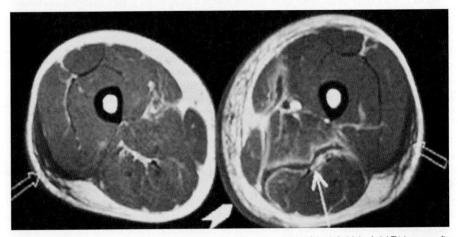

Fig. 48.3 MRI findings for a patient with necrotizing fasciitis and myositis of the left thigh. Axial T1 images after contrast injection demonstrate increased soft tissue enhancement and gas in the soft tissues (thin white arrow). Thick white arrow points to thickening of the skin with subcutaneous fat infiltration Normal skin is noted for comparison on the right side (black arrow). (From Malghem J, Lecouvet FE, Omoumi P, et al: Necrotizing fasciitis: contribution and limitations of diagnostic imaging, *Joint Bone Spine* 80(2):146–154, 2013; with permission.)

The patient is given a dose of vancomycin, piperacillin-tazobactam, and clindamycin, and is taken to the operating room for radical wide debridement of his left thigh. In the operating room, extensive, murky, dishwater-like fluid and necrotic subcutaneous tissue are encountered. Cultures are obtained, and tissue sent for pathologic analysis. All involved tissue is removed and debrided. The wound is left open and packed, and he is taken to the surgical intensive care unit (SICU) postoperatively.

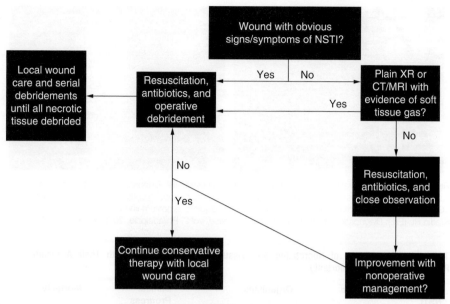

Fig. 48.4 Algorithm for the management of NSTIs.

What Is the Pathophysiology of NSTIs?

Necrosis in patients with NSTIs extends rapidly beyond the involved skin to include the underlying soft tissue, fascia, and muscle far from the visible wound. For this reason, radical debridement and, usually, serial debridements are required.

In general, the infection starts with any form of trauma or break in the skin. This results in bacterial inoculation and microvascular thrombosis due to bacterial toxin release. The resultant hypoxia leads to ischemia and necrosis. The ischemic environment promotes bacterial overgrowth and rapid spread through soft tissues.

The literature supports two anatomic entities: necrotizing fasciitis and necrotizing myositis. The former is characterized by epidermal, dermal, subcutaneous, and fascial involvement. Fascia has a poor blood supply, allowing for rapid spread of infection along the fascial plane. The muscle is spared, as it has better perfusion. In rare instances, the muscle may become involved, resulting in necrotizing myositis. This may present with later signs of skin involvement and hence a worse clinical outcome.

CLINICAL PEARL (STEPS 2/3)

NSTIs result in obliterative vasculitis early in their course (Fig. 48.5A). As the disease progresses, there is liquefactive necrosis of the subcutaneous tissue and fascia with neutrophilic infiltration (see Fig. 48.5B). Infection spreads horizontally along the fascial planes. Vertical spread to underlying muscle typically occurs late in the progression of disease.

How are NSTIs classified?

NSTIs are classified as type I–IV based on the pathogen(s) involved (Table 48.2). Type I is the most common. It accounts for 70% of infections and is polymicrobial. It often involves both aerobic (e.g., *Escherichia coli, Klebsiella, Enterobacter,* and *Proteus* sp.) and anaerobic bacteria (e.g., *Clostridium, Bacteroides,* and *Peptostreptococcus*). Polymicrobial infections are most common in diabetics, those with vascular disease, or those with preexisting immune or wound healing deficiencies.

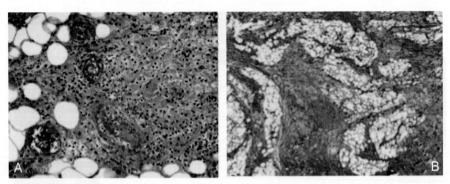

Fig. 48.5 (A) Obliterative thrombosis of several small vessels. (B) Extensive liquefactive necrosis of the subcutaneous adipose tissues with a dense neutrophilic infiltrate dissecting between the septa. (From Demicco EG, Kattapuram SV, Kradin RL, Rosenberg AE: Infections of joints, synovium-lined structures, and soft tissue. In Kradin RL (Ed.): *Diagnostic pathology of infectious disease,* vol 2, Philadelphia, 2018, Elsevier, pp 418–420.)

TABLE 48.2 ▪ **Types of Necrotizing Soft Tissue Infections (NSTIs) With Their Associated Pathogens and Risk of Mortality**

Types of NSTI	Cause	Organisms	Clinical Progress	Mortality
Type I (70%–80%)	Polymicrobial	Mixed anaerobes & aerobes	Indolent, better prognosis	Dependent on underlying comorbidities
Type II (20%–30%)	Monomicrobial	Usually GAS, Staph aureus possible	Aggressive	> 30%
Type III (more common in Asia)	Marine related	Vibrio species	Seafood ingestion or water contamination	30%–40%
Type IV (Fungal)	Trauma	Candida – Immunocompromised Zygomycetes- immunocompetent	Aggressive	> 50%

From Bonne, S. S., Kadri, S.: Evaluation and management of necrotizing soft tissue infections. Infect Dis Clin North Am, vol 31, 2017, pp 497–511.

Type II NSTIs are typically more aggressive than type I and are monomicrobial. Often, Group A *Streptococcus* (GAS) causes these infections, and 60% of patients will also present with bacteremia. GAS is typically the implicated pathogen in necrotizing myositis, and patients may show no evidence of skin changes until there has been extensive soft tissue or muscle destruction. The mortality in these cases may reach as high at 70%, so a high index of clinical suspicion is always required.

Type III cases are less common and are caused by *Vibrio* species. Type IV NSTIs are due to fungal infection. Both Type III and IV, though rare, have exceedingly high mortality rates.

NSTIs can also be classified by their anatomic location. For example Fournier's gangrene is necrotizing fasciitis of the perineum. It can spread rapidly to the anterior abdominal wall, genitalia, and gluteal muscles. In the head and neck region, there is Ludwig's angina, an infection of the submandibular fascial spaces, usually due to an odontogenic source. Airway management and infection control are critical in these patients. NSTIs in the head and neck region in general have the potential to spread to the mediastinum as well.

BASIC SCIENCE PEARL (STEPS 1/2/3)

Group A Streptococcus (GAS) can be a particularly aggressive pathogen because of a number of virulence factors. M protein is a bacterial surface protein that assists in attachment to host cells and inhibits phagocytosis. GAS also secretes exotoxins that damage endothelium, causing microvascular thrombosis and stimulating the release of cytokines. Exotoxin A and M protein are important mediators of toxic shock syndrome, which can cause cardiomyopathy and cardiovascular collapse.

The patient is hypotensive and tachycardic upon admission to the SICU postoperatively and requires a norepinephrine drip. He is resuscitated with isotonic fluid and broad-spectrum antibiotic. He is weaned off the vasopressors within 24 hours but requires a continuous insulin infusion for persistently elevated blood sugars. The patient returns to the operating room in 48 hours after the initial procedure for a second debridement. There is more murky dishwater fluid and necrotic tissue encountered, but it is not as extensive as during the first procedure. All involved tissue is removed, down to healthy muscle. The area is irrigated and negative pressure wound therapy is initiated.

What Are Some Adjuvant Therapies Used in the Management of NSTIs?

Surgical debridement and appropriate antibiotics remain the most critical therapy for NSTIs. Additional supportive therapy and particularly proper fluid resuscitation should not be overlooked, as an adequately debrided patient can easily die of inadequate resuscitation.

Fluid management in this population is of extreme importance. Damage to capillaries occurs from circulating toxins and the patient's inflammatory response, leading to capillary leak and often a need for substantial resuscitative crystalloid or albumin.

Given the gravity of these infections, severe septic shock is not uncommon. Vasopressor support is a frequent requirement, and the patient may require considerable pharmacologic intervention to maintain tissue perfusion. After appropriate fluid resuscitation, norepinephrine is recommended to accomplish this. This is followed by vasopressin up to 0.03 U/min or titrated epinephrine.

Target parameters for resuscitation commonly include a central venous pressure (CVP) of 8 to 12 mm Hg, mean arterial pressure (MAP) of greater than or equal to 65, urine output of at least 0.5 mL/kg/hr and systemic venous oxygen saturation (SCVO2) of 70% or higher. These measurements should be accomplished through invasive monitoring such as central venous catheters and/or arterial cannulation or through newer advanced noninvasive techniques as appropriate.

Beyond supportive ICU care, other adjuncts to surgery and antibiotics are controversial and have varying degrees of evidence supporting their use. One of these adjuncts is hyperbaric oxygen therapy. Although hyperbaric oxygen has demonstrated some value in wound healing and is believed to suppress bacterial growth (including that of *Clostridium* sp.) through increased arterial oxygen tension, its use in NSTIs remains unproven, and it is not at present considered a primary treatment for these infections.

Intravenous administration of immunoglobulin (IVIG) to counteract bacterial toxins has also come in and out of favor, as has plasmapheresis for removal of toxins and inflammatory mediators. Current recommendations do not support the use of either for NSTIs. In a similar fashion, there has been some study of recombinant activated protein C, which has antiinflammatory effects and may reduce death in sepsis. It remains unproven in NSTIs and may cause increasing bleeding in a patient population that will likely need repeated operative evaluation and intervention.

The patient undergoes serial dressing changes and remains on intravenous antibiotics. He is extubated on the third postoperative day and transferred out of the SICU on the fifth postoperative day. He is discharged home later that week with appropriate control of his diabetes and comorbidities. His wound heals by secondary intention over the ensuing weeks.

BEYOND THE PEARLS

- The term *necrotizing soft tissue infection (NSTI)* encompasses a variety of organism types. All cause rapid and life-threatening tissue destruction, particularly in patients with impaired immune function.
- High clinical suspicion is critical to identifying NSTIs early and preserving both tissue and life.
- Clinical scoring systems such as the LRINEC score may aid in identifying NSTI. Tissue crepitus or bullae are often a hallmark of the disease, and imaging showing fascial gas patterns is typically diagnostic. However, reliance on these signs alone may, unfortunately, lead to the miss of a life-threatening infection in the absence of surgical exploration. Exploration should never be delayed if clinical suspicion exists.
- Although newer therapy modalities exist, only appropriate antibiotics, early surgical debridement, and appropriate supportive care are known to change outcomes.

Suggested Readings

Bonne, S., & Kadri, S. (2017). Evaluation and management of necrotizing soft tissue infections. *Infect Dis Clin North Am*, *31*, 497–511.

Demicco, E. G., Kattapuram, S. V., Kradin, R. L., & Rosenberg, A. E. (2018). Infections of joints, synovium-lined structures, and soft tissue. In R. L. Kradin (Ed.), *Diagnostic pathology of infectious disease* (Vol. 2, pp. 418–420). Philadelphia: Elsevier.

Howell, G., & Rosengart, M. (2011). Necrotizing soft tissue infections. *Surg Infect*, *12*(3), 185–190.

Hussein, Q., & Anaya, D. (2013). Necrotizing soft tissue infections. *Crit Care Clin*, *29*, 795–806.

Shiroff, A. M., Herlitz, G. N., & Gracias, V. (2014). Necrotizing soft tissue infections. *J Intensive Care Med*, *29*(3), 138–144.

Stevens, D. L., & Bryant, A. E. (2017). Necrotizing soft tissue infections. *New Engl J Med*, *377*, 2253–2265.

Rhodes, A., Evans, L. E., Alhazzani, W., et al. (2017). Surviving sepsis campaign: International guidelines for management of sepsis and septic shock 2016. *Intensive Care Med*, *43*(3), 304–377.

Transplant Surgery

Transplant Surgery

CHAPTER 49

Cirrhosis in a 45-Year-Old Male

Meera Gupta ■ Susanna M. Nazarian ■ Roberto Gedaly

A 45-year-old male with history of nonalcoholic fatty liver disease (NAFLD), obesity, hyperlipidemia, and diabetes presents to the emergency room with new onset confusion, distended abdomen, and abdominal pain. The patient has been gradually more fatigued, having a poor appetite, and has lost approximately 50 pounds over the last year. He worked as a truck driver until two years ago and has been quite sedentary for more than 10 years. He admits to drinking approximately 1 to 2 beers per month. He is on no hepatotoxic medications, and he denies any family history of liver disease or malignancies in his family. His wife mentions that his primary care physician had previously expressed concern for the patient developing cirrhosis, but he has never followed through on laboratory or imaging studies to evaluate these concerns.

What Are the Causes of Liver Disease?

There are more than 100 causes of liver disease. Some of the more common causes of end-stage liver disease are summarized in Table 49.1. The most common causes of liver disease among adults in the United States are acquired and include hepatitis C, alcoholic liver disease, and nonalcoholic fatty liver disease. Viral hepatitis is the most common cause of cirrhosis worldwide, accounting for at least 50% of cases. The patient's history, including age, other demographics, and social risk factors, is important in helping narrow the differential diagnosis as to the etiology of a patient's liver disease.

BASIC SCIENCE PEARL (STEP 1)

The liver has eight segments that comprise three major lobes: right, left, and caudate lobes. The left hepatic lobe contains segments 2 to 4, the right lobe contains segments 5 to 8, and the caudate lobe is considered segment 1. The gallbladder resides in the gallbladder fossa along the inferior aspect of the liver, bordering segments 4 and 5 (Fig. 49.1). The cystic duct drains into the common bile duct within the porta hepatis. The hepatoduodenal ligament, or porta hepatis, contains the hepatic artery and bile duct anteriorly and the portal vein posteriorly. There are two major sources that supply blood to the liver: the portal vein and the hepatic artery. The portal vein provides approximately 65% to 75% of the liver's total blood supply and originates from the junction of the superior mesenteric vein and splenic vein behind the neck of the pancreas. The common hepatic arteries supplies 25% to 35% of the liver's blood supply and originates from the celiac trunk of the aorta, becoming the proper hepatic artery after the takeoff of the right gastric and gastroduodenal arteries. Although a smaller proportion of the liver's blood supply comes from the hepatic artery, the artery is the major source of oxygenated blood which is necessary to maintain bile duct integrity and hepatocyte function. The extrahepatic arterial anatomy of the liver is commonly aberrant with accessory (extra) or replaced (originating from a different source) arteries supplying the liver.

TABLE 49.1 ■ Causes of Liver Disease

Hereditary/Genetic	Biliary atresia
	Alagille syndrome
	Wilson's disease
	Hemochromatosis
	Alpha-1-antitrypsin deficiency
	Glycogen storage disease
	Hereditary amyloidosis
	Cystic fibrosis
Infectious	Viral hepatitis
	Parasitic hepatitis
Cholestatic	Primary sclerosing cholangitis
	Primary biliary cirrhosis
	TPN cholestasis
	Other biliary outflow obstruction
Autoimmune	Autoimmune hepatitis
	Sarcoidosis
Toxic	Alcoholic liver disease
	Fatty liver disease/NASH
	Drug-induced, Tylenol overdose
Primary Liver Cancer	Hepatocellular carcinoma
	Cholangiocarcinoma
	Angiosarcoma
	Hemangiosarcoma
Congestive	Budd Chiari syndrome
	Heart failure
Other	Idiopathic/cryptogenic cirrhosis

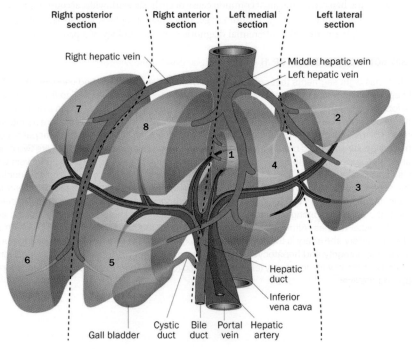

Fig. 49.1 Liver anatomy. (Redrawn from Siriwardena AK, Mason JM, Mullamitha S, et al: Management of colorectal cancer presenting with synchronous liver metastases. *Nat Rev Clin Oncol* 11:446–459, 2014.)

What are the Essential Functions of the Liver?

The liver is considered the largest internal organ and the main metabolic workshop for the body. It is responsible for the synthesis of new proteins, including immune factors, clotting factors, and angiotensinogen, to raise the blood pressure when signaled by renin and for producing bile to aid in fat, cholesterol, and vitamin (A, D, E, K) absorption. The liver takes up, stores, and processes nutrients from food and delivers them to the body when there is metabolic demand. It also stores glycogen, the precursor of glucose. During periods of early hypoglycemia, glycogen is converted to glucose by the liver before being released into the bloodstream to maintain glucose control. Finally, the liver metabolizes and removes waste products such as fat, cholesterol, medications, and toxins.

What Is Cirrhosis?

Chronic liver disease and cirrhosis is the 12th most common cause of death in the United States, leading to approximately 40,000 deaths each year. The liver can regenerate and recover after an initial insult such as an acute infection or a short-term course of hepatotoxic medications. But, in the setting of chronic injury, such as alcohol or nonalcoholic fatty liver disease (NAFLD), the liver's natural ability to regenerate hepatocytes becomes pathologic, resulting in oxidative stress, inflammation and cell damage, destruction of the vascular and biliary trees, marked fibrosis, and a nodular and scarred parenchyma. A cirrhotic liver can be classified as **micronodular, macronodular**, or **mixed** based on its macroscopic appearance. A **micronodular** pattern is described as nodules smaller than 3 mm in size, uniformly distributed, in which the liver is typically normal in size or slightly enlarged. The **macronodular** pattern consists of nodules larger than 3 mm in size, with architectural distortion of the portal tracts and variable septal thickness. The mixed nodular livers have both micronodular and macronodular patterns.

On examination, the patient's temperature is 97.8°F, pulse rate 80 bpm, blood pressure 98/58, respiration rate 16/min, and oxygen saturation 97% on room air. His body mass index (BMI) is 36. The patient has no jugular venous distension (JVD) and has normal heart and lung sounds. Positive findings on examination include jaundice, temporal and proximal muscle wasting, spider angiomata, a moderately distended abdomen with positive fluid shift, hepatosplenomegaly, and 2+ lower extremity edema.

What Are the Clinical Findings of Cirrhosis?

Liver disease affects homeostasis in many ways. When the liver is impaired, levels of clotting factors, including factors I (fibrinogen), II (prothrombin), V, VII, VIII, IX, X, XI, and XIII, as well as protein C, protein S, and antithrombin, may be insufficient. This lack of synthesis leads to a relative coagulopathy and results in a rise in serum international normalized ratio (INR) and the risk of easy bruising and bleeding. Additionally, the diseased liver cannot properly serve as a filter using Kupffer cells to clear antigens and particulate matter from the portal system. In conjunction with low white blood cell counts from hypersplenism, this leads to an immunologically weakened state with increased risk of infection, including spontaneous bacterial peritonitis. A sick liver cannot produce albumin efficiently, leading to a decrease in the intravascular oncotic pressure and movement of fluid into the interstitial space (third space), causing edema and ascites. The body becomes catabolic, leading to the breakdown of skeletal muscle, which induces weight loss, and the patient becomes wasted and debilitated. Lack of oncotic pressure decreases the body's ability to transport fatty acids, nutrients, and steroid hormones. The cirrhotic patient is often hypotensive due to lack of angiotensinogen, despite high renin levels. The diseased liver cannot break down toxins, metabolites, and medications, resulting in elevated ammonia levels and other centrally acting products. Over time, this leads to the development of hepatic encephalopathy (confusion, memory loss, difficulty concentrating, hypersomnolence) and asterixis (flapping motion of outstretched, dorsiflexed hands). With the distortion of the biliary architecture, the cirrhotic patient cannot excrete bile efficiently, leading to clinical jaundice, scleral icterus, and pruritus. Physical findings of cirrhosis are described in Table 49.2.

Portal hypertension occurs in approximately 80% of cirrhotics and is defined as a portal pressure exceeding the normal range of 3 to 7 mm Hg. A clinically significant hepatic venous pressure gradient is 10 mm Hg or higher, and, in many advanced cirrhotics can rise to 20 to 30 mm Hg. This is largely due to increased resistance to portal blood flow by the liver. As a result of portal venous congestion, the cirrhotic patient develops splenomegaly with sequestration of platelets, thrombocytopenia, engorgement of vascular beds resulting in esophageal and gastric varices, rectal hemorrhoids, ascites, edema, and hepatic hydrothorax. Spontaneous bacterial peritonitis is a complication of portal hypertension and ascites, occurring in up to 10% of patients. It may be related to bacterial translocation from the gut in the setting of a depressed immune system and previous gastrointestinal bleed. Hepatorenal syndrome (HRS) refers to the development of acute renal failure in the patient with advanced liver disease. HRS is felt to arise from shunting of blood away from the kidneys in these patients due to splanchnic vasodilation. Doppler ultrasound of the kidneys will reveal renal vasoconstriction with high resistive indices and an elevated serum renin level. The medical treatment for HRS has included fluid resuscitation and diuretics, with poor response. The use of albumin, systemic vasopressors, transjugular intrahepatic portosystemic shunts (TIPS), and molecular adsorbent recirculatory system (MARS) as a modified renal replacement therapy has shown improved outcomes.

TABLE 49.2 ■ **Physical Findings of Cirrhosis**

Examination Findings	Incidence
Palpable liver	96%
Esophageal or gastric varices	25%–70%
Thrombocytopenia	15%–70%
Jaundice/scleral icterus	68%
Ascites and edema	66%
Spider angiomas	49%
Dilated abdominal wall veins	47%
Palpable spleen	46%
Testicular atrophy	45%
Palmar erythema	24%
Noninfectious fever	22%
Hepatic encephalopathy	18%
Gynecomastia	15%

From Marvin MR, Emond JC: Cirrhosis and portal hypertension: physical findings in cirrhosis. In Mulholland MW, Lillemoe KD, Doherty GM, et al, editors: *Greenfield's surgery: scientific principles & practice*, ed 5, Philadelphia, 2010, Wolters Kluwer.

TABLE 49.3 ▪ Child-Turcotte-Pugh Classification for Severity of Cirrhosis

Clinical and Laboratory Criteria	Points[a]		
	1	2	3
Encephalopathy	None	Mild to moderate (grade 1 or 2)	Severe (grade 3 or 4)
Ascites	None	Mild to moderate (diuretic responsive)	Severe (diuretic refractory)
Bilirubin (mg/dL)	< 2	2–3	> 3
Albumin (g/dL)	> 3.5	2.8–3.5	< 2.8
Prothrombin time			
Seconds prolonged	< 4	4–6	> 6
Internalized normal ratio	< 1.7	1.7–2.3	> 2.3

[a]Child-Turcotte-Pugh class obtained by adding score for each parameter (total points).
Class A: 5 to 6 points (least severe liver disease)
Class B: 7 to 9 points (moderately severe liver disease)
Class C: 10 to 15 (most severe liver disease)

CLINICAL PEARL (STEPS 2/3)

The severity of cirrhosis and its associated prognosis can be quantified using the Child-Turcotte-Pugh Classification (Table 49.3), with class C representing the most severe liver disease. Overall 1-year survival is 100% for patients with Class A disease but is only 80% and 45% for patients with Class B and C disease, respectively. A more complex calculation using serum creatinine, bilirubin, and international normalized ratio (INR) generates the model for end-stage liver disease (MELD) score, which has potential values between 6 and 40. The MELD score also predicts a patient's likelihood of mortality.

CLINICAL PEARL (STEPS 2/3)

It is important for all general surgeons to understand the risks of surgery for patients with liver disease. The decision to operate on patients with cirrhosis should always be considered seriously, and preoperative planning should involve the medicine and anesthesia teams. A discussion regarding the possibilities of liver decompensation, treatment, and consideration for liver transplantation should take place with patients and their families. Major perioperative risk depends on the clinical setting (e.g. emergency procedures), type of procedure, and severity of illness. The overall mortality risk among patients undergoing non-hepatic intraabdominal surgery, as stratified by Child-Pugh classes A, B, and C cirrhosis, are 10%, 17%, and 63%, respectively. Postoperative ascites, in the absence of active infection, can be managed with drains, diuretics, and potentially TIPS.

What Is the Workup and Management of a Patient With Cirrhosis?

The workup of the patient with end-stage liver disease should include laboratory tests including comprehensive metabolic panel, complete blood count, coagulation panel, hepatitis serologies, alpha-fetoprotein for hepatocellular carcinoma screening, CA 19-9 for cholangiocarcinoma screening, and immune markers to test for autoimmune pathologies. Tests, such as serum transferrin saturation, ferritin, ceruloplasmin, copper, or genetic testing, are needed to diagnose other, less frequent illnesses such as hemochromatosis, Wilson's disease, and other genetically predisposed diseases. An abdominal ultrasound assesses liver echotexture, the presence of liver masses, the size of the liver and spleen, and the presence of portal vein thrombosis. Patients often undergo computed tomography (CT) or magnetic resonance imaging (MRI) liver protocol scans as part of the workup of cirrhosis. These scans are more sensitive and specific in diagnosing portal vein thrombosis and primary liver cancers. Liver biopsy is often not required unless there is uncertainty in the diagnosis of a particular lesion.

Management goals of the end-stage liver disease patient include carefully treating their decompensations and, if failing to recover, bridging them to transplant. The treatment of hepatic encephalopathy includes bowel-cleansing medications to reduce ammonia production and absorption in the gut and nutrient supplementation. Lactulose acts on the distal ileum and colon, where it enhances the uptake of ammonia by intestinal bacteria, as well as excretion of ammonia through its cathartic activity. Antibiotics, such as rifaximin, metronidazole, and neomycin, have also been used to lower the concentration of ammonia-forming bacteria in the gut. Esophageal and gastric varices are medically managed with beta blockade, nitrates, and acid reduction. Patients with moderate or severe varices, with or without bleeding, may undergo prophylactic endoscopic banding, which has been shown to provide better long-term outcomes compared with endoscopic sclerotherapy. In the current era of successful hepatitis C therapy with medications such as ledipasvir/sofosbuvir or glecaprevir/pibrentasvir, more patients are being effectively treated. Patients can now be treated before transplant. For patients with posttreatment relapse, transplant can be performed with hepatitis C re-treatment thereafter.

Patients with advanced liver disease are often nutritionally depleted, and supplemental enteral or parenteral nutrition should be considered. Volume status should be optimized as large-volume paracentesis with albumin resuscitation may be necessary for patients with hemodynamic or respiratory distress due to large volume ascites. Hyponatremia develops from arterial vasodilation, leading to activation of the renin-angiotensin-aldosterone and sympathetic nervous systems. This results in a release of antidiuretic hormone, which causes retention of free water and relative decrease in total body sodium. Medical treatment of hyponatremia in these patients consists of free water restriction, vasopressin receptor inhibitors and careful use of diuretics. It is important to correct the sodium slowly to prevent the development of central pontine myelinolysis or osmotic demyelination syndrome (ODS). The risk of ODS is highest among patients with serum sodium lower than 130 meq/L who undergo rapid correction in the peritransplant period. It is important to closely monitor the patient's electrolytes, including potassium and magnesium, cardiac function, and volume status in the setting of all of the previously mentioned medical therapies. In some circumstances, when medical treatment fails, the patient may require renal replacement therapy for HRS.

On laboratory analyses the patient's albumin is 2.1, total bilirubin 3.5, AST 89, ALT 78, creatinine 1.4, INR 2.0, and sodium 128. His hemoglobin (Hgb) is 8.3, and his white blood cell count 8.0. His alpha-fetoprotein (AFP) is 3.0 ng/mL (normal in adults is less than 10.0 ng/mL), and hepatitis serologies are negative. Right-upper quadrant ultrasound reveals moderate perihepatic ascites and a nodular-appearing liver. The patient is therefore considered a class C cirrhotic and has a calculated MELD score of 27. The patient and his wife are counseled regarding the prognosis of his disease. They state that one of their neighbors had liver cancer and underwent a liver transplant; they wonder if the patient is a transplant candidate.

What Are the Indications for Liver Transplant? How Are Patients Listed for Transplantation?
Liver transplantation is warranted for those with significant compromise of basic hepatic function and complications from portal hypertension. Patients with acute liver failure are also given

consideration when medical management has failed. Candidates for liver transplantation are typically listed on the transplant waiting list once their calculated MELD score becomes 15 or greater.

In some instances the severity of a patient's liver disease may not be adequately captured by the biologic MELD score. Some of these patients receive MELD exception point approval by the regional review board. A common indication for MELD exception includes hepatocellular carcinoma (HCC) provided that a patient's tumor burden falls within Milan criteria, which emerged from the initial classic study in 1996 to establish which patients with HCC would be appropriate candidates for liver transplantation. The Milan criteria grant exception to patients with solitary tumors $<=$ 5cm or 2–3 tumors none exceeding 3cm and no evidence of vascular invasion and/or extra-hepatic spread. Other conditions that warrant MELD exception are hepatopulmonary syndrome, portopulmonary hypertension, familial amyloid polyneuropathy, primary hyperoxaluria, cystic fibrosis, hilar cholangiocarcinoma, ischemic cholangiopathy after prior liver transplant, and hepatic artery thrombosis within 2 weeks of liver transplantation.

Some patients with hepatocellular carcinoma and well-preserved liver function who are not candidates for liver transplant may undergo hepatic resection. The risk of recurrent or de novo HCC within 2 years without additional treatment remains 50%. In order to limit the magnitude of a liver operation for a patient with HCC who may subsequently go on to liver transplantation, there are several less invasive locoregional modalities that have been developed to treat and hopefully downstage HCC in an attempt to bridge patients to transplant. Interventional radiology has developed many such successful options, including transcatheter chemoembolization (TACE), percutaneous ethanol injection, cryoablation, radiofrequency ablation, and, more recently, focused arterial injection of the isotope yttrium-90 (Y-90) to control tumor progression. Liver transplantation for cholangiocarcinoma is performed only under strict inclusion criteria at select centers and includes an extensive workup to characterize the extent of disease before liver transplant, including staging laparoscopy after neoadjuvant chemotherapy and radiation.

Liver Transplantation

1. Make a "chevron" incision, a bilateral subcostal incision with upper midline extension.
2. Mobilize the native liver from the diaphragm and retroperitoneum.
3. Isolate the portal structures (hepatic artery, portal vein, and bile duct) and ligate them with suitable length for tension-free anastomoses to the allograft.
4. Remove the native liver.
5. Prepare the liver allograft on the back table (assuring that blood vessels and bile duct are suitable for anastomosis).
6. Begin allograft implantation by sewing the donor vena cava to the recipient vena cava (bicaval, Fig. 49.2) or the donor vena cava to the recipient hepatic vein cuff (piggyback).
7. Perform portal vein and hepatic artery anastomoses.
8. Reperfuse the allograft and assure hemostasis.
9. Perform bile duct anastomosis:
   - Duct-to-duct (typical)
   - Duct-to-Roux-en-Y limb of jejunum (patients with primary sclerosing cholangitis or child with biliary atresia and previous Kasai procedure).

What Are the Important Aspects of Postoperative Management of the Liver Transplant Recipient?
Expert perioperative management of liver transplant patients is essential for their recovery and successful long-term outcome. Patients generally have invasive monitoring such as Swan-Ganz catheters to measure pulmonary arterial pressures, arterial lines, large-bore intravenous lines,

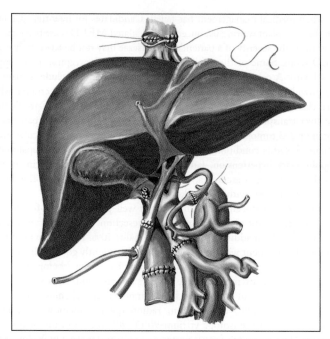

Fig. 49.2 Liver transplantation with bicaval technique. (Redrawn from Vilarinho S, Lifton RP: Liver transplantation: from inception to clinical practice, *Cell* 150(6):1096–1099, 2012.)

and nasogastric tubes for decompression. This facilitates close monitoring and the provider's ability to treat the patient during the operation, especially allograft reperfusion, and thereafter. Reperfusion of the liver allograft can lead to serious consequences including acute right heart failure, pulmonary embolus, and cardiac arrhythmia. Specially trained liver anesthesiologists are aware of these potential events and work with the surgical team to treat the recipient before and during reperfusion. Postoperatively, the patient requires close monitoring in the intensive care unit (ICU) for at least the first 24 to 48 hours. Center-specific posttransplant protocols are utilized by providers to monitor allograft recovery during the early postoperative period. These protocols include serial laboratory studies, including comprehensive metabolic panels, blood counts, coagulation studies, and arterial blood gases. Early signs of liver recovery include the normalization of electrolytes, stability of blood counts, improvement in mental status and successful extubation, and production of bile.

Vigilant assessment for signs of allograft rejection and initiation of immunosuppression are important aspects of postoperative care. See Chapter 50 for a discussion of rejection and immunosuppressive drugs.

What Are the Potential Complications of Liver Transplantation?

Complications after liver transplantation are common and are often associated with the difficulty of the operation. Examples of increased complexity are retransplantation cases, pediatric transplants, or those needing vascular reconstruction, or Roux-en-Y hepaticojejunostomy. Other factors associated with liver transplant complications include the underlying compromised functional and nutritional status of the recipient as well as the allograft quality (donor characteristics and degree of procurement or reperfusion injury). Late, and even early, signs and symptoms of postoperative complications may also be overlooked due to immunosuppression. For example, fever, leukocytosis, or pain may be absent in the presence of an infectious or inflammatory complication. Major complications that must be recognized after liver transplant include surgical bleed, hepatic artery thrombosis, acute renal insufficiency or failure, biliary leak or stricture, neurologic complications (strokes, seizures, infections, encephalopathy), hepatic vein or inferior vena cava stenosis, portal vein thrombosis, sepsis, and primary allograft nonfunction.

Posttransplant biliary anastomotic leaks and strictures are the most common surgical complications, occurring in approximately 10% to 30% of recipients, and are often managed with endoscopic retrograde cholangiopancreatography (ERCP).

Hepatic artery thrombosis (HAT) is a feared complication; which has an occurrence of 1% to 2% among adult recipients in experienced transplant centers. Risk factors for HAT include small arterial size (seen with pediatric or living donor liver transplant; arterial size less than 3 mm), arterial size mismatch, need for arterial reconstruction, CMV status, early acute rejection, and recipient smoking status. The diagnosis of HAT should be suspected and evaluated immediately if there is an acute rise in liver enzymes, worsening hepatic function (rise in INR and bilirubin, change in mental status), intrahepatic abscesses and fevers, and biliary complications. When any of these signs or symptoms is identified, a Doppler ultrasonography or CT angiogram of the liver should be done emergently to examine intrahepatic and extrahepatic arterial flow. If the diagnosis is made early (within a few days), arterial flow may be restored with reexploration and arterial reconstruction. Hepatic arterial thrombosis that occurs months to years later may manifest with biliary strictures and/or hepatic abscesses and requires intervention. However, salvage of arterial flow in this case is usually not feasible.

Postoperative hemorrhage is identified by the presence of a dropping hematocrit and bloody fluid in the drains within the early postoperative period and occurs 5% to 15% of the time. This is usually due to both the extensive surgical dissection and the relatively coagulopathic state of the recipient as the new liver graft recovers and regains function, but is also related to the extensive dissection.

Primary allograft nonfunction is rare (less than 1%) and occurs when the transplanted liver fails to function, leading to death in the absence of retransplantation. Factors associated with primary nonfunction include prolonged warm and cold ischemic times, allograft steatosis, donor age, and need for complex vascular reconstruction.

CLINICAL PEARL (STEPS 2/3)

Major complications from liver transplant requiring urgent intervention include bile leak or stricture, hepatic artery thrombosis, hemorrhage, and primary nonfunction. Early hepatic artery thrombosis requires retransplantation in around 50% of the cases.

What Is Graft-Versus-Host Disease?

Graft-versus-host disease (GVHD) is an immune phenomenon that requires the presence of immunocompetent cells in the transplanted graft, an immunocompromised host, and donor cells that have the ability to recognize the recipient's antigen as "foreign." Pathogenesis of GVHD follows when there is allograft tissue damage and donor T lymphocytes are shed. Proinflammatory cytokines (IL-1, TNF-alpha) and the recipient's antigen-presenting cells then activate donor T lymphocytes. The donor's T lymphocytes mount an alloreactive response to the recipient's tissues. Effector T lymphocytes migrate to the skin, gut, and bone marrow to cause direct damage and recruitment of other immune cells. GVHD is common after hematopoietic cell transplantation (HCT) but rarely occurs after solid organ transplantation. Typical onset occurs within 8 weeks from transplant, and clinical manifestations include rash (94.2%), fever (66.6%), diarrhea (54%), and pancytopenia (54%). Although GVHD after liver transplant has an incidence of 0.1% to 2%, it carries an extremely high mortality risk (greater than 75%). The diagnosis of GVHD is made by biopsy of the affected tissue.

What Are the Outcomes and Special Considerations After Liver Transplantation?

There have been 151,193 liver transplants performed in the United States from January 1, 1988 to May 31, 2017, with an increase in number annually. In 2016 there were 7841 liver transplants, with 7496 harvested from deceased donors and 345 donated by living donors. Over the years, outcomes after liver transplantation have improved. One-year survival after liver transplant is 85% for adults and 90% for children. Annual mortality rate after transplant is approximately 3%. Long-term outcomes after liver transplantation depends on the severity of medical illness and level of care (ICU, hospital, or home) before the transplant, repeat transplantation, the underlying disease, and the experience of the transplant center (higher-volume centers have higher adjusted overall patient survival rates).

Pediatric and adult living donor liver transplantation grew after the success of living donor kidney transplant and deceased donor split liver transplantation. With the success of partial adult liver living donation (often segments 2/3) in the pediatric population, adult-to-adult living transplantation techniques were developed to safely resect and implant whole lobe allografts for selected liver recipients. To date, almost 5% of all liver transplants in the United States are from living donors. Preparation of the living donor and recipient operation is complex and involves medical, surgical, and anesthesia teams. Advanced imaging including MRI and volumetric CT scans of the donor liver that are necessary to determine favorable anatomy for splitting the liver, adequate volumes of the anticipated donor allograft and remnant, and volume requirement for the recipient and to evaluate the need for vascular reconstruction. Similar to the recipient selection, a multidisciplinary transplant committee is involved with donor selection with an additional donor advocate member, who is a necessary part in determining overall eligibility for living donor transplantation. Overall, living donor liver transplantation is a viable option with good outcomes and is performed at select centers in the United States.

The patient undergoes pretransplant evaluation (complete with radiographic and laboratory workup) and is reviewed by the multidisciplinary transplant board. He is deemed appropriate for liver transplantation. After several months on the transplant wait list, he undergoes a deceased-donor liver transplantation. He follows a typical postoperative course, is started on immunosuppressive agents along with antimicrobial prophylaxis, and is discharged from the hospital without complications. He sees his transplant team in the office 1 week later. His incisions are healing well, he is tolerating his medication regimen without difficulty, and his laboratory values are within normal limits. He and his wife are educated on posttransplant surveillance and continued office visits with medical and surgical providers.

BEYOND THE PEARLS

- Up to 50% of patients with liver disease have no underlying symptoms. Cirrhosis ensues from chronic liver stress and injury. With repeated bouts of inflammation, the liver will attempt to regenerate, which leads to fibrosis and eventually cirrhosis.
- The liver is responsible for many functions and is considered the metabolic factory of the body. A diseased liver will not store or process nutrients, build protein or clotting factors, or metabolize and eliminate toxins in the bloodstream.
- Patients with cirrhosis who experience added stress may decompensate by developing ascites, edema, encephalopathy, jaundice, coagulopathy, malnutrition and weight loss, upper or lower gastrointestinal bleeding from varices, and hepatorenal syndrome.
- Minimally invasive management, including TIPS, ERCP, endoscopy with banding and sclerotherapy, and locoregional therapy by IR and radiation oncology for HCC, has facilitated medical management of patients with end-stage liver disease.

- More than 70% of all cases of primary liver cancer occur in patients with cirrhosis. Milan criteria were developed to offer a curative option with transplantation for patients with HCC. Patients can undergo locoregional therapy with TACE, ablation, or Y-90 for downstaging or tumor control while they await transplantation.

- Major complications from liver transplant that require urgent intervention include bile leak or stricture, hepatic artery thrombosis, hemorrhage, and primary nonfunction. Primary nonfunction and most early hepatic artery thrombosis cases require immediate retransplantation.

- Medication reconciliation is paramount when a patient with history of transplant presents with new or worsening chronic complaints. Medication changes or adjustments in immunosuppression may be necessary if a patient is being considered for an elective operation or procedure.

- Graft-versus-host disease is rare among solid organ transplant recipients, with symptoms affecting organs with high cell turnover: skin, gut, and bone marrow. Mortality is extremely high, with limited success from current available therapies.

- Liver transplantation is curative for end-stage liver disease as well as select patients with hepatocellular carcinoma and cholangiocarcinoma, with overall 1-year survival more than 85%.

Suggested Readings

Akbulut, S., Yimaz, M., & Yimaz, S. (2012). Graft-versus-host disease after liver transplant: A comprehensive literature review. *World J Gastroenterol, 18*(37), 5240–5248.

Levitsky, J., Goldberg, D., Smith, A. R., et al. (2017). Acute rejection increases risk of graft failure and death in recent liver transplant recipients. *Clin Gastroenterol Hepatol, 15*(4), 584–593.

Ma, C., Crippin, J. S., Chapman, W. C., Korenblat, K., Vaccharajani, N., Gunter, K. L., et al. (2013). Parenchymal alterations in cirrhotic livers in patients with hepatopulmonary syndrome of portopulmonary hypertension. *Liver Transpl, 19*(7), 741–750.

Neef, H., Mariaskin, D., Spangenberg, H. C., Hopt, U. T., & Makowiec, F. (2011). Perioperative mortality after non-hepatic general surgery in patients with liver cirrhosis: An analysis of 138 operations in the 2000s using Child and MELD scores. *J Gastrointest Surg Jan, 15*(1), 1–11.

Oh, C. K., Sawyer, R. G., Pelletier, S. J., et al. (2004). Independent predictors for primary non-function after liver transplantation. *Yonsei Med J, 45*(6), 1155–1161.

CHAPTER 50

End-Stage Renal Disease in a 46-Year-Old Female

Ahmad Safra ■ Ashesh P. Shah

> A 46-year-old Caucasian female with past medical history of type 2 diabetes mellitus and essential hypertension, which have progressively resulted in chronic kidney disease, presents to the transplant center for evaluation. She has no other medical history, has undergone no previous surgeries, and is currently taking aspirin, a beta blocker, and an ACE inhibitor. She was referred to the center by her nephrologist who says that she will require dialysis soon and recommended her for evaluation for potential kidney transplantation.

What Are the Major Causes of Chronic Kidney Disease?

The clinical etiology of kidney disease has been classically classified into three major categories including prerenal, intrinsic renal, or postrenal. A prolonged process in any of these categories may result in chronic kidney disease (CKD), leading to end-stage renal disease (ESRD), which requires renal replacement therapy. Examples of chronic conditions leading to CKD are outlined in Table 50.1.

Diabetes and hypertension are responsible for two-thirds of all cases of chronic kidney disease.

Diabetic nephropathy occurs in type 1 and type 2 diabetes mellitus, which can lead to multiple pathological changes in the kidney (Fig. 50.1 and 50.2), eventually leading to microalbuminuria and renal failure. Chronic hypertension can lead to nephrosclerosis involving vascular, glomerular, and tubulointerstitial components of the renal parenchyma.

What Is the Epidemiology of Chronic Kidney Disease and How Is It Classified?

Chronic kidney disease is a major challenge in public health worldwide. In the United States, it is estimated that 660,000 people are being treated for kidney failure. Of those, 468,000 are dialysis patients. In 2013, 117,000 new cases of kidney failure were reported in the United States; the majority of those patients are between 45 and 64 years of age, and the estimated annual Medicare spending to treat kidney failure in the United States exceeds $31 billion.

Chronic kidney disease is classified into five stages based on the glomerular filtration rate (GFR) as shown in Table 50.2.

> The patient is accompanied to the office by her husband who states, "I will donate one of my kidneys if I am a match!" She comes with recent laboratory analyses that show her GFR is 28 mL/min/1.73m^2. The patient and her husband are eager to undergo evaluation, as she wants to avoid initiating dialysis if possible.

TABLE 50.1 ■ **Chronic Conditions Leading to Chronic Kidney Disease**

Prerenal Azotemia	Intrinsic Renal Azotemia	Postrenal Azotemia
Heart failure	Nephrosclerosis	Nephrolithiasis
Cirrhosis	Glomerulonephritis	Benign prostatic hyperplasia
Renal artery atherosclerosis	Vasculitis	Chronic ureteral obstruction
	Interstitial nephritis	Bladder carcinoma
	Polycystic kidney disease	Retroperitoneal fibrosis
	Nephrocalcinosis	
	Sarcoidosis	
	Nephrotoxic drugs	
	Radiographic contrast dyes	

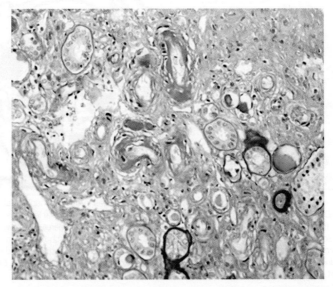

Fig. 50.1 Benign nephrosclerosis. A characteristic feature of hypertensive arteriosclerosis is the reduplication or multiplication of the internal elastic lamina, which can be observed with elastic stains or at the time of the immunofluorescence studies. Zhou M, Netto GJ, Epstein JI: Benign nephrosclerosis. In *High-Yield Uropathology*. Philadelphia: Elsevier, 2012, pp. 254-255.

What Does the Workup for Renal Transplantation Entail?

Referral of patients with CKD to a transplant center is generally recommended when their GFR falls below 30 mL/min/1.73m^2. Although they are usually not on renal replacement therapy at this point, the early referral allows for full evaluation and complete testing of patients who are considered candidates for renal transplantation. The extensive workup is aimed at identifying comorbid conditions that would complicate transplantation and the required postoperative immunosuppression.

The initial evaluation begins with a detailed history and physical examination of the patient. It is important to rule out comorbid conditions which could be contraindications to kidney transplant or could substantially affect survival following transplantation, such as cardiopulmonary disease, malignancies, current infections, or a history of peripheral vascular disease. Eliciting a history of

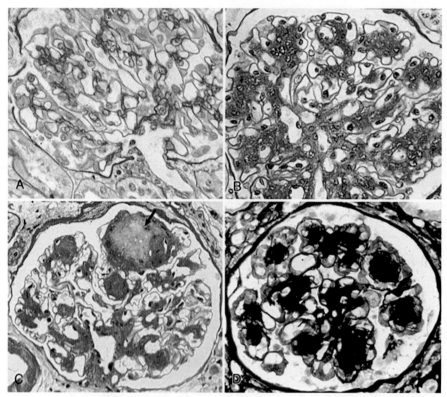

Fig. 50.2 Diabetic nephropathy. Light microscopy of structural changes in diabetic nephropathy. (A) Normal glomerulus. (B) Diffuse glomerular lesion: widespread mesangial expansion. (C) Nodular lesion as well as mesangial expansion: there is a typical Kimmelstiel-Wilson nodule at the top of the glomerulus *(arrow)*. (A, B, and C, Periodic acid–Schiff reaction). (D) Nodular lesion: methenamine silver staining shows the marked nodular expansion of mesangial matrix. Tang S, Sharma K: Pathogenesis, clinical manifestations, and natural history of diabetic kidney disease. In *Comprehensive Clinical Nephrology*, 6th ed. Philadelphia: Elsevier, 2019, pp. 357–375.e1.

TABLE 50.2 ■ **Stages of chronic kidney disease as defined by glomerular filtration rate (GFR).**

Stage	GFR (mL/min/1.73 m^2)
1	>90 (normal)
2	60–89
3	30–59
4	15–29
5	<15

prior surgeries, especially on the abdomen, is very important for operative planning. Additionally, the patient's body mass index (BMI) should be assessed, as obesity can be a challenge in performing the operation. Related to antigenic considerations, previous pregnancies, history of blood transfusion, and prior transplants can make transplant candidates more sensitized to human leukocyte antigens (HLA) which increases the positivity of crossmatch to potential donors, decreasing the likelihood of HLA matching to a wide variety of donors.

The physical examination should be performed with attention paid to the end organ effects of the medical comorbidities that caused the patient's renal failure. Additionally, the examination should include an assessment of arterial pulses in the lower extremities that can help identify aortoiliac atherosclerotic disease. Any suspicion of aortoiliac disease warrants further testing because the renal graft is typically anastomosed to the iliac vessels.

Furthermore, history and physical examination should identify any active infection, malignancy, or substance abuse, all of which are considered absolute contraindications to transplantation. Other contraindications include uncontrolled psychiatric disorders and ongoing treatment noncompliance, both of which are risks for noncompliance with the postoperative immunosuppressive regimen and ultimate graft loss.

Laboratory studies should include complete blood count, comprehensive metabolic panel, pregnancy test, blood type, coagulation studies, parathyroid hormone, hemoglobin A1C, serologic testing for viral infections including human immunodeficiency virus (HIV), cytomegalovirus (CMV), hepatitis B and C, measles, mumps, and rubella. HLA and panel reactive antibody assay are needed to detect previous sensitization that might affect waiting time on the transplant list.

Further testing should focus on identifying any of the contraindications to transplant mentioned previously. Patients should undergo all recommended cancer screenings: colonoscopy should be performed for all patients over the age of 50; prostate-specific antigen (PSA) should be performed on men; Pap smear and breast examination for all women; and mammography for all women over 40 years old. An electrocardiogram (ECG), chest radiograph, and purified protein derivative (PPD) test should also be obtained.

What Are the Available Sources of Kidneys for Transplantation?

Patients who need kidney transplantation have one of two options: renal allografts from either live or deceased donors. All potential transplant recipients should be counseled about the value of live kidney donation at the time of their initial evaluation. Living donors are usually healthy individuals who can be related or unrelated and known (family or friend) or unknown (altruistic donor) to the recipient. Those individuals undergo detailed screening and testing, which also include HLA and major histocompatibility complex (MHC) type I and II. In case of mismatch, paired kidney donation can be organized among multiple institutions or within the same institution for organ transplantation between groups of donors and recipients who are matches.

Once all the testing results are obtained, the candidacy of the potential renal transplantation recipient is discussed among a multidisciplinary team, including transplant surgeons, transplant nephrologists, psychiatrists, social workers, and transplant coordinators. If the patient is deemed a candidate for transplantation, he or she is added to the transplant waiting list. Patients should be evaluated periodically when on the list to verify their continued candidacy and to rule out any emerging contraindications that might mandate temporary or permanent removal from the transplant waiting list. This list is managed by the United Network for Organ Sharing (UNOS). A newly implemented kidney allocation system characterizes donors on a percent scale using the kidney donor profile index and allocates the 20% of deceased donor kidneys with the greatest expected posttransplant longevity to the 20% of candidates with the best expected posttransplant survival; kidneys that are not accepted are then offered to the remaining 80% of candidates.

Patients should be counseled that recipients of live donor kidney transplants have a better 10-year survival and better early and late graft function compared with recipients of deceased donor kidney transplants. The half-life of live donor kidney transplant is about 14 years compared with 9 years for deceased donor kidney transplant. Patients who have no potential living donors are placed on the waiting list for deceased donors.

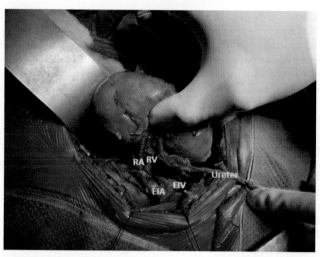

Fig. 50.3 Renal transplantation with implantation of the allograft in the right lower quadrant, shown after completion of vascular anastomosis and reperfusion. (RA: renal artery; RV: renal vein; EIA: external iliac artery; EIV: external iliac vein.)

No further comorbidities are elicited in the patient's history. Her physical examination reveals vital signs that are within normal limits, normal cardiopulmonary and abdominal examinations, and palpable distal pulses in her bilateral lower extremities. She undergoes a complete workup and is determined to be a transplant candidate by the multidisciplinary transplant team. Laboratory analyses determine that there is serologic mismatch between her and her husband, and he is therefore not a potential donor. The patient is added to the transplant list. Six months later, the patient's renal function has deteriorated to a GFR of 16 mL/min/1.73m². She presents for reevaluation, is matched with an altruistic donor, and is scheduled for transplantation two weeks later.

Renal Transplantation

1. Place the patient supine, induce general anesthesia, and insert central venous line and a three-way Foley catheter (used for instillation of saline into the bladder at the time of ureteral implantation).
2. Make a curvilinear incision medial to the anterior superior iliac spine, inferomedially to just above the pubic tubercle on the same side (the so-called Gibson incision).
3. Divide subcutaneous tissue and abdominal muscle lateral to the rectus abdominus.
4. Identify and expose the iliac artery and vein, and anastomose the renal allograft artery and vein, respectively, using end-to-side anastomoses.
5. Reperfuse the renal allograft and assure hemostasis (Fig. 50.3).
6. Implant the allograft ureter into the bladder (the ureterocystostomy); there are several techniques for performing this step.

What Are the Important Aspects of Postoperative Management After Renal Transplantation?
There are many important considerations in the postoperative care of the renal transplant recipient, many of which focus on optimizing allograft function. It is important to avoid hypotension in the postoperative period in order to maximize blood flow to the renal allograft. Urine output should be closely monitored, and an equivalent volume replaced as intravenous crystalloid each

TABLE 50.3 ■ Summary of Immunosuppressant Drug Classes and Mechanisms of Action

Drug Class and Examples	Mechanism of Action
Corticosteroids Prednisone Methylprednisone	Inhibit inflammatory response and cytokine production
Antimetabolites Azathioprine Mycophenolate mofetil	Interfere with DNA synthesis
Calcineurin inhibitors Cyclosporine Tacrolimus	Inhibit T-cell activation by inhibition of calcineurin phosphatase
mTOR inhibitors Sirolimus	Inhibit T-cell activation by inhibition of IL-2
Antibodies Thymoglobulin	Deplete B and T cells

hour. The central venous pressure should be monitored, which helps in assessing volume status and the need for additional fluid resuscitation. Urine output is also monitored to detect whether there is immediate, delayed, or slow graft function. Sudden drops in the urine output can be related to a blood clot blocking the Foley catheter, therefore flushing the catheter should be the first step in management. If the patient is still not making urine after a period of good urine output, Doppler ultrasound should be obtained immediately to check for renal vascular thrombosis, which mandates emergent surgical exploration to salvage the renal graft.

Immunosuppressant regimens vary but often begin with steroids preoperatively and continue immediately postoperatively (Table 50.3). Daily laboratory testing should be obtained as pancytopenia can be a side effect of the immunosuppression medications. Prophylactic antibiotics are initiated preoperatively and often continue also.

BASIC SCIENCE PEARL (STEPS 1/2/3)

Immunosuppressive regimens for solid organ transplantation begin with induction agents at the time of transplant and continue with maintenance drugs. Table 50.3 outlines these drugs and their uses.

What Are Potential Complications After Renal Transplantation?

Renal transplantation can be complicated by several conditions, which can be transient and amenable to intervention, or permanent and result in graft loss. The most feared complication is allograft rejection, the causes of which are outlined in Table 50.4. Potential early postoperative complications include wound infections, renal arterial or venous thrombosis, stricture at the arterial or venous anastomosis, ureteral obstruction and stent malfunction, urine leak, perinephric hematoma or seroma, acute rejection, and gastrointestinal complications. Late complications can include renal artery stenosis, lymphocele, ureteral stricture, calculus disease, chronic rejection, opportunistic infections, neoplasms as a result of immunosuppression, and posttransplantation lymphoproliferative disorder. Appropriate studies such as laboratory analysis, radiographic studies such as allograft ultrasound, and biopsy, if indicated, should be obtained for any suspected complication to try to identify it as early as possible. Treatment should always focus on optimizing patient and graft survival. Allograft nephrectomy may be at times mandated for some post-transplant complications. A patient's candidacy for retransplant should always be evaluated after allograft nephrectomy in hopes of avoiding the initiation of dialysis.

TABLE 50.4 ■ Types of Transplant Rejection and Pathophysiology

Type	Mechanism	Timing	Hypersensitivity Type
Hyperacute	Preformed antibodies	Immediate	II
Acute	T cells mediate parenchymal cell death (cellular); antibody-mediated damage to graft vasculature (humoral)	Weeks–months	IV
Chronic	T cell–mediated deposition of smooth muscle and parenchymal fibrosis	Months–years	III/IV

The patient undergoes live donor renal transplant and the renal allograft begins producing urine in the operating room. Postoperatively, she is maintained on intravenous fluids and her urine output is monitored hourly. Immunosuppression and antibacterial prophylaxis are started, which she tolerates well. Her urinary catheter is removed on postoperative day three. The transplant team reviews the patient's new medication regimen with both her and her husband and they are given anticipatory guidance about warning signs of infection or rejection. She is discharged to home with instructions for follow up in one week.

Beyond the Pearls

– Renal transplantation is the most common solid organ transplantation in the United States.
– Two thirds of cases of chronic kidney disease are caused by diabetes and/or hypertension.
– Renal allografts can be procured from living or deceased donors.
– In addition to the ABO blood type, human leukocyte antigen (HLA) subtype matching is an important factor in decreasing the chance of allograft rejection.
– Renal allografts are typically placed in the iliac fossa and anastomosed to the iliac artery and vein. Native kidney explantation is rarely required.
– Immunosuppression is required for the prevention of allograft rejection, but also increases the risk of opportunistic infections for which prophylactic antimicrobials are important.

Suggested Readings

Abramowicz, D., Cochat, P., Claas, F. H., et al. (2015). European Renal Best Practice Guideline on kidney donor and recipient evaluation and perioperative care. *Nephrol Dial Transplant, 30*, 1790–1797.
Jha, V., Garcia-Garcia, G., Iseki, K., et al. (2013). Chronic kidney disease: Global dimension and perspectives. *Lancet, 20*(9888), 260–272.
Kasiske, B. L., Cangro, C. B., Hariharan, S., et al. (2001). The evaluation of renal transplantation candidates: Clinical practice guidelines. *Am J Transplant, 1*(Suppl 2), 3–95.

Pediatric Surgery

CHAPTER 51

Jaundice in a 1-Month-Old Male

Shannon N. Acker ■ Jonathan P. Roach

A 30-day-old former term male is referred for evaluation of jaundice. The child's mother reports that the baby had jaundice at birth with bilirubin up to 20, but this improved with phototherapy. The baby is otherwise healthy, is tolerating breast milk feeds without vomiting or diarrhea, and is growing normally. Over the past 2 days, the mother noted jaundice again that is now worsening. She also reports that his stools are getting lighter and his urine is getting darker. He has no known exposure to hepatitis. On examination, the vital signs are within normal limits, and the baby is well developed and well nourished. Examination is notable for scleral icterus. The abdomen is soft, liver is palpable 3 cm lower than the costal margin, liver span is 6 cm; the liver is firm, and there is no evidence of ascites. There are no rashes or skin lesions, but the baby is diffusely jaundiced. Acholic stools are visualized in two diapers.

What Is the Differential Diagnosis for Jaundice in a Newborn?

The most common cause of jaundice in the newborn is physiologic jaundice due to high bilirubin load and immature elimination system. Physiologic jaundice is more common in breast-fed infants and usually does not require any specific treatment. In contrast to physiologic jaundice, pathologic jaundice should be suspected if any of the following are present: jaundice within the first 24 hours of life; total bilirubin greater than 12 to 15mg/dL in an otherwise healthy term infant; jaundice that persists after 14 days; or conjugated hyperbilirubinemia. Causes of conjugated hyperbilirubinemia include infectious, genetic, metabolic, or undefined abnormalities that lead to either mechanical obstruction of bile flow or functional impairment of bile secretion. The most common causes that require involvement of a pediatric surgeon are biliary atresia and choledochal cysts (Fig. 51.1).

What Is the Standard Workup to Evaluate Jaundice in a Neonate?

Laboratory investigation is required for prolonged or severe hyperbilirubinemia. For a baby presenting with jaundice at older than 14 days it is essential to obtain a fractionated serum bilirubin. Further evaluation of the patient should include assessment of stool color, hepatic synthetic function, urine and serum bile acids, alpha1-antitrypsin assessment, thyroxine and TSH, sweat chloride and mutation analysis, Coombs test, urine and serum amino acids, and urine reducing substances, as well as testing for hepatitis and communicable congenital bacterial infections. After laboratory evaluation, an abdominal ultrasound should be obtained to exclude a choledochal cyst and to evaluate the liver and biliary tree. At times this is followed by hepatobiliary scintigraphy to document bile duct patency or obstruction, however this is infrequently required. Liver biopsy is the final step in the workup to evaluate for biliary atresia or suggest to determine other causes.

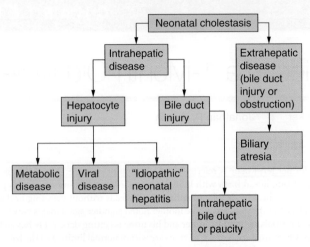

Fig. 51.1 Conceptual overview of the evaluation of neonatal cholestasis. There may be some overlap between intrahepatic and extrahepatic causes of cholestasis. Patients with biliary atresia may have some degree of intrahepatic disease, and patients with idiopathic disease may be found to have a viral or metabolic cause in the future.

BASIC SCIENCE PEARL (STEP 1)

Bilirubin is conjugated to glucuronic acid within hepatocytes by the enzyme glucuronyltransferase (Fig. 51.2). Conjugated bilirubin, also known as direct bilirubin, is excreted from hepatocytes to either be stored in the gallbladder or excreted into the gastrointestinal tract. Conjugated bilirubin can be deconjugated by gut bacteria to urobilinogen, which can be reabsorbed into the circulation and reexcreted in the bile—the so-called enterohepatic circulation.

CLINICAL PEARL (STEPS 2/3)

In contrast to unconjugated hyperbilirubinemia, an elevation in the conjugated bilirubin level is always pathologic and should be evaluated. Additionally, any hyperbilirubinemia that persists after day 14 of life is pathologic. The most important step in the evaluation of these infants is to differentiate neonatal hepatitis, which implies intrahepatic cholestasis, from an extrahepatic biliary obstruction such as biliary atresia or choledochal cyst.

On further workup, laboratory studies are notable for a normal complete blood count and no evidence for immune reactivity against erythrocytes (direct and indirect Coombs test). The synthetic function of the liver is normal with normal PT and INR as well as total protein and albumin. The alpha-1-antitrypsin level is also normal. Total bilirubin is 9.4 mg/dL (elevated) with a total conjugated bilirubin of 4.8 mg/dL (elevated). The AST and ALT are elevated at 740 and 582 U/L. The GGT is also elevated at 162 U/L. An abdominal ultrasound reveals a liver that is normal in size and contour without intrahepatic ductal dilation along with a contracted gallbladder. The common bile duct is normal, and there is no evidence of a choledochal cyst. Echocardiogram and spine radiographs are also normal.

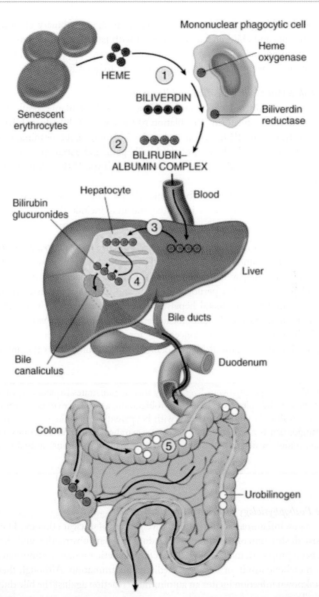

Fig. 51.2 Bilirubin metabolism. Biliverdin, a breakdown product of heme from senescent erythrocytes, is reduced to bilirubin, which is conjugated to glucuronic acid by hepatocytes. Conjugated bilirubin is excreted as a component of bile through the biliary tree and is deconjugated to urobilinogen by gut bacteria. (From Thiese ND: Liver and gallbladder. In Kumar V, Abbas AK, Aster JC, editors: *Robbins and Cotran pathologic basis of disease*, ed 9, Philadelphia, 2015, Elsevier, pp 821–881.)

What Is the Typical Presentation of a Choledochal Cyst?

Choledochal cysts are congenital bile duct anomalies that present as dilations of either the intrahepatic or extrahepatic biliary tree. The classic triad of a choledochal cyst includes right upper quadrant pain, jaundice, and a palpable mass; this triad is present in only 30% of children at presentation. Based on the severity and portions of the biliary tree affected, they can present anytime from childhood to adulthood, and presentation can vary from signs of biliary obstruction to vague abdominal pain. Infants and children can also present with jaundice with or without either a palpable right upper quadrant mass or a cystic lesion seen on ultrasound. Prenatal diagnosis is becoming more common as prenatal ultrasound is utilized more frequently.

How Are Choledochal Cysts Classified and Treated?

Choledochal cysts are categorized into types I to V based on the Todani classification (Fig. 51.3). Type I include cystic (Ia) or fusiform (Ib) dilation of the common bile duct (CBD). Type II are diverticula of the CBD. Type III are choledochoceles (dilation of the terminal CBD within the duodenal wall). Type IV include dilation of the intrahepatic and extrahepatic bile ducts (IVa) or extrahepatic bile duct dilation and a choledochocele (IVb). Type V (Caroli disease) includes only intrahepatic ductal dilation.

Treatment of choledochal cysts varies based on severity. Due to risk of developing cholangiocarcinoma, complete surgical excision is indicated and may include the need for liver transplant depending on the degree of intrahepatic involvement.

What Is the Next Step in the Workup of Pediatric Patients With Obstructive Jaundice?

Neonates with obstructive jaundice should undergo percutaneous liver biopsy to evaluate for biliary atresia. Findings on liver biopsy that suggest biliary atresia include bile ductular proliferation, presence of bile plugs, and portal or perilobular edema and fibrosis. The basic hepatic architecture remains intact. In contrast, in neonatal hepatitis, there is distortion of the lobular architecture, infiltration with inflammatory cells, and focal hepatocellular necrosis with no change in the bile ductules. If biopsy findings are concerning for biliary atresia or biliary atresia cannot be ruled out, this should be followed by a cholangiogram to fully assess the architecture of the biliary tree.

The patient undergoes a percutaneous liver biopsy that demonstrates hepatocytic, canalicular, and biliary cholestasis with bile plugs and bile duct proliferation, as well as marked hepatocytic reactive changes and portal fibrosis. After discussion with his parents, he is taken to the operating room where a cholangiogram is attempted, but no patent extrahepatic ductal structures, including the gallbladder, are found. A diagnosis of biliary atresia is made and communicated to the patient's parents.

What Is the Pathophysiology of Biliary Atresia?

Biliary atresia is a rare inflammatory fibroobliterative process of unclear etiology. The inflammation causes progressive destruction of the biliary tree leading to biliary obstruction and cirrhosis. Various etiologies have been proposed, including viral infection, genetic mutation, abnormal duct remodeling, vascular or metabolic insult, or immune-mediated inflammation. Although there is some evidence that an unknown infection incites an autoimmune reaction against the bile duct, the ultimate cause remains unknown.

How Is Biliary Atresia Classified?

Biliary atresia is classified into one of three categories based on the macroscopic appearance (Fig. 51.4). Type I is atresia of the CBD. Type IIa is atresia of the common hepatic duct. Type IIb is atresia of the CBD and the common hepatic duct. Type III is atresia of all extrahepatic bile ducts up to the porta hepatis. Type III is the most common form, accounting for 90% of cases.

What Is the Recommended Operative Intervention for Biliary Atresia?

A hepatoportoenterostomy, or Kasai procedure, is the standard treatment for biliary atresia. The goal of the operation is to promote bile drainage from the liver. The procedure involves making

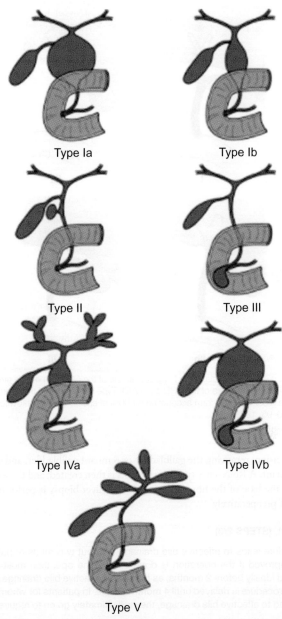

Type Ia

Type Ib

Type II

Type III

Type IVa

Type IVb

Type V

Fig. 51.3 Todani classification of choledochal cysts. Type I include cystic (Ia) or fusiform (Ib) dilation of the CBD. Type II are diverticulum of the CBD. Type III are choledochoceles (dilation of the terminal CBD within the duodenal wall). Type IV include dilation of the intrahepatic and extrahepatic bile ducts (IVa) or extrahepatic bile duct dilation and a choledochocele (IVb). Type V (Caroli disease) include only intrahepatic ductal dilation. (From Todani T, Watanabe Y, Narusue M, et al: Congenital bile duct cyst: classification, operative procedure, and review of 37 cases including cancer arising from choledochal cyst, *Am J Surg* 134:263–269, 1977.)

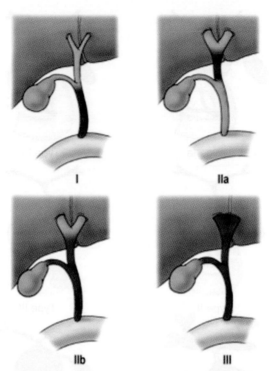

Fig. 51.4 Classification of biliary atresia. Type I involves atresia of the CBD. Type IIa is atresia of the common hepatic duct (CHD). Type IIb is atresia of the CBD and CHD. Type III is atresia of the entire extrahepatic biliary system. Type III is the most common form accounting for 90% of cases. (From Lefkowitch JH: Biliary atresia, *Mayo Clin Proc* 73:90–95, 1998.)

a right subcostal incision, removing the gallbladder or remnant gallbladder, and excising the extra-hepatic biliary remnant. A Roux-en-y type anastomosis is then created, and the jejunal limb is anastomosed widely to the base of the fibrous ductal plate. A liver biopsy is performed if this had not been accomplished preoperatively.

CLINICAL PEARL (STEPS 2/3)

The Kasai procedure leads to effective bile drainage in about two-thirds of patients. However, outcomes are improved if the operation is done earlier. The operation must be done before 90 days of life and ideally before 2 months, as the rate of effective bile drainage drops off to less than 10% if the procedure is delayed until 4 months of age. In patients for whom the Kasai operation does not lead to effective bile drainage, they will ultimately go on to require liver transplant.

CLINICAL PEARL (STEPS 2/3)

A recent prospective study comparing the use of high-dose steroids plus surgery with surgery alone demonstrated that the addition of steroids did not significantly improve bile drainage among infants with biliary atresia. The use of steroids is no longer recommended in this population.

What Is the Expected Outcome After the Kasai Operation?

After the Kasai operation, approximately two-thirds of patients will obtain satisfactory biliary drainage. Usually the bilirubin level normalizes 3 to 4 weeks after surgery, and the stool color changes within the first 2 weeks. Among the children who establish biliary drainage, half will continue to have good bile drainage and will likely keep their native liver long term. However, the other half will have ongoing inflammation and fibrosis leading to liver failure. This group will ultimately require liver transplantation. This occurs at a mean age of 5.4 years. The remaining third of patients will never establish bile flow after the Kasai procedure, and these children require liver transplant before age 2.

After informed consent, the patient undergoes a hepatoportoenterostomy (Kasai procedure). Pathology from the biliary remnant showed a diminutive gallbladder and biliary tree with ductal fibroobliterative changes consistent with extrahepatic biliary atresia. He recovers well and is set up for regular follow-up with the pediatric liver team.

BEYOND THE PEARLS

- Jaundice that persists after day 14 of life in a newborn is pathologic and needs to be evaluated.
- If biliary atresia is suspected, thorough evaluation should be undertaken quickly, as long-term survival with the native liver in place is significantly improved if the Kasai operation is performed before day 60 of life.
- Despite timely therapy, two-thirds of infants who undergo a Kasai will ultimately require liver transplant due to poor bile drainage from the native liver, leading to cirrhosis and portal hypertension.
- Choledochal cysts should be resected at the time of diagnosis, as they carry a risk of malignant degeneration.
- Children with a history of a choledochal cyst remain at increased risk of cholangiocarcinoma, even after complete cyst excision, and must be followed throughout their life.

Suggested Readings

Bezerra, J. A., Spino, C., Magee, J. C., et al. (2014). Use of corticosteroids after portoenterostomy for bile drainage in infants with biliary atresia: The START randomized clinical trial. *JAMA*, *311*(17), 1750–1759.

Gonzales, K. D. & Lee, H. (2012). Choledochal cyst in pediatric surgery. In A. G. Coran (Ed.), *Pediatric Surgery* (7th ed., pp. 1331–1339). New York: Saunders.

Liem, N. T. & Holcomb, G. W. (2014). Choledochal cyst and gallbladder disease. In G. W. Holcomb, III, J. P. Murphy, D. J. Ostlie, & S. D. St. Peter (Eds.), *Ashcraft's Pediatric Surgery* (6th ed., pp. 593–606). New York: Saunders.

Nightingale, S., Stormon, M. O., O'Loughlin, E. V., et al. (2017). Early posthepatoportoenterostomy predictors of native liver survival in biliary atresia. *J Pediatr Gastroenterol Nutri*, *64*(2), 203–209.

Sanchez-Valle, A., Kassira, N., Varela, V. C., et al. (2017). Biliary atresia: Epidemiology, genetics, clinical update, and public health perspective. *Adv Pediatr*, *64*(2), 285–305.

Serinet, M. O., Wildhaber, B. E., Broue, P., et al. (2009). Impact of age at Kasai operation on its results in late childhood and adolescence: A rational basis for biliary atresia screening. *Pediatrics*, *123*(5), 1280–1286.

Shneider, B. L., Brown, M. B., Haber, B., et al. (2006). A multicenter study of the outcome of biliary atresia in the United States, 1997 to 2000. *J Pediatr*, *148*(4), 467–474.

Yamataka, A., Cazares, J., & Miyano, T. (2014). Biliary atresia. In G. W. Holcomb, III, J. P. Murphy, D. J. Ostlie, & S. D. St. Peter (Eds.), *Ashcraft's Pediatric Surgery* (6th ed., pp. 580–592). New York: Saunders.

CHAPTER 52

Abdominal Wall Defect in a Newborn Female

Emily C. Alberto ■ Erin Teeple

A 22-year-old pregnant female, gravida 1 para 0, is referred for prenatal consultation after her routine 20-week ultrasound demonstrated concern for abdominal wall defect. Her pregnancy to this point has been unremarkable, with expected weight gain and all other prenatal visits revealing no abnormality. Neither she nor her husband has a personal or family history of congenital anomalies.

What Is the Differential Diagnosis for Abdominal Wall Defect on Prenatal Ultrasound?
There are several congenital anomalies that must be considered when there is suspicion for an abdominal wall defect on prenatal ultrasound.

An **omphalocele** is identifiable by a membranous sac protruding from the abdomen that is in continuity with the umbilical cord (Fig. 52.1). At around 6 weeks of gestation, the majority of the embryonic gut is within the coelom. At around 10 weeks of gestation, the gut returns to the abdominal cavity, rotates, and fixates. If the lateral folds of the embryo fail to completely migrate to the midline at the umbilicus, a defect remains that allows for persistence of the intestines and liver into the thin membranous sac, resulting in an omphalocele.

As the initial insult occurs early in gestation, omphalocele is often associated with other structural abnormalities, the most common being cardiac anomalies. Therefore prenatal echocardiography is recommended. Expecting mothers must also be counseled about associated chromosomal trisomies, including 13, 18, and 21. There are also associated constellations of defects in pleuroperitoneal fold migration such as failure of fusion of the cranial fold resulting in **pentalogy of Cantrell** (omphalocele, anterior diaphragmatic hernia, sternal cleft, ectopia cordis, and structural heart defect) as well as failure in the caudal fold resulting in bladder and cloacal exstrophy (Fig. 52.2).

Gastroschisis is another abdominal wall defect that can be identified on prenatal ultrasound (Fig. 52.3). It differs from omphalocele in that the externalized organs are not contained in a sac and, instead, are directly exposed to the amniotic fluid (Fig. 52.4). This results in thickened and edematous bowel loops shortly after delivery. Additionally, whereas an omphalocele is a midline defect, gastroschisis typically occurs to the right of the umbilical cord and is thought to be due to a weakness at the site of the obliterated right umbilical vein. Gastroschisis has a better prognosis than that of omphalocele most likely because the instigating insult occurs later in gestation resulting in fewer associated anomalies. The most common associated anomaly in gastroschisis is intestinal atresia.

Umbilical cord hernia is a midline defect covered in a membranous sac but much smaller than an omphalocele (less than 4 cm). This results from a failure of the midgut to return to the intraabdominal cavity at around 10 to 12 weeks of gestation. There are rarely any associated anomalies.

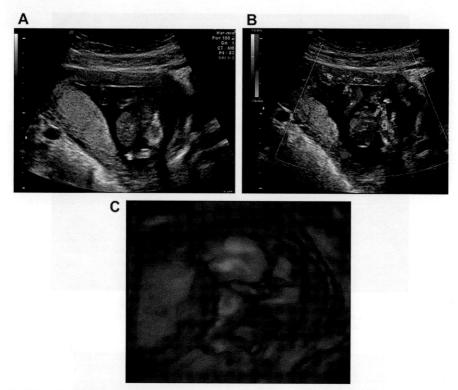

Fig. 52.1 Ultrasound image of fetus with omphalocele. (A) The omphalocele on two-dimensional (2D) ultrasound image; (B) the omphalocele on color Doppler image; and (C) the omphalocele on 3D ultrasound image, using the surface rendering mode. (From Liang Y-L, Kang L, Tsai P-Y, et al: Prenatal diagnosis of fetal omphalocele by ultrasound: A comparison of two centuries. Taiwanese Journal of Obstetrics and Gynecology Volume 52, Issue 2, June 2013, Pages 258–263.)

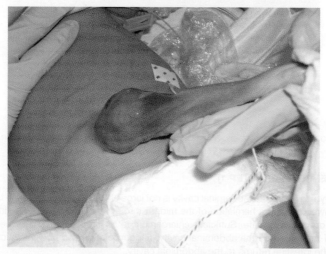

Fig. 52.2 Neonate with omphalocele.

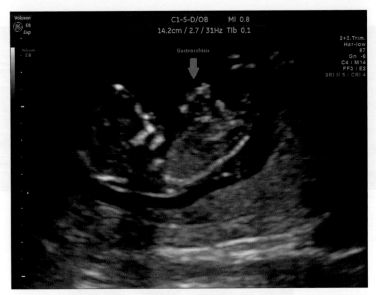

Fig. 52.3 Ultrasound of fetus with gastroschisis. From Oakes MC, Porto M, Chung JH: Advances in prenatal and perinatal diagnosis and management of gastroschisis. Seminars in Pediatric Surgery Volume 27, Issue 5, October 2018, Pages 289–299.

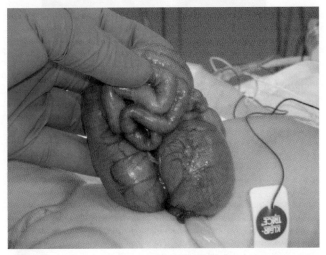

Fig. 52.4 Neonate with gastroschisis. Note lack of sac. Stomach, small intestine, and colon are in defect.

BASIC SCIENCE PEARL (STEP 1)

As the embryo develops, the abdominal cavity is not large enough to accommodate the enlarging liver and bowel, causing a herniation of the midgut through the umbilical ring during about the sixth week of intrauterine life. Sufficient enlargement is accomplished by 10 weeks, allowing for return of the midgut to the abdominal cavity. Midgut rotation and bowel fixation is accomplished as the intestine returns to the abdominal cavity.

How Should Women Be Counseled Regarding Expectations and Method of Delivery After a Prenatal Diagnosis of an Abdominal Wall Defect Is Made?

Once the diagnosis of omphalocele is made, it is important that multidisciplinary prenatal counseling occurs regarding what to expect both before and after birth. Much of these expectations revolve around concurrent anomalies discovered during prenatal investigation, particularly congenital heart defects and chromosomal anomalies. Additionally, most women will undergo serial ultrasound surveillance of the abdominal wall defect as the pregnancy progresses.

One element of prenatal counseling that must be addressed for both omphalocele and gastroschisis is the method of delivery. There is no proven benefit of Cesarean delivery over vaginal delivery. Unless there are other obstetric reasons for pursuing Cesarean section, mothers can be allowed to deliver vaginally.

Although there is controversy surrounding preterm delivery, most believe that the risks of immaturity outweigh the theoretic potential benefit of early delivery, including less edema of tissues in the abdominal wall defect. Women should be encouraged to carry as long as they and their obstetrician deem safe for baby and mother. The mother should be encouraged to routinely monitor fetal activity and contact her obstetrician with a change, as decreased fetal movement may indicate a problem with *in utero* bowel that could be salvaged by early delivery.

The woman should be counseled that, although she does not need to deliver at a center with a pediatric surgeon on site, she needs to deliver at a hospital that can rapidly provide immediate care for the infant and its associated anomalies and transfer to an institution with pediatric surgical availability.

CLINICAL PEARL (STEPS 2/3)

Omphaloceles have a higher incidence of associated anomalies. For this reason, their prognosis is worse overall than other abdominal wall defects. Women can be encouraged to deliver vaginally despite a known abdominal wall defect. Infants with giant omphaloceles may warrant Cesarean section to prevent shoulder dystocia.

The woman has spontaneous rupture of membranes at 37 weeks gestation but ultimately undergoes emergent Cesarean section for nonreassuring fetal heart tones. Upon delivery, a neonatology team, which includes a pediatric surgeon, is called to the delivery room to evaluate the male infant. On examination, Apgar scores are 8 and 9 at 1 and 5 minutes, respectively, and an abdominal wall defect with an intact peritoneal sac is seen, which measures 6 cm and both liver and bowel are inside the intact sac (Fig. 52.5).

How Should the Infant Be Managed in the Immediate Postnatal Period?

For any infant with an abdominal wall defect, immediate focus should be on stabilizing the infant, including airway management, intravenous access, and fluid resuscitation, before addressing the abdominal wall defect. Early echocardiogram is important as are other studies to investigate associated anomalies. To mitigate fluid and temperature loss as ongoing stabilization occurs, the lower half of the infant can be placed in a clear plastic bag (i.e., a "bowel bag"). This allows for visual monitoring of the exteriorized bowel during resuscitation as well as reduction in evaporative heat and fluid loss.

Initial management specific to **omphalocele** focuses on protecting the sac. Care is taken not to rip or tear the sac with manipulation of the baby. In both gastroschisis and omphalocele, attempts are made at reducing the abdominal viscera as much as safely possible. To facilitate this, an orogastric tube is placed and meconium is evacuated from the anus. Dependent on the size of the defect, the clinical condition of the infant, and the contents of the defect, the child is then

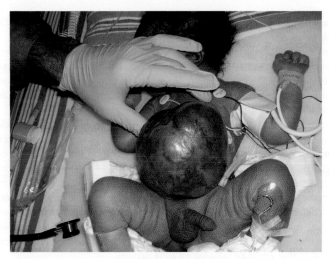

Fig. 52.5 Neonate with giant omphalocele. Note the intact peritoneal sac.

considered for primary closure or delayed repair. In the case of a giant omphalocele, antiseptic top-ical agents such as Betadine are used to create an eschar on the sac. This is followed by a moist dressing and finally an elastic wrap around the torso and omphalocele sac to stabilize and compress the intrasac contents. It is important to reduce torque on the omphalocele as shifting the contents can cause ischemic injury to the bowel or liver.

Gastroschisis requires similar management in the immediate postnatal period including airway management, establishment of intravenous access, and fluid and temperature regulation. Neonates with gastroschisis can also be placed in a bowel bag as resuscitation and investigation occur. The exposed bowel, which will typically initially appear normal, will become thickened and edematous shortly after birth. The fascial defect should be palpated and the extraabdominal contents examined. If there is concern for ongoing ischemia due to compression of the fascia on visceral blood supply, the fascial defect should be enlarged to allow for reperfusion of the bowel. After initial stabilization, the bowel should be covered with an impermeable dressing that allows for serial reduction of the bowel within the abdomen over the first week of life. Recently, there has been the advent of a spring-loaded silo device that uses a circular spring that is deployed under the fascia and a cylindrical silastic silo that holds the extraabdominal contents (Fig. 52.6). The silo is serially squeezed and secured, slowly reducing the contents over the first few days of life. Once all the abdominal contents are successfully reduced, consideration is then given to operative versus "sutureless" closure.

CLINICAL PEARL (STEPS 2/3)

The most important early treatment for infants with abdominal wall defects includes regulation of temperature, fluid resuscitation, and airway stabilization. Initially placing a clear plastic bag over the lower half of the infant, including the abdominal wall defect, reduces fluid and temperature loss and allows for monitoring of the liver and bowel for ischemia during initial resuscitation.

What Is the Operative Management of Omphalocele?

Depending on the size of the omphalocele, attempts should be made to reduce the organs into the abdomen. Similar to a spring-loaded silo, the sac can be serially squeezed and secured, reducing the organs within the abdominal wall (Fig. 52.7). If the organs can be reduced, primary closure can be performed. If the organs cannot fully be reduced due to respiratory distress or lack of abdominal

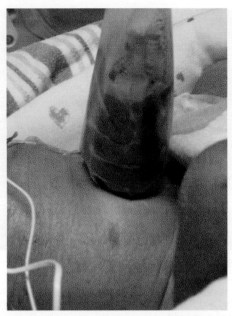

Fig. 52.6 Neonate with gastroschisis defect covered by spring-loaded silo. Note that the bowel has been serially reduced within the abdomen by placement of surgical ties at top of silo.

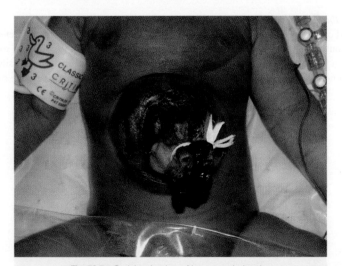

Fig. 52.7 Serial reduction of large omphalocele.

domain, consideration can be given to alternative methods of closure such as the use of prosthetic mesh (Fig. 52.8). The skin only can be closed, knowingly leaving a fascial defect but providing coverage for abdominal contents. This allows the child to grow and return at a later date for fascial closure once abdominal domain has been established. If the abdominal contents can be reduced but the fascia cannot be safely closed, synthetic mesh can be placed to create a fascial closure, knowing that it will have to be removed and native fascia closed at a later date. Lastly, if the abdominal

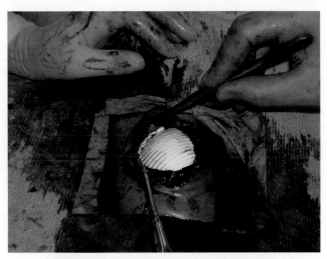

Fig. 52.8   Closure of fascial defect with prosthetic mesh.

contents cannot be reduced and the skin is not sufficient to close over the defect, consideration must be given to leaving the sac intact and "painting" it with a topical antiseptic to create an eschar. The child can then be allowed to grow and return for definitive excision of sac along with fascial and skin closure.

What Is the Operative Management of Gastroschisis?

The method of closure is dependent on the size of the defect as well as surgeon preference. After the bowel contents are reduced, the fascia can be closed primarily in the operating room or non-operatively in the neonatal nursery. If the fascial defect is small and the bowel easily reduced, a sutureless or nonoperative closure can be performed (Fig. 52.9). This occurs after the contents have

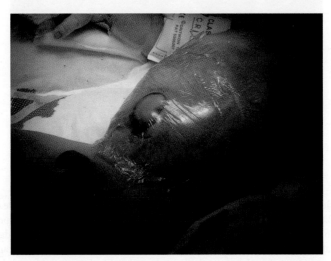

Fig. 52.9   Sutureless closure in which the intraabdominal contents have been reduced, and the umbilical cord has been used to seal the defect. Occlusive dressing remains in place.

been reduced using a silo. The preserved umbilical cord is then placed over the fascial defect and secured with a dressing that is left in place for a number of days. After removal of the dressing, the wound is allowed to heal by secondary intention utilizing the remnant umbilical cord that is spread over the defect and allowed to granulate in over time. Other approaches include a primary fascial closure and utilization of prosthetic mesh.

What Are the Long-term Outcomes After Abdominal Wall Repair?

Survival rate of gastroschisis is upward of 90% with a primary fascial closure rate of around 80%. Due to poor motility associated with gastroschisis, median time to feed was 30 days with median length of stay around 45 days. This was longer if there was an associated atresia. Omphalocele has a 20% mortality rate due mostly to associated anomalies. Late concerns for both are small bowel obstruction, malrotation, and psychological distress about lack of an umbilicus.

CLINICAL PEARL (STEPS 2/3)

The majority of omphalocele and gastroschisis survivors have excellent quality of life with minimal recurrent medical difficulties related to their abdominal wall defect.

The infant is resuscitated and assessed for other congenital anomalies not detected prenatally. Due to the large abdominal wall defect and significant contents of the sac, the omphalocele sac is painted with dilute Betadine solution and wrapped in a nonadhesive covering followed by gauze and an elastic wrap to keep the viscera upright. The neonate's parents are taught how to care for the omphalocele, and they are eventually discharged home. The sac is ultimately excised, and the fascia closed primarily.

BEYOND THE PEARLS

- Abdominal wall defects may be diagnosed on prenatal ultrasound and prompt investigation into the presence of other congenital anomalies.
- Omphaloceles are more likely than gastroschisis to be associated with other congenital anomalies.
- Omphaloceles are defects of abdominal organs contained within a membranous sac. In contrast, abdominal organs have no covering in gastroschisis and are instead exposed to amniotic fluid *in utero* or to the environment after birth.
- The treatment modalities for abdominal wall defects center around resuscitation of the neonate, protection of the abdominal organs that are contained within the defect, reduction of the defect (typically over time), and ultimate repair of the abdominal wall (often in a delayed fashion).

Suggested Readings

Koivusalo, A., Lindahl, H., & Rintala, R. J. (2002). Morbidity and quality of life in adult patients with a congenital abdominal wall defect: A questionnaire survey. *J Pediatr Surg, 37*, 1594–1601.

Minkes, R. K. (2005). Abdominal wall defects. In K. T. Oldham et al. (Eds.), *Principles and practice of pediatric surgery.* Lippincott Williams & Wilkins.

Riboh, J., Abrajano, C. T., Garber, K., et al. (2009). Outcomes of sutureless gastroschisis closure. *J Pediatr Surg, 44*, 1947.

CHAPTER 53

Hypoxemia and Labored Breathing in a Newborn

Natalie Tully ■ Celeste Hollands

A nurse in the newborn nursery calls the neonatology team to evaluate a 6-hour-old male due to tachypnea and grunting respirations. He was born at 37 weeks gestation to a 28-year-old gravida 2 para 1 mother via normal spontaneous vaginal delivery and weighs 2.8 kg. Appropriate prenatal care and monitoring occurred throughout the pregnancy. Because the pregnancy was uneventful, the obstetrician and patient elected not to perform an ultrasound. On physical examination, he appears to be a normal term male but is cyanotic, tachypneic, and dyspneic, despite 100% oxygen via mask. On examination, his abdomen is soft and nondistended. The baby is transferred to the neonatal intensive care unit (NICU).

What Is the Differential Diagnosis for Hypoxia and Dyspnea in a Newborn?

There are myriad pathologies that can result in respiratory distress in a neonate. Acute and congenital causes exist. Common acute causes include meconium aspiration or neonatal pneumonia; congenital causes can include congenital diaphragmatic hernia (CDH) and tracheoesophageal fistula (TEF). Other, less common etiologies for hypoxia and dyspnea are in Table 53.1.

What Are the Primary Physical Examination Findings in Determining the Etiology of a Newborn's Respiratory Distress?

When a newborn is in clear respiratory distress, the primary concern, even before an in-depth physical examination, should be stabilization with supplemental oxygen. On physical examination the infant will likely show a dusky or cyanotic complexion; however, this is not absolute, as the hypoxia present may not be sufficient to result in cyanosis, and this examination finding can be complicated by patient skin color. Findings of tachypnea and grunting respirations should draw immediate concern and prompt a thorough cardiopulmonary examination. In CDH, there will likely be reduced breath sounds on the side of the hernia defect—there may or may not be bowel sounds appreciable. In TEF, there will likely not be appreciable auscultatory changes. Also critically important is a thorough abdominal examination, which includes inspection for scaphoid or distended status, auscultation for presence of bowel sounds in all four quadrants of the abdomen, and palpation to determine whether the abdomen is firm or soft.

What Are the Diagnostic Modalities Utilized for Evaluation of the Etiology of Respiratory Distress in a Newborn?

After complete physical examination the next steps in evaluating a newborn with respiratory distress should include ordering an urgent chest radiograph (CXR), arterial blood gas, oxygen saturation

TABLE 53.1 ■ Potential Etiologies and Associated Physical Examination Findings for Hypoxia and Dyspnea in a Newborn

	Pathology	Physical Examination Findings
Infectious/ Physiologic	Pneumonia	Fever, tachypnea, costal retraction, lethargy, crackles or rhonchi on auscultation
	Neonatal respiratory distress syndrome	Nasal flaring, intercostal and subcostal retractions, accessory respiratory muscle use
	Transient tachypnea of the newborn	Tachypnea, nasal flaring, mild intercostal and subcostal retractions, and expiratory grunting
	Persistent pulmonary hypertension	Tachypnea, cyanosis, systolic tricuspid insufficiency murmur
Congenital	Congenital diaphragmatic hernia	Dependent on amount of herniated abdominal contents
		Barrel-shaped chest, scaphoid abdomen, absence of breath sounds on the ipsilateral side
		Displaced heartbeat in left-sided CDH
	Congenital heart disease	Wide variety of cardiac murmurs, decreased breath sounds or crackles may be present
	Tracheoesophageal fistula	Dependent on presence of concomitant esophageal atresia
		Intrauterine polyhydramnios, excessive secretions that cause drooling, choking, respiratory distress, and feeding difficulty, gastric distension, reflux
Traumatic	Meconium aspiration	Meconium-stained nails, umbilical cord, and/or vernix, grunting, nasal flaring, barrel-shaped chest, accessory respiratory muscle use
	Pneumothorax/Air leak	Asymmetric chest expansion, decreased breath sounds, shifted point of maximal cardiac impulse

monitoring, and a complete blood count with differential. Placement of an orogastric (OGT) or nasogastric (NGT) tube before the CXR can be very helpful.

The CXR in a neonate with TEF may show an air-filled upper pouch. It is pretty standard to attempt to pass on OGT/NGT in infants with this clinical scenario. Figs. 53.1 and 53.2 show the OGT/NGT terminating in the air-filled upper pouch. Most surgeons would consider this diagnostic of esophageal atresia (EA). The surgeon will often remove the OGT/NGT and reattempt passage to confirm the diagnosis. Sometimes a contrast study through the tube is preferred to confirm the diagnosis and rule out esophageal perforation with OGT/NGT as the reason for lack of advancement of the tube and to rule out upper pouch fistula if bronchoscopy is not planned intraoperatively.

The CXR in neonates with CDH, on the other hand, demonstrate bowel (typically air-fluid levels) in the pleural space. It may also show the OGT/NGT above where the diaphragm should be signifying that the stomach may also be in the chest.

The infant continues on supplemental oxygen and is found to have a PO_2 of 43 mm Hg on arterial blood gas. The NICU team attempts placement of an orogastric tube, but they meet resistance when attempting to advance the tube. A chest radiograph is obtained (Fig. 53.3) that reveals that the tube is in what appears to be a blind esophageal pouch. The surgical team is consulted for evaluation and after an attempt at reinsertion of the tube diagnoses the patient with esophageal atresia. Given the air seen in the infant's stomach on radiographs, they note that the infant also likely has a distal tracheoesophageal fistula. The surgeon has a discussion related to treatment options with the infant's parents, who give informed consent for operative treatment.

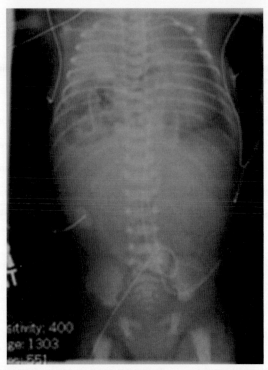

Fig. 53.1 Right-sided CDH with herniated bowel in the right chest. (From the personal teaching collection of Celeste Hollands, who gives permission to use these images in this chapter and retains copyright.)

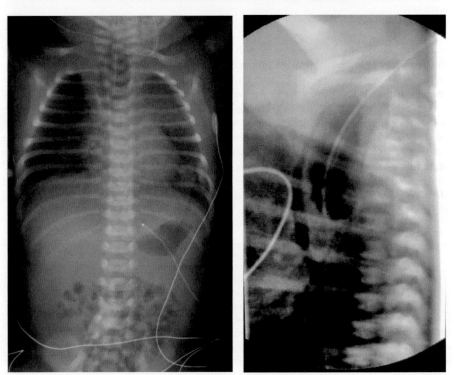

Fig. 53.2 Anterior *(left)* and lateral *(right)* chest radiographs showing an orogastric tube and air in an upper esophageal pouch. The anterior chest radiograph shows gas in the GI tract compatible with esophageal atresia with tracheoesophageal fistula. (From the personal teaching collection of Celeste Hollands, who gives permission to use these images in this chapter and retains copyright.)

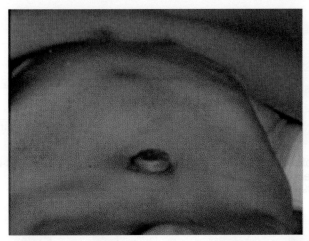

Fig. 53.3 Scaphoid abdomen of infant with CDH with herniated intestinal contents. (From the personal teaching collection of Celeste Hollands, who gives permission to use these images in this chapter and retains copyright.)

CLINICAL PEARL (STEPS 2/3)

Two of the classic examination findings in CDH and TEF are not always appreciable—only in a significant CDH will enough abdominal contents herniate into the thorax to produce a scaphoid abdomen (see Fig. 53.3), or one in which the abdomen has a sucked-in appearance. Only in more serious cases of TEF will there be abdominal distension due to gastric air trapping.

CLINICAL PEARL (STEPS 2/3)

A key point to elucidate in the patient history when considering EA/TEF and CDH as a diagnosis is the presence or absence of polyhydramnios in utero.

BASIC SCIENCE PEARL (STEP 1)

The diaphragm is formed from the fusion of the pleuroperitoneal canals in the 8th week of gestation. This model has been challenged recently, and it is likely that there are a multitude of etiologies leading to CDH that include failure of muscular ingrowth in addition to failure of pleuroperitoneal canal fusion. Regardless, if the diaphragm is not completely closed before the bowel returns to the abdominal cavity in the 10th week of gestation, it may herniate into the chest. The right hemidiaphragm is typically closed before the left, and therefore most CDH occurrences are seen on the left side.

How Are Tracheoesophageal Fistulae Categorized?

There are many anatomic variants of anomalies of the esophagus and trachea, some of which have fistulous connections between the two, and others that do not. Fig. 53.4 illustrates these anatomic variants. All of these anomalous anatomic variants demonstrate esophageal atresia (EA, a blind-ending esophageal pouch) with the exception of the H-type TEF, and only one variant presents without a fistula at all. It should be noted that the most common variant is esophageal atresia with a distal TEF. Although contrast studies are often necessary to differentiate these anatomic variants from one another, the presence of air within the stomach can help rule out variants without a distal TEF.

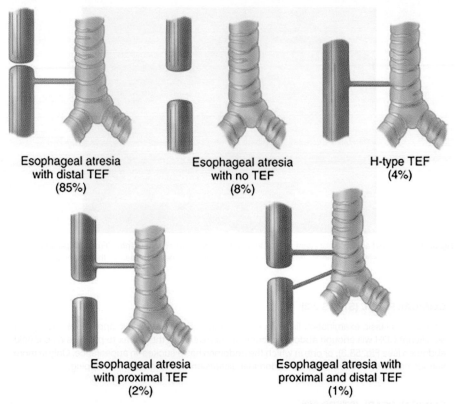

Esophageal atresia
with distal TEF
(85%)

Esophageal atresia
with no TEF
(8%)

H-type TEF
(4%)

Esophageal atresia
with proximal TEF
(2%)

Esophageal atresia with
proximal and distal TEF
(1%)

Fig. 53.4 Types of tracheoesophageal fistulae and their relative frequency. (Redrawn from Marcdante KJ, Kliegman RM: Esophagus and stomach. In *Nelson essentials of pediatrics*, Philadelphia, 2019, Elsevier, pp 480–487.)

What Are the Treatment Options for Neonates With Tracheoesophageal Fistulae?

The goal in management of neonates that are diagnosed with tracheoesophageal fistulae is to restore continuity of the esophagus and abolish its connection to the airway. When surgical options are being considered, neonates must be managed with airway support as dictated by clinical respiratory status, an orogastric tube to suction in the upper pouch of the esophagus, and nutritional support as dictated by defect type, severity, gestational age, and birthweight.

Most TEF patients are treated by surgical division of the fistula and primary anastomosis of the esophagus. In infants with a long-gap (greater than 3 cm) esophageal atresia, a primary repair would be placed under significant tension, so there are several approaches to managing these patients. Primary repair can be delayed until the proximal and distal ends of the esophagus can grow, stretch, or hypertrophy to a point at which the gap is 2 cm or less. For those patients whose native esophagus cannot be used, the stomach, small intestine, or colon can be substituted. In patients with a fistula, it is divided right on the trachea, and a primary repair of the trachea is performed. There are several acceptable approaches to this repair that include access via right posterolateral thoracotomy, right thoracoscopy, or transthoracic extrapleural approach (Foker technique). Postoperatively, the patient may be sedated and ventilated for several days to allow for healing. Subsequent stricture of the repair may need to be treated with balloon dilation.

What Are the Treatment Options for Neonates With Congenital Diaphragmatic Hernia?

The goals in management of neonates with a congenital diaphragmatic hernia are to repair the hernia defect and to reestablish normal anatomy with the stomach and bowel in the abdominal cavity. Preoperative management should include supportive cardiopulmonary treatment with intubation/ventilation as clinically indicated, blood pressure support via fluids and inotropes, and surfactant administration.

Surgical repair of the hernia defect is typically delayed 48 to 72 hours after birth in order to allow for stabilization of the infant. The surgical approach is dictated by patient factors and the anatomy of the defect and can be either open (via thoracotomy or laparotomy), thoracoscopic, or laparoscopic. Regardless of the approach, the abdominal contents are reduced from the chest into the abdomen and the hernia defect is closed either primarily using suture (small defects) or with a patch (large defects). Consideration must be made of the increased abdominal pressure given reduction of hernia contents into the abdomen. The abdominal approach allows the surgeon to leave the abdomen open or to close skin only leaving an incisional hernia that can be closed at a later date in order to prevent increased pressure on the diaphragm that interferes with ventilation and/or abdominal compartment syndrome.

BASIC SCIENCE PEARL (STEP 1)

Pulmonary surfactant is a substance secreted by type II pneumocytes high in lipids and proteins that serves to lower alveolar surface tension and prevent alveolar collapse during exhalation.

BASIC SCIENCE PEARL (STEPS 1/2/3)

Remember that esophageal atresia with tracheoesophageal fistula can be part of the VACTERL (Vertebral, Anal, Cardiac, TEF, Renal, and Limb) association, and it is critically important to evaluate the neonate for concomitant malformations due to this association.

What Are the Potential Complications of Surgical Repair of Tracheoesophageal Fistula and Congenital Diaphragmatic Hernia?

Perioperative complications of both TEF and CHD repair include infection and hemorrhage. Repairs of TEF may be acutely complicated by anastomotic leak, esophageal stricture, recurrent fistula, gastric reflux, and delayed gastric emptying. Specific to CHD, rare complications include chylothorax and persistent pulmonary hypertension, the latter of which is the most serious complication and is difficult to manage.

Late complications of TEF repair include dysphagia, GERD, esophagitis, asthma, Barrett esophagus, and esophageal cancer, whereas those of CHD include neurologic sequelae, spinal and chest wall abnormalities, recurrent hernia, patch failure, hernia recurrence, and chronic respiratory disease.

The infant is taken to the operating room where a right thoracotomy and extrapleural approach is used to identify a blind upper esophageal pouch and distal tracheoesophageal fistula (Fig. 53.5). The fistula is ligated, and the esophageal atresia is repaired using a primary anastomosis given a gap between proximal and distal ends of 1 cm. The infant does well postoperatively, is discharged to home from the hospital 10 days postoperatively, and suffers no short-term complications.

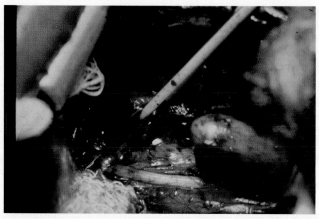

Fig. 53.5 Esophageal atresia with distal tracheoesophageal fistula. The proximal pouch is to the right and is distended with a bougie dilator to aid identification and dissection. The distal tracheoesophageal fistula is seen on the left encircled by the yellow vessel loop before entering the trachea. (From the personal teaching collection of Celeste Hollands, who gives permission to use these images in this chapter and retains copyright.)

BEYOND THE PEARLS

- Avoid intubating an infant with TEF, as it will precipitate gastric distention with no way of reducing the stomach, which can catastrophically end in gastric perforation.
- The most common type of TEF is esophageal atresia with distal TEF.
- Infants with CDH often experience a "honeymoon" period, wherein they do not manifest pulmonary hypertension (due to lung hypoplasia) for up to 72 hours after birth. This grants the surgeon a few days to stabilize the infant before definitive repair.
- Ensure the sidedness of the infant's aortic arch is definitively identified in patients with TEF to determine the side of thoracotomy.
- Infants with CDH have a significant chance of having intestinal malrotation and should be evaluated for the nonrotation type of intestinal malrotation. This can be done at the time of operation if performed from the abdomen or evaluated radiographically if thoracic approach is planned.

Suggested Readings

Foker, J. E., Linden, B. C., Boyle, E. M., Jr., & Marquardt, C. (1997). Development of a true primary repair for the full spectrum of esophageal atresia. *Ann Surg, 226*(4), 533–543.

Holcomb, G. W., III., Rothenberg, S. S., KMA, Bax, Martinez-Ferro, M., et al. (2005). Thoracoscopic repair of esophageal atresia and tracheoesophageal fistula a multi-institutional analysis. *Ann Surg, 242*(3), 422–430.

Losty, P. D. (2014). Congenital diaphragmatic hernia: Where and what is the evidence? *Seminars in Pediatric Surgery, 23*(5), 278–282. https://doi.org/10.1053/j.sempedsurg.2014.09.008.

CHAPTER 54

Bilious Vomiting in a 1-Week-Old Male

Stephanie Rakestraw ■ Loren Berman

A 1-week-old male is brought to the emergency department by his parents. He was born full term at normal weight and discharged home on day 1. He has been vomiting for the last 12 hours. His parents report that he has lost interest in feeding since the vomiting began. No other people in the home are reported to be sick.

What Is the Differential Diagnosis for Vomiting in a Neonate?

As the child is only 1 week old, acute and congenital causes are primary considerations in the differential diagnosis (Table 54.1). Acute considerations include gastroenteritis, gastroesophageal reflux disease, and toxin ingestion. Congenital conditions include intestinal obstruction, inborn errors of metabolism, and adrenal insufficiency. A thorough history should be taken to determine duration, pattern, and type of vomiting. Bilious vomiting in a child is a medical emergency and usually indicates distal intestinal obstruction. Nonbilious vomiting may still be emergent. Potential causes for each are outlined in Table 54.2. Bilious vomiting in a neonate should be assumed to be malrotation with midgut volvulus until proven otherwise.

What Are the Primary Physical Examination Techniques to Evaluate Vomiting?

A thorough physical examination should be undertaken in order to assess the acuity of the infant and for any signs related to the cause for the vomiting. In infants, checking the fontanelle and mucous membranes allows for a quick assessment of the patient's volume status. An abdominal examination should be performed to assess for masses, tenderness, and distension. Anorectal examination can also provide insight into potential etiologies of distal intestinal obstruction. Part of the physical examination is assessing the quality of the vomit if possible.

An emergent upper gastrointestinal (GI) series will make the diagnosis. Immediate surgery without any imaging is also an option in a sick child. Getting the child to the OR quickly will maximize the chances of bowel salvage.

What Is the Relevant Anatomy of Malrotation?

In normal development, the gut exits the abdomen, rotates 270 degrees around the superior mesenteric artery, then returns to the abdomen during development. Upon return, the gut fixes itself to the peritoneal wall via the mesentery. Malrotation results from any deviation in the normal 270-degree rotation, and results in mesenteric attachment to the bowel in improper locations, or failure of fixation (Fig. 54.2A–C). Failure of fixation predisposes patients to volvulus because the mesentery has a very narrow base rather than the broad base that is formed with normal fixation. Most of the time, volvulus presents with one to three clockwise rotations around the narrow base of the mesentery. In a healthy child without malrotation, the right colon is fixed to the retroperitoneum. In children with malrotation, Ladd's bands are connections between the cecum and the retroperitoneum that pass over the duodenum and may cause duodenal obstruction.

TABLE 54.1 ■ **Differential Diagnosis in Vomiting Neonate**

	Pathology	Physical Examination Findings
Acute	Gastroenteritis	Mild abdominal distention, normal bowel sounds
	Gastroesophageal reflux disease	Effortless regurgitation
	Toxin ingestion	Alterations in neurologic status
Congenital	Intestinal obstruction	Distended, tender abdomen, absent or high-pitched bowel sounds
	Inborn errors of metabolism	Alterations in neurologic status
	Adrenal Insufficiency	Ambiguous genitalia (more so in females), hyperkalemia

TABLE 54.2 ■ **Causes of Bilious and Nonbilious Vomiting in a Neonate**

	Pathology
Bilious vomit	Intestinal atresia
	Malrotation with volvulus
	Intussusception
Nonbilious vomit	Pyloric stenosis
	Pyloric duplication
	Upper duodenal stenosis
	Gastric volvulus

What Are the Clinical Findings of Malrotation With a Volvulus?

Bilious emesis is the classic presentation. The patient may also present with hematochezia (indicating bowel ischemia), tachycardia, hemodynamic instability secondary to hypovolemic or septic shock, or peritonitis. A malrotation with a volvulus may appear on an abdominal radiograph with a misplaced duodenum or cecum, a gasless abdomen, a "corkscrew duodenum," or a "double bubble" sign with duodenal obstruction. It is possible to have a normal-appearing abdominal radiograph, however, so a normal study does not rule out volvulus in a child with bilious emesis. Malrotation cannot be definitively diagnosed on a plain film, and an upper GI series is the study of choice for definitive diagnosis. In a sick child with an acute abdomen, if clinical suspicion is high enough, it may be appropriate to forego any imaging and take the patient straight to the operating room. Time is of the essence in restoring intestinal blood flow, and imaging may cause unnecessary delays.

Arterial blood gasses can also point the physician toward a diagnosis of bowel ischemia. Metabolic acidosis, particularly lactic acidosis, combined with abdominal pain and distention is concerning for bowel ischemia and should increase clinical suspicion for a volvulus. However, the absence of lactic acidosis does not rule out a volvulus, and imaging should still be obtained. In addition, lactic acidosis can be present as a result of global poor perfusion related to sepsis or other inflammatory process and does not always signify bowel ischemia.

After a thorough history and physical examination, it is appreciated that the child has bilious vomiting, a tender abdomen, and absent bowel sounds, indicating intestinal obstruction. An abdominal radiograph and upper gastrointestinal series are ordered. The patient's upper GI series shows a malrotation with midgut volvulus, noted by failure of small intestine to cross back over the left side of the abdomen where the ligament of Treitz should be positioned, and the corkscrew pattern of the contrast in the proximal small bowel (Fig. 54.1). After a discussion with the patient's parents, he is scheduled for emergent surgery.

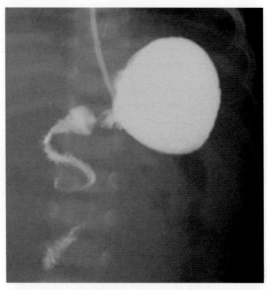

Fig. 54.1   Upper GI series showing midgut rotation with a volvulus and corkscrew sign of the duodenum.

BASIC SCIENCE PEARL (STEPS 1/2/3)

The ligament of Treitz, also known as the suspensory muscle of the duodenum, is the soft tissue division between the duodenum and jejunum and offers a point of fixation for the rotating bowel during development. The connective tissue also marks the location of the superior mesenteric and celiac arteries.

CLINICAL PEARL (STEPS 2/3)

Upper GI is the best imaging study for diagnosis of malrotation. This is defined by failure of contrast to cross back over the midline to the left abdomen after it exits the pylorus in the right abdomen. On lateral view, the duodenum should course posteriorly into the retroperitoneum, but with malrotation it courses anteriorly.

Do All Patients With Malrotation Require Surgery?

Patients can live with malrotation and remain asymptomatic, possibly not even being aware of their condition. However, malrotation with a volvulus is a surgical emergency and requires immediate surgery to preserve blood supply to the bowel. Delaying diagnosis or intervention for a volvulus can result in bowel ischemia, necrosis, septic shock, and death.

Malrotation may cause intermittent volvulus that can present subacutely with intermittent vomiting or feeding intolerance. Infants and children with these symptoms should have a workup that includes an upper GI contrast study to evaluate for malrotation. If malrotation without volvulus is seen on imaging, regardless of whether the patient is having symptoms, the patient should undergo surgery to reduce the risk of volvulus.

What Surgery Is Used to Treat Malrotation?

Treatment for malrotation is dependent on whether the patient presents with volvulus and on the status of the bowel appreciated during surgery. If the bowel is healthy and has adequate blood flow

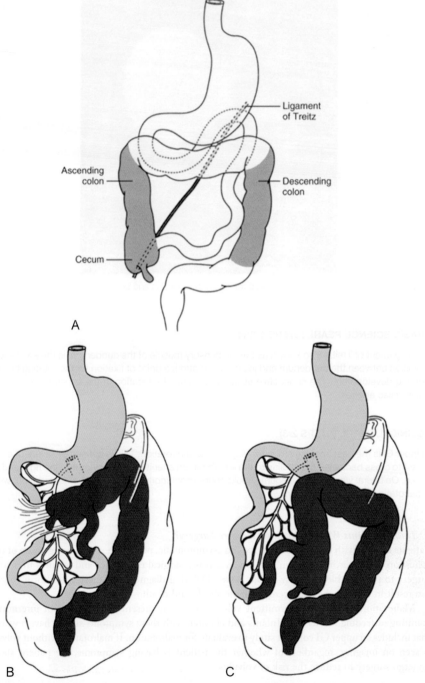

Fig. 54.2   (A) Normal rotation. (B) Malrotation with Ladd's bands. (C) Nonrotation of intestine. Prearterial regions are lightly shaded; postarterial regions are darkly shaded.

with no signs of ischemia or necrosis, the Ladd's procedure is performed (see below). If the bowel is questionable, detorsion can be performed, and the bowel can be rechecked in 12 to 24 hours to determine the need for future care. If the bowel is necrotic or not able to be salvaged, anastomosis or fecal diversion can be performed. Regardless of procedure, children are started on IV fluids and antibiotics preoperatively. A nasogastric tube should be placed to decompress the stomach.

The Ladd's procedure has been the standard of care since 1936 and significantly reduces mortality of patients with malrotation. A laparoscopic approach can be considered in children who are hemodynamically stable and without an acute volvulus, and may be associated with faster progression to normal diet and discharge. However, an open approach has been thought to create adhesions, reducing the risk of recurrent volvulus.

For the open Ladd's, a right upper quadrant or an upper midline incision is made. The bowel is eviscerated for inspection (Fig. 54.3A). The volvulus is found and detorsion is performed, often requiring two to three complete, counterclockwise twists to return blood flow. An assessment of anatomy and bowel health is then performed to determine future steps (Fig. 54.3B). If the bowel is considered viable, the Ladd's procedure continues. Ladd's bands between the cecum and right retroperitoneum, overlying the duodenum, are divided, and the mesentery is widened. Additionally, an appendectomy is performed. The bowel is then oriented in a position of nonrotation, with the descending colon on the left. Surgical fixation is not performed, as adhesions will form, adhering the bowel to the retroperitoneum.

A laparoscopic Ladd's procedure involves the same steps but is approached through umbilical and lateral ports. The laparoscopic approach is only performed when there is no indication of volvulus or bowel ischemia.

What Are the Potential Complications of the Open Ladd's Procedure?

Perioperative complications If the bowel is deemed nonviable, an anastomosis or ostomy is performed at the discretion of the surgeon. Preserving as much bowel as possible is a priority. Children can also experience postoperative ileus, intussusception, and small bowel obstruction. The most common complication associated with the Ladd's procedure is postoperative ileus and feeding intolerance, although this usually resolves over time without specific intervention.

Long-term complications Particularly if bowel segments are removed, patients can experience short bowel syndrome. Adhesions may form, causing adhesive small bowel obstruction. Recurrent volvulus, although rare, may occur. Overall mortality rate after surgery is 3% to 9%, with a higher incidence in patients with necrotic bowel necessitating resection.

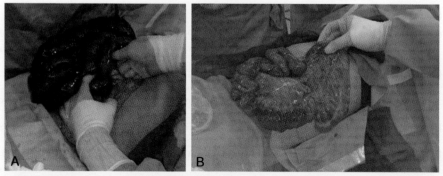

Fig. 54.3 (A) Bowel with compromised blood supply from a midgut volvulus. Bowel is from an older child than described in the case. (B) Bowel inspection after detorsion and suctioning of hemorrhagic contents. Bowel is from an older child than described in the case.

What Are the Potential Complications of the Laparoscopic Ladd's Procedure?

Perioperative complications Overall complication rates are lower with the laparoscopic Ladd's procedure than with the open Ladd's, but complications are similar. No difference in postoperative bowel obstruction was noted between laparoscopic and open Ladd's procedures. The laparoscopic Ladd's procedure has also been associated with a faster progression to full enteral feeding and a shorter length of stay than open Ladd's.

Long-term complications Laparoscopic Ladd's procedures are associated with a higher rate of recurrent volvulus than open Ladd's. It is believed that this is a result of the laparoscopic Ladd's procedures creating fewer adhesions than open Ladd's, allowing the bowel to remain mobile.

CLINICAL PEARL (STEPS 2/3)

There is a residual risk of midgut volvulus even after Ladd's procedure, but a child presenting with bilious emesis who has had a Ladd's procedure is more likely to have an adhesive obstruction than recurrent volvulus.

The patient undergoes an open exploration, the point of volvulized small bowel is found, and the volvulus is reduced. The bowel is pink and viable, so the operative team proceeds with a Ladd's procedure without bowel resection. The infant tolerates the procedure well and is able to take full feeds within the next several days. He is discharged from the hospital, and the parents are given anticipatory guidance and instructions for follow-up in 2 weeks.

BEYOND THE PEARLS

- The differential diagnosis for vomiting in a neonate includes both acute and congenital causes.
- Due to caloric and hydration needs, severe vomiting in a neonate needs to be evaluated.
- Whether the vomit is bilious or nonbilious provides clues as to where along the gastrointestinal tract the problem may be.
- Malrotation can be silent or present as subacute with intermittent abdominal pain and vomiting or acute with severe abdominal pain and vomiting.
- The Ladd's procedure divides points of abnormal anatomic bowel fixation caused by malrotation during development and orients the bowel in a position of nonrotation.

Suggested Readings

Catania, V. D., Lauriti, G., Pierro, A., & Zani, A. (2016). Open versus laparoscopic approach for intestinal malrotation in infants and children: A systematic review and meta-analysis. *Pediatr Surg Int, 32*(12), 1157–1164.

Christison-Lagay, E., & Langer, J. C. (2014). Intestinal rotation abnormalities. In M. M. Ziegler, R. G. Azizkhan, D. Allmen & T. R. Weber (Eds.), *Operative pediatric surgery* (2nd ed). New York: McGraw-Hill. http://accesssurgery.mhmedical.com.proxy1.lib.tju.edu/content.aspx?bookid=959 & sectionid=53539609.

Hackam, David J., et al. (2015). "Pediatric Surgery." In F. Charles Brunicardi, et al. (Eds.) *Schwartz's Principles of Surgery* (10th ed). New York, NY: McGraw-Hill.

Huntington, J. T., Lopez, J. J., Mahida, J. B., Ambeba, E. J., Asti, L., Deans, K. J., & Minneci, P. C. (2017). Comparing laparoscopic versus open Ladd's procedure in pediatric patients. *J Pediatr Surg, 52*(7), 1128–1131. https://doi.org/10.1016/j.jpedsurg.2016.10.046.

Juvekar, N. M., Deshpande, S. S., Pratap, U., & Jagtap, R. R. (2011). Patankar SP: Perioperative management of a neonate presenting with midgut volvulus and obstructed infracardiac total anomalous pulmonary venous connection. *Ann Card Anaesth, 14*, 62–65. https://doi.org/10.4103/0971-9784.74407.

CHAPTER 55

Abdominal Pain, Vomiting, and Fever in a 3-Year-Old Female

Matthew M. Boelig ■ Gary W. Nace

A 3-year-old female with no significant past medical history presents to the emergency department with 48 hours of abdominal pain, distention, and vomiting. She has had several episodes of non-bloody, nonbilious emesis over the last day, as well as fevers and anorexia. She has not eaten since yesterday and is urinating less frequently. On examination, her abdomen is distended and diffusely tender to palpation with no palpable mass or hernia. Her vital signs include a temperature of 101.2°F, heart rate of 145 bpm, blood pressure 100/60 mm Hg, and respiratory rate 22/minute.

What Is the Differential Diagnosis for Abdominal Pain, Emesis, and Fevers in This Age Group? The differential diagnosis of abdominal pain, emesis, and fevers in young children is broad and features surgical and medical pathologies (Table 55.1). It is critical to quickly discern which children require an acute intervention. A thorough history and physical examination is the best way to begin.

What Are Important Clinical Symptoms or Signs of Appendicitis, Intussusception, and Midgut Volvulus?

APPENDICITIS

Although less common in this age group, appendicitis may be particularly challenging to diagnose in younger children based on history and physical examination alone. Children less than 3 years old generally present with appendiceal perforation (> 80%). Delays in diagnosis, secondary to lack of clear history and examination, may increase the risk of perforation and subsequent morbidity and mortality. Few children present with the classic signs/symptoms of periumbilical pain that migrates to the right lower quadrant (RLQ), McBurney's point tenderness (located one-third of the distance between the anterior superior iliac spine and the umbilicus), fever, and anorexia. Other classical examination findings that may be absent in children are reviewed in Chapter 5. Small children have limited ability to "wall off" an appendiceal perforation—likely secondary to their diminutive omentum—and they more commonly present with diffuse purulent peritonitis and an associated ileus. Other oft-encountered symptoms include diarrhea and dysuria, which seem to be more frequent with appendicitis within the pelvis.

Over the years, investigators have attempted to develop more quantitative clinical scoring systems to predict the presence of appendicitis. The pediatric appendicitis score (PAS) is a scoring system that has undergone prospective validation and may be useful to guide decision making as far as imaging and surgical consultation in patients aged 3 to 18 (Table 55.2). A PAS score of 1 to 3 is considered low risk, 4 to 6 moderate risk, and 7 to 10 high risk.

TABLE 55.1 ■ **Differential Diagnosis of Abdominal Pain, Vomiting, and Fever in Children**

Surgical	Medical
• Acute appendicitis (simple or perforated)	• Pancreatitis
• Ileocolic intussusception	• Gastroenteritis
• Midgut volvulus	• Inflammatory bowel disease
• Meckel's diverticulum—diverticulitis with or without perforation, torsion, lead point for intussusception	• Urinary tract infection
• Enteric duplication cyst with torsion or volvulus	• Pelvic inflammatory disease
• Choledochal cyst with obstruction or cholangitis	
• Bowel obstruction (e.g., incarcerated inguinal hernia, Ladd's bands, omphalomesenteric duct remnant causing obstruction)	
• Ovarian torsion	

TABLE 55.2 ■ **Pediatric Appendicitis Score (PAS)**[a]

PAS Element	Point(s) on PAS Scale
Cough/percussion tenderness (i.e., pain with coughing or hopping)	2
RLQ tenderness	2
Anorexia	1
Fever	1
Nausea/Emesis	1
Migration of Pain	1
Leukocytosis (white blood cell count > 10,000 cells/uL)	1
Polymorphonuclear neutrophilia	1

[a]The pediatric appendicitis score (PAS) is a prospectively validated scoring system used to guide the diagnosis of acute appendicitis in patients aged 3 to 18. Less than 4 = Low risk; 4 to 6 = Moderate risk; higher than 6 = High risk.
(From Samuel M: Pediatric appendicitis score, *J Pediatr Surg* Jun;37(6):877–881, 2002.)

INTUSSUSCEPTION

There are many common clinical findings between children presenting with appendicitis and those with intestinal intussusception, which occurs when a portion of intestine (intussusceptum) telescopes, in an antegrade fashion, into the lumen of a contiguous piece of intestine (intussuscipiens). The majority of symptomatic intussusceptions in children are ileocolic (terminal ileum telescopes into the colon) and hence present with symptoms in the right lower quadrant (Fig. 55.1). Ileocolic intussusceptions usually have a benign etiology. The favored hypothesis is that, after a viral illness, hypertrophied Peyer's patches in the distal ileum can serve as a lead point for intussusception. However, in about 10% of cases, and more commonly in children 3 years of age and older, there is a pathologic lead point (e.g., Meckel diverticulum, appendiceal inflammation, enteric duplication cyst, lipoma, lymphoma, polyp). Although no definitive guidelines exist, most experts recommend that children older than 5 should have evaluation for pathologic lead points. Patients presenting diffuse abdominal tenderness and a generalized septic appearance should be evaluated for a complication associated with intussusception, such as bowel necrosis and perforation.

Ileocolic intussusception has a peak incidence between 5 to 10 months of age, exhibits a 2:1 male-to-female predominance, and occurs more frequently in the fall and winter months when

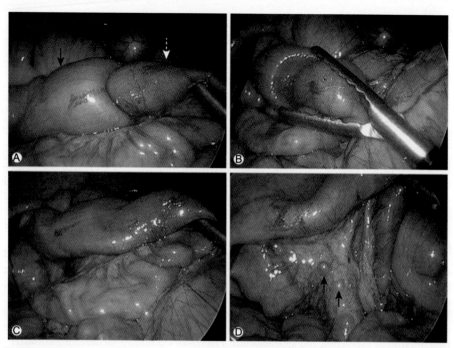

Fig. 55.1 Ileocolic intussusception, laparoscopic view. (A) Intussusceptum *(white arrow)* telescoping into the intussuscipiens *(black arrow).* (B) Laparoscopic grasper seen reducing the intussusception. (C) Complete reduction of intussusception. (D) Mesenteric lymphadenopathy *(black arrows).* (From Maki AC, Fallat ME: Intussusception. In Holcomb GW, Murphy JP, Ostlie DJ, St. Peter SD, editors: *Ashcraft's pediatric surgery*, ed 6, Philadelphia, 2014, Elsevier, pp 531–538.)

upper respiratory and gastroenteric viral illnesses are more prevalent. The classic presentation is a triad of severe, episodic (colicky) abdominal pain, vomiting, and "currant jelly" stool (indicative of ischemia and mucosal sloughing). This triad is rare and occurs less than 25% of the time. One may also be able to palpate a mass in the right upper quadrant, whereas the RLQ may feel scaphoid/empty (Dance sign). Delayed presentation or delays in diagnosis can have devastating consequences and lead to bowel ischemia, necrosis, and perforation. These patients may present with frank peritonitis and shock.

MIDGUT VOLVULUS

A diagnosis that requires consideration in any young child presenting with vomiting is malrotation with midgut volvulus. Malrotation and midgut volvulus are discussed in detail in Chapter 54.

Any bowel obstruction in a young child should have a surgical consultation. In this particular patient, there should be concern for intestinal compromise, especially if bilious emesis was the first/primary symptom.

BASIC SCIENCE PEARL (STEP 1)

Peyer's patches are aggregates of lymphoid tissue found in the ileum. Similar to any lymphoid tissue, Peyer's patches become hypertrophied when reactive as part of an immune response. This hypertrophy has been linked to both appendicitis and intussusception as the inciting blockage of the appendiceal base or lead point, respectively.

CLINICAL PEARL (STEP 2/3)

In young children (especially less than 3 years old), the diagnosis of appendicitis can be very difficult and requires a high index of suspicion. In older children and adults, acute appendicitis can be diagnosed quite accurately by performing a thorough history and physical examination. Selective use of laboratory data (e.g., white blood cell count with differentiation) and imaging (ultrasonography first, with magnetic resonance imaging [MRI] or computed tomography [CT] if equivocal) is indicated when there is a moderate level of suspicion and when more data is required to make a diagnosis.

What Initial Studies and/or Laboratory Tests Should Be Ordered?

In the stable patient without peritonitis, one should proceed with obtaining relevant laboratory analyses and imaging. A complete blood count (CBC) with differential, C-reactive protein (CRP), and complete metabolic panel (CMP) are obtained. Appendicitis usually features a leukocytosis and a left shift (i.e., increased immature forms of neutrophils). Labs may be normal in the setting of ileocolic intussusception, although leukocytosis and bandemia may be a sign of intestinal ischemia or perforation.

Abdominal ultrasonography (US) should be the initial imaging modality in cases of suspected appendicitis or ileocolic intussusception. When visualized, the appendix appears as a blind-ending tubular structure on US. In the setting of acute appendicitis, it may be dilated (> 6 mm), thickened, and noncompressible (Fig. 55.2A). Ovarian pathology may also be diagnosed in female patients. When the appendix is not visualized (due to bowel gas or obese body habitus), specific "secondary signs" have been demonstrated to be associated with appendicitis, particularly fluid collection, free fluid, mesenteric hyperemia, and appendicolith. The classic US finding for ileocolic intussusception is a "target sign" (see Fig. 55.2B), and the intussusceptum may actually be visualized within the colon.

CT with intravenous contrast is highly sensitive and specific (97% and 99%, respectively) in diagnosing appendicitis but exposes children to ionizing radiation (Fig. 55.3). Abdominal MRI, where available, is both sensitive and specific for appendicitis and often useful in the setting of equivocal US findings; however, MRI is expensive and requires the patient to remain immobile for a considerable duration of time. A contrast rectal enema may be a useful diagnostic adjunct in children with ileocolic intussusception. Consider obtaining cross-sectional imaging in older children or recurrent intussusception to assess for a pathologic lead point.

Upper gastrointestinal series (UGI) to the ligament of Treitz should be obtained without delay (before blood work and other imaging) in neonates, infants, and toddlers who present with new bilious emesis (see Chapter 54).

CLINICAL PEARL (STEP 2/3)

Bilious emesis in an infant or toddler is abnormal and should be considered a surgical emergency until proven otherwise. The initial study of choice is an UGI, allowing the contrast to pass to the ligament of Treitz. This study identifies abnormal fixation of the duodenojejunal junction, a sign of intestinal malrotation, which is a risk factor for midgut volvulus due to the narrow attachment of the small bowel mesentery to the retroperitoneum. In the setting of volvulus, there is typically corkscrewing of the proximal jejunum or a tapering "beak sign" with an abrupt contrast cutoff. If the child is too unstable for a fluoroscopy study or if there is a high suspicion and UGI is not available, an emergent exploration may be indicated.

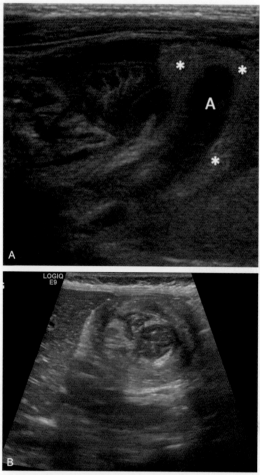

Fig. 55.2 Ultrasound images of (A) acute appendicitis (*marks echogenic, thickened periappendiceal fat; A = appendix). (B) Target sign. (A, from Trout AT, Sanchez R, Ladino-Torres MF: Reevaluating the sonographic criteria for acute appendicitis in children: a review of the literature and retrospective analysis of 246 cases, *Acad Radiol* Nov;19(11):1382–1394, 2012. B, from Padilla BE, Moses W: Lower gastrointestinal bleeding & intussusception, *Surg Clin North Am* Feb;97(1):173–188, 2017.)

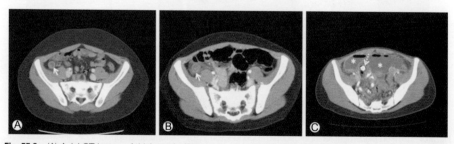

Fig. 55.3 (A) Axial CT image of thickened, dilated appendix *(white arrow)* in the setting of acute appendicitis. (B) Axial CT image demonstrating inflamed, dilated appendix *(white arrow)* with fluid and inflammatory changes medially in the setting of early perforation. (C) Axial CT image of perforated appendicitis with abscesses *(asterisks)* and a large fecalith *(dotted arrow)*. (From Sullins VF, Lee SL: Appendicitis. In Holcomb GW, Murphy JP, Ostlie DJ, St. Peter SD, editors: *Ashcraft's pediatric surgery*, ed 6, Philadelphia, 2014, Elsevier, pp 568–579.)

Initial laboratory values are significant for a leukocytosis (white blood cell count 24,000/uL) and an elevated C-reactive protein of 12.0 mg/dL. Targeted abdominal ultrasound shows that the appendix is dilated to 1.5 cm with an appendicolith at the base. There is a periappendiceal abscess measuring 5 x 4 x 4 cm.

What Is the Surgical Management of Acute Appendicitis?

Appendicitis is the most common abdominal surgical emergency in the pediatric population. As discussed, the diagnosis of appendicitis is not always obvious, and most institutions use a combination of scoring models, laboratory work, and judicious imaging to arrive at a diagnosis.

Acute appendicitis has traditionally been managed with surgery (60,000–80,000 annually in the United States). Nonoperative management with antibiotics has been investigated rigorously in adults, but there are few prospective trials in children. Of the few trials that have been conducted, nonoperative management leads to a success rate of 70% to 85% at 1 year, but long-term results are unknown. Treatment failure or recurrence was not associated with higher rates of complicated appendicitis in these studies. The presence of an appendicolith was highly predictive of failure of nonoperative management. With few exceptions, healthy children presenting with acute appendicitis should be managed surgically.

Traditional (three-port) laparoscopic appendectomy (Fig. 55.4) is the most common operative intervention for acute appendicitis, but alternatives include transumbilical laparoscopic appendectomy (laparoscopic externalization of the appendix through a single umbilical incision followed by open excision) and single-incision laparoscopic surgery (SILS). When open surgery is performed, a McBurney (oblique) or Rocky-Davis (transverse) type incision is performed in the RLQ.

CLINICAL PEARL (STEP 2/3)

Preoperative antibiotics are indicated in the management of uncomplicated appendicitis, with target organisms being skin and bowel flora. Many antibiotic combinations are used, though cephalosporins and metronidazole are the most common. Initiation of prophylactic antibiotics within 1 hour of the time of incision has been shown to decrease postoperative infection. Postoperative antibiotics are not required in the management of uncomplicated appendicitis.

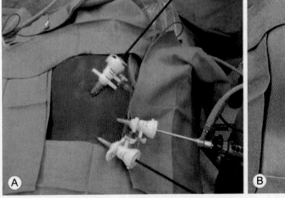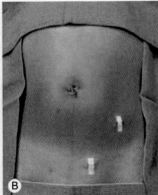

Fig. 55.4 (A) Port placement for laparoscopic appendectomy. (B) Postoperative appearance. (From Sullins VF, Lee SL: Appendicitis. In Holcomb GW, Murphy JP, Ostlie DJ, St. Peter SD, editors: *Ashcraft's pediatric surgery*, ed 6, Philadelphia, 2014, Elsevier, pp 568–579.)

What Is the Management of Complicated Appendicitis?

Complicated appendicitis denotes the presence of appendiceal perforation with or without abscess. Suppurative and gangrenous appendicitis—diagnoses that can only be made during surgery—are not perforated and can be managed like uncomplicated appendicitis with no antibiotics after surgery. Patients with complicated appendicitis should initially be managed with intravenous fluid resuscitation and antibiotics. Patients who present with perforated appendicitis and large, well-demarcated abscesses should be drained percutaneously and subjected to a trial of nonoperative management with IV antibiotics.

Ultimately, decisions regarding surgery and timing are nuanced and there are no consensus guidelines. Options include operative exploration, intravenous antibiotics with or without percutaneous drainage with interval appendectomy (6–10 weeks later), or intravenous antibiotics with or without percutaneous drainage without interval appendectomy. Nonoperative management with interval appendectomy, particularly in the setting of a well-demarcated abscess, appears to be safe and effective. There is a paucity of prospective evidence regarding whether foregoing interval appendectomy after an episode of complicated appendicitis is safe.

What Is the Management of Ileocolic Intussusception?

As discussed, ileocolic intussusception in infants and toddlers is typically not associated with a pathologic lead point. The etiology is likely due to enlarged Peyer's patches in the terminal ileum after a viral illness, so anatomic or pathologic lead points are unusual. Enteroenteric intussusceptions diagnosed on US are typically observed and managed conservatively and occur in the setting of viral illness.

Air contrast enema, performed under fluoroscopic or ultrasound guidance, is the intervention of choice in a child with ileocolic intussusception and the absence of peritonitis. Pneumatic reduction is usually attempted before the injection of water-soluble contrast. Reflux of air or contrast into the terminal ileum confirms successful reduction. Recurrence rate after successful air contrast enema reduction is approximately 5%, with one-third occurring within 24 hours of reduction. Early recurrences are managed with repeat air contrast enemas. After successful reduction, the patient remains NPO for a period of time (6 hours at our institution) and then can initiate a clear liquid diet. They are observed in the hospital for 24 hours before discharge to ensure tolerance of oral intake and to monitor for recurrence. Recent studies have suggested that it is safe to observe and discharge children from the Emergency Department after successful fluoroscopic guided enema reduction of an ileocolic intussusception. Surgical consultation should be obtained in all patients with ileocolic intussusception, regardless of the management protocol.

When air contrast enema is ineffective at ileocolic intussusception reduction, surgical reduction should be attempted. Risk factors associated with the failure of therapeutic enema include the presence of free fluid on US, evidence of intestinal obstruction, and location of the distal tip of the intussusceptum beyond the splenic flexure. Laparoscopy is the preferred initial approach, and the swollen intussusceptum is gently delivered from the intussuscipiens. One must carefully inspect the bowel for viability and lead points (e.g., Meckel's diverticulum) and excise/resect if present. Surgical exploration may also be indicated in the setting of multiple recurrent intussusceptions (same admission or spaced out), although there are no consensus guidelines for this. Surgery should always be performed when there is evidence of intestinal perforation or peritonitis.

The patient is started on intravenous antibiotics (metronidazole and ceftriaxone), and a percutaneous drainage catheter is placed into the periappendiceal abscess by interventional radiology. The patient is admitted to the surgical service and is permitted to take oral intake as tolerated. Her fevers subside within 48 hours and symptoms of pain and nausea significantly improve. The drain output decreases after 5 days, and the drain is removed. She is transitioned to oral antibiotics and discharged home on a 14-day course. She is scheduled for follow-up with the surgeon in 2 weeks to assess her clinical recovery and discuss timing of interval appendectomy.

BEYOND THE PEARLS

- The differential diagnosis of abdominal pain, vomiting, and fever in children is broad and includes surgical and medical entities.
- Acute appendicitis is diagnosed via a combination of history, physical examination findings, clinical scores, and selective imaging (ultrasonography being the mainstay). Acute appendicitis should be managed surgically because of the high recurrence rates with intravenous antibiotics alone.
- Perforated appendicitis is managed via percutaneous drainage and IV antibiotics when there is a well-demarcated abscess. Interval appendectomy may be safely performed 6 to 10 weeks later.
- Ileocolic intussusception typically occurs between 5 to 10 months of age and should be managed initially with air contrast enema under fluoroscopic guidance. Surgery is performed in the setting of failed enema reductions, multiple recurrences, or perforation with peritonitis.
- Midgut volvulus is a surgical emergency and should be ruled out expeditiously in any newborn or infant presenting with new-onset bilious emesis. The initial study of choice is an upper gastrointestinal series to assess for malrotation and associated volvulus. Surgical detorsion and a Ladd's procedure are performed emergently.

Suggested Readings

Gonzalez, D. O., Deans, K. J., & Minneci, P. C. (2016). Role of non-operative management in pediatric appendicitis. *Semin Pediatr Surg, 25*(4), 204–207.

Langer, J. C. (2017). Intestinal rotation abnormalities and midgut volvulus. *Surg Clin North Am, 97*(1), 147–159.

Partain, K. N., Patel, A., Travers, C., et al. (2016). Secondary signs may improve the diagnostic accuracy of equivocal ultrasounds for suspected appendicitis in children. *J Pediatr Surg, 51*(10), 1655–1660.

Pepper, V. K., Stanfill, A. B., & Pearl, R. H. (2012). Diagnosis and management of pediatric appendicitis, intussusception, and Meckel diverticulum. *Surg Clin North Am, 92*(3), 505–526.

Samuel, M. (2002). Pediatric appendicitis score. *J Pediatr Surg, 37*(6), 877–881.

Gondek, A. S., Riaza, L., Cuadras, D., et al. (2018). Ileocolic intussusception: Predicting the probability of success of ultrasound guided saline enema from clinical and sonographic data. *J Pediatr Surg, 53*(4), 599–604. https://doi.org/10.1016/j.jpedsurg.2017.10.050. Apr. Epub 2017 Nov 15.

Note: Page numbers followed by *f* indicate figures, *t* indicate tables, and *b* indicate boxes.